Study Guide for

Maternity & Pediatric Nursing

SECOND EDITION

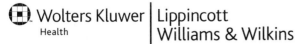
Wolters Kluwer | Lippincott
Health | Williams & Wilkins

Philadelphia • Baltimore • New York • London
Buenos Aires • Hong Kong • Sydney • Tokyo

Acquisitions Editor: Patrick Barbera
Product Manager: Helene T. Caprari
Editorial Assistant: Zackary Shapiro
Design Coordinator: Holly McLaughlin
Illustration Coordinator: Brett MacNaughton
Manufacturing Coordinator: Karin Duffield
Prepress Vendor: S4Carlisle Publishing Services

Second edition

9 8 7 6 5 4 3 2 1

Printed in China

ISBN 978-1-4511-5156-5

Care has been taken to confirm the accuracy of the information presented and to describe generally accepted practices. However, the authors, editors, and publisher are not responsible for errors or omissions or for any consequences from application of the information in this book and make no warranty, expressed or implied, with respect to the currency, completeness, or accuracy of the contents of the publication. Application of this information in a particular situation remains the professional responsibility of the practitioner; the clinical treatments described and recommended may not be considered absolute and universal recommendations.

The authors, editors, and publisher have exerted every effort to ensure that drug selection and dosage set forth in this text are in accordance with the current recommendations and practice at the time of publication. However, in view of ongoing research, changes in government regulations, and the constant flow of information relating to drug therapy and drug reactions, the reader is urged to check the package insert for each drug for any change in indications and dosage and for added warnings and precautions. This is particularly important when the recommended agent is a new or infrequently employed drug.

Some drugs and medical devices presented in this publication have Food and Drug Administration (FDA) clearance for limited use in restricted research settings. It is the responsibility of the health care provider to ascertain the FDA status of each drug or device planned for use in his or her clinical practice.

LWW.com

Preface

This Study Guide was developed by Kim Cooper and Kelly Gosnell, to accompany the second edition of *Maternity & Pediatric Nursing* by Susan Scott Ricci, Terri Kyle, and Susan Carman. The Study Guide is designed to help you practice and retain the knowledge you have gained from the textbook, and it is structured to integrate that knowledge and give you a basis for applying it in your nursing practice. The following types of exercises are provided in each chapter of the Study Guide.

SECTION I: ASSESSING YOUR UNDERSTANDING

The first section of each Study Guide chapter concentrates on the basic information of the textbook chapter and helps you to remember key concepts, vocabulary, and principles.

- *Fill in the blanks*
  Fill in the blank exercises test important chapter information, encouraging you to recall key points.

- *Labeling*
  Labeling exercises are used where you need to remember certain visual representations of the concepts presented in the textbook.

- *Matching*
  Matching questions test your knowledge of the definition of key terms.

- *Sequencing*
  Sequencing exercises ask you to remember particular sequences or orders, for instance testing processes and prioritizing nursing actions.

- *Short answers*
  Short answer questions will cover facts, concepts, procedures, and principles of the chapter. These questions ask you to recall information as well as demonstrate your comprehension of the information.

SECTION II: APPLYING YOUR KNOWLEDGE

The second section of each Study Guide chapter consists of case study-based exercises that ask you to begin to apply the knowledge you have gained from the textbook chapter and reinforced in the first section of the Study Guide chapter. A case study scenario based on the chapter's content is presented, and then you are asked to answer some questions, in writing, related to the case study. The questions cover the following areas:
- Assessment
- Planning nursing care
- Communication
- Reflection

SECTION III: PRACTICING FOR NCLEX

The third and final section of the Study Guide helps you practice NCLEX-style questions while further reinforcing the knowledge you have been gaining and testing for yourself through the textbook chapter and the first two sections of the study guide chapter. In keeping with the NCLEX, the questions presented are multiple choice and scenario based, asking you to reflect, consider, and apply what you know and to choose the best answer out of those offered.

ANSWER KEYS

The answers for all of the exercises and questions in the Study Guide are provided at the back of the book, so you can assess your own learning as you complete each chapter.

We hope you will find this Study Guide to be helpful and enjoyable, and we wish you every success in your studies toward becoming a nurse.

The Publishers

Table of Contents

CHAPTER 1

Perspectives on Maternal and Child Health Care

Learning Objectives

- Analyze the key milestones in the history of maternal, newborn, and child health and health care.
- Examine the evolution of maternal, newborn, and pediatric nursing.
- Compare the past definitions of health and illness with the current definitions, as well as the measurements used to assess health and illness in children.
- Assess the factors that affect maternal and child health.
- Differentiate the structures, roles, and functions of the family and how they affect the health of women and children.
- Evaluate how society and culture can influence the health of women, children, and families.
- Appraise the health care barriers affecting women, children, and families.
- Research the ethical and legal issues that may arise when caring for women, children, and families.

SECTION I: ASSESSING YOUR UNDERSTANDING

Activity A FILL IN THE BLANKS

1. A _____ is a lay birth assistant who provides quality emotional, physical, and educational support to the woman and family during childbirth and the postpartum period.

2. The _____ is considered the basic social unit.

3. Under certain conditions, a minor can be considered _____ and can make health care decisions independently of parents.

4. The ability to apply knowledge about a client's culture to adapt his or her health care accordingly is known as cultural _____.

5. _____ is the measure of prevalence of a specific illness in a population at a particular time.

6. More children and adolescents die from _____ injuries than from any other cause.

7. Children's medical records are only shared with legal parents, _____, or others, with written authorization by the parents.

8. The resiliency model of family stress and family adjustment and the adaptation response model identify the element of risk and _____ factors that aid a family in achieving positive outcomes.

9. _____ refers to a basic human quality involving the belief in something greater than oneself and a faith that affirms life positively.

10. Children's temperament is categorized into three major groups: _____, difficult, and slow to warm up.

Match the cultural group in Column A with the characteristic in Column B.

Column A

_____ **1.** Asian Americans

_____ **2.** African Americans

_____ **3.** Native Americans

_____ **4.** Hispanics

Column B

a. Childbirth is viewed as a normal, natural process; entire family may be present during birth

b. Bed rest maintained for the first 3 days postpartum

c. Breast-feeding withheld for the first 2 to 3 days after birth

d. Quiet stoic appearance of woman during labor

1. Using the boxes provided below, put the following characteristic approaches in the evolution of maternal and newborn nursing in the proper chronologic order.

   a. The assistance of certified nurse midwives and doulas grew in popularity as a choice in childbirth.

   b. "Granny midwives" handled the normal birthing process for most women; infant and maternal mortality rates were high.

   c. "Natural childbirth" practices advocating birth without medication and focusing on relaxation techniques were introduced.

   d. Physicians attended about half the births, with midwives caring for women who could not afford a doctor.

   □ → □ → □ → □

2. Using the boxes provided below, place the letter of each of the following stages of Duvall's developmental theory into their proper sequence.

   a. Family with school-aged children

   b. Marriage

   c. Family with adolescents

   d. Childbearing stage

   e. Middle-aged parents

   f. Family with preschool children

   g. Family in later years

   h. Family with young adults

   □ → □ → □ → □ → □ → □ → □ → □

Briefly answer the following.

1. How do the risk factors for cardiovascular disease differ between men and women?

   _____

   _____

   _____

2. What are considered the major risk factors for developing breast cancer?

   _____

   _____

   _____

3. What is meant by maternal mortality rate?

   _____

   _____

   _____

4. What are the predictors of infant mortality?

   _____

   _____

   _____

5. How has the Women, Infants, Children program supported the health of women and children?

   _____

   _____

   _____

6. When using positive reinforcement discipline strategies, what three characteristics of feedback are pivotal for success?

_____

_____

_____

SECTION II: APPLYING YOUR KNOWLEDGE

Activity E CASE STUDY

Isabella Gonzales is a 6-year-old female with a history of cerebral palsy. She was born at 28 weeks and is currently admitted to the hospital due to difficulty breathing secondary to pneumonia. Her parents, Jose and Angelina, are very active in her care. Isabella lives at home with her parents and two brothers, Sergio and Tito.

1. Discuss the barriers to health care that the Gonzales may encounter.

_____

_____

_____

2. What cultural aspects would you need to keep in mind when providing care for this family?

_____

_____

_____

SECTION III: PRACTICING FOR NCLEX

Activity F NCLEX-STYLE QUESTIONS

Answer the following questions.

1. A female client who has just given birth has been reading health reports and is alarmed at the high rate of infant mortality. She seems anxious about the health of her child and wants to know ways to keep her baby from getting an infection. Which of the following instructions should the nurse offer?

   a. Place the infant on his or her back to sleep

   b. Breastfeed the infant

   c. Feed the infant foods high in starch

   d. Feed the infant liquids frequently

2. A group of nurses are running a campaign initiated by the Maternal and Child Health Bureau to educate women about better maternal and infant care. Which of the following measures should they advocate for the prevention of neural defects in infants?

   a. Take folic acid supplements

   b. Take vitamin E supplements

   c. Perform mild exercises during pregnancy

   d. Regularly eat citrus fruits during pregnancy

3. A nurse is caring for a client who wishes to undergo an abortion. The nurse has concerns because abortion is against her personal convictions, and this is interfering with her professional duty. Which of the following should the nurse do to follow ANA's code of ethics for nurses?

   a. Provide emotional support to the client while caring for her

   b. Not allow her personal convictions to interfere with her profession

   c. Involve the client's family in convincing the client against an abortion

   d. Make arrangements for alternate care providers

4. A female client who has just given birth arrives in a health care facility and asks the nurse about how to prevent sudden infant death syndrome (SIDS). Which of the following instructions should the nurse provide?

   a. Drape the infant in warm clothes

   b. Feed a mixture of salts, sugar, and water

   c. Provide very soft bedding

   d. Place the infant on his or her back to sleep

5. A nurse is caring for a critically ill female client who has recently been diagnosed with advanced lung cancer. Which of the following reasons could have contributed to the late detection and diagnosis?

   a. Women have a stronger resistance against lung cancer

   b. Lung cancer has no early symptoms

   c. Lung cancer is considered more deadly in men than in women

   d. Lung cancer is more challenging to diagnose in women than in men

6. It is important to be able to measure the health status of a group of people or a nation so that the number of people who die prematurely will decrease over time. How does the United States measure the health status of its people?

   a. Tracks the incidence of violent crime

   b. Examines health disparities between ethnic groups

   c. Examines mortality and morbidity data

   d. Identifies specific national health goals related to maternal and infant health

7. The nurse is caring for an Arab-American woman. Which approach would be most successful?

   a. Inquiring about folk remedies used

   b. Coordinating care through the client's mother

   c. Dealing exclusively with the husband

   d. Promoting preventive health care

8. The nurse is caring for a client with end-stage breast cancer. When she takes chemotherapy medication into the client's room, the client states, "I'm too tired to fight any more. I don't want any more medication that may prolong my life." The client's husband is at the bedside and states, "No! You have to give my wife her medication. I can't let her go." What action by the nurse is most appropriate?

   a. Giving the medication

   b. Explaining to the husband that his wife has the right to refuse medication and care

   c. Encouraging the client to heed her husband's wishes

   d. Stating that she has to give the medication unless the doctor orders the medication stopped

9. The nurse is talking with the mother of a 2-year-old girl during a scheduled visit. Which of the following least supports the emphasis on preventive care?

   a. Reminding that child will imitate parents

   b. Explaining how to toddler proof the house

   c. Describing self-care for brushing teeth

   d. Explaining how to teach self hand washing

10. The nurse is updating the records of a 10-year-old girl who had her appendix removed. Which of the following actions could jeopardize the privacy of the child's medical records?

    a. Changing identification and passwords monthly

    b. Letting another nurse use the nurse's log-in session

    c. Closing files before stepping away from computer

    d. Printing out confidential information for transmittal

11. The nurse is assessing a 9-year-old boy during a back-to-school check up. Which of the following findings is a factor for childhood injury?

    a. Records show child weighed 2,450 g at birth

    b. Mother reports she has abused alcohol and drugs

    c. The parents adopted the boy from Guatemala

    d. Mother reports the child is hostile to other children

12. During a well-child visit, a mother laughingly reports that her 10-year-old child's teacher has recommended a mental health evaluation for the child. What response by the nurse is most appropriate?

    a. "<MCA>Your child is too young to be concerned with mental health problems"

    b. "Mental health issues in children are pretty rare"

    c. "Does anyone in your family have mental health problems? "

    d. "What types of issues is the teacher concerned about?"

13. The parents of a 12-year-old client preparing to undergo surgery explain to the nurse that their religious beliefs do not allow for blood transfusions. What initial action by the nurse is most appropriate?

    a. Explain to the parents that the surgeon will make the final decision in the event a blood transfusion is needed by the child

    b. Ask the child what their preference will be

    c. Contact the hospital attorney

    d. Document the parents' requests

14. A nurse is caring for a 31-year-old pregnant female client who is subjected to abuse by her partner. The client has developed a feeling of hopelessness and does not feel confident in dealing with the situation at home, which makes her feel suicidal. Which of the following nursing interventions should the nurse offer to help the client deal with her situation?

    a. Counsel the client's partner to refrain from subjecting his partner to abuse

    b. Help the client understand the legal impact of her situation to protect her

    c. Provide emotional support to empower the client to help herself

    d. Introduce the client to a women's rights group

15. A recently licensed nurse is orienting to a Pediatric unit in an acute care facility. The nurse is discussing causes of infant mortality with her preceptor. Which of the following should be included as the leading cause of infant mortality?

    a. Cardiac disease

    b. Respiratory infection

    c. Congenital anomalies

    d. SIDS

16. A group of women are attending a community presentation discussing the health concerns of women. Which of the following will be included as the leading cause of death for women?

    a. Lung cancer

    b. Cancers of the reproductive system

    c. Cardiovascular disease

    d. HIV infection

17. The nursing instructor is discussing culture with a group of nursing students. Which of the following should be included in the discussion of this topic? Select all that apply.

    a. Personal space

    b. Race

    c. Primary language spoken

    d. Level of education

    e. Religious beliefs

18. The nurse is reviewing the family history information in a newly admitted client's chart. The nurse notes the client lives with his parents and grandparents. Which term best describes the client's family structure?

    a. Blended family

    b. Communal family

    c. Binuclear family

    d. Extended family

CHAPTER 2

Core Concepts of Maternal and Child Health Care and Community-Based Care

Learning Objectives

- Identify the core concepts associated with the nursing management of women, children, and families.
- Examine the major components and key elements of family-centered care.
- Explain the different levels of prevention in nursing, providing examples of each.
- Give examples of cultural issues that may be faced when providing nursing care.
- Provide culturally competent care to women, children, and families.
- Outline the various roles and functions assumed by the nurse working with women, children, and families.
- Demonstrate the ability to use excellent therapeutic communication skills when interacting with women, children, and families.
- Explain the process of health teaching as it relates to women, children, and families.
- Examine the importance of discharge planning and case management in providing nursing care.
- Explain the reasons for the increased emphasis on community-based care.
- Differentiate community-based nursing from nursing in acute care settings.
- Identify the variety of settings where community-based care can be provided to women, children, and families.

SECTION I: ASSESSING YOUR UNDERSTANDING

Activity A FILL IN THE BLANKS

1. The collaborative process of assessment, planning, application, coordination, follow-up, and evaluation of the options needed to meet an individual's needs is referred to as _____.

2. _____ communication, also referred to as body language, includes attending to others and active listening.

3. _____ may be defined as a "specific group of people, often living in a defined geographical area, who share a common culture, values, and norms."

4. _____ prevention involves avoiding the disease or condition before it occurs through health promotion activities, environmental protection, and specific protection against disease or injury.

5. Cultural _____ involve participating in cross-cultural interactions with people from culturally diverse backgrounds.

6. _____ literacy is the ability to read, understand, and use health care information.

Activity B MATCHING

Match the health care facility in Column A with the service provided in Column B.

Column A

_____ **1.** Counseling centers

_____ **2.** Wellness centers

_____ **3.** Wholeness healing centers

_____ **4.** Educational centers

Column B

a. Provide health lecture instruction on breast self-examination and computers for research

b. Provide acupuncture, aromatherapy, and herbal remedies

c. Offer stress reduction techniques

d. Offer various support groups

Activity C SEQUENCING

Using the boxes below, place the steps used to provide education to clients and families in the correct sequence.

1. Intervening to enhance learning

2. Planning education

3. Evaluating learning

4. Documenting teaching and learning

5. Assessing teaching and learning needs

☐ → ☐ → ☐ → ☐ → ☐

Activity D SHORT ANSWERS

Briefly answer the following.

1. What are the three levels of care provided by maternal and pediatric nurses?

_____

_____

_____

2. Describe the components of case management.

_____

_____

_____

3. What techniques can the nurse use to enhance learning?

_____

_____

_____

4. What are the four main purposes of documenting childcare and education?

_____

_____

_____

5. What do discharge planning and case management contribute to in the community setting?

_____

_____

_____

6. What is the focus of community health nursing?

_____

_____

_____

7. What is a birthing center?

_____

_____

_____

SECTION II: APPLYING YOUR KNOWLEDGE

Activity E CASE STUDY

Consider this scenario and answer the questions.

A couple in their late 20s is expecting their first child. They are touring the labor and delivery suite at the hospital they have chosen for the birth. The nurse who is conducting the tour refers to giving "family centered care" and using "evidence-based nursing" on their unit.

1. During the question and answer period, the couple asks what "family-centered care" is. How would the nurse respond to this couple's question?

_____

_____

_____

2. The couple then asks what the nurse means by "evidence-based nursing" and how that affects the two of them and their newborn. What is the nurse's best response?

_____

_____

_____

SECTION III: PRACTICING FOR NCLEX

Activity F **NCLEX-STYLE QUESTIONS**

Answer the following questions.

1. A nurse is working in a community setting and is involved in case management. Which activity would the nurse most likely be involved with?
   a. Helping a grandmother to learn a procedure
   b. Assessing the sanitary conditions of the home
   c. Establishing eligibility for a Medicaid waiver
   d. Scheduling speech and respiratory therapy services

2. Which of the following is a key element for providing family-centered care?
   a. Communicating specific health information
   b. Being in control of the way care is given
   c. Limiting health information to that which is absolutely necessary
   d. Avoiding cultural issues by providing care in a standardized fashion

3. The nurse is educating the family of a 2-year-old Asian American boy with asthma about the disorder and its treatment. The parents speak no English. Which action, involving an interpreter, can jeopardize the family's trust?
   a. Allowing too little appointment time for the translation
   b. Using a person who is not a professional interpreter
   c. Asking the interpreter side questions not meant for the family
   d. Using a relative to communicate with the parents

4. Nurses play important roles in a variety of community settings. Which of the following goals is common to all community settings?
   a. Removing or minimizing health barriers to learning
   b. Promoting the health of a specific group of clients
   c. Determining initially the type of care a client needs
   d. Ensuring the health and well-being of clients and their families

5. A nurse is working with a family to ensure effective therapeutic communication. The development of which of the following would be least important?
   a. Trust
   b. Respect
   c. Empathy
   d. Literacy

6. A nurse is conducting a teaching session with a child and his family. Which techniques would help to facilitate their learning? Select all that apply.
   a. Use medical terminology emphasize the importance of the information
   b. Limit each teaching session to about 10–15 minutes
   c. Focus on the "need-to-know" information first
   d. Repeat the information about 4–5 times.
   e. Avoid using videos that can distract the learners

7. A community health nurse is engaged in primary prevention activities. Which of the following would be applicable? Select all that apply.
   a. Drug education program for schools
   b. Smoking cessation programs
   c. Poison prevention education
   d. Cholesterol monitoring
   e. Fecal occult blood testing

8. While interviewing a woman who has come to the clinic for a check-up, the woman tells the nurse that she places objects in her environment so that they are in harmony with chi. The nurse interprets this as which of the following?
   a. Reflexology
   b. Feng Shui

   c. Therapeutic touch

   d. Aromatherapy

9. You are working with an interpreter to gather information from a family. Which of the following would be most important?

   a. Positioning the interpreter between you and the family

   b. Assuming the interpreter is the content expert

   c. Allowing additional time to compensate for the translation

   d. Talking directly to the interpreter

10. You are working with the parents of young child and teaching them how to care for their son. You would integrate knowledge of which of the following when developing the teaching plan?

   a. Adults are very problem-focused

   b. Adults value dependent learning

   c. Adults value the future

   d. Adults desire delayed need satisfaction

11. A nurse is working on developing cultural competence. Which of the following would the nurse do first?

   a. Become sensitive to the values, beliefs, and customs of one's own culture

   b. Obtain knowledge about various worldviews of different cultures

   c. Assess each client's unique cultural values, beliefs, and practices

   d. Engage in cross-cultural interactions with people from diverse cultural groups

12. A 4-year-old child is brought to the clinic by his parents for evaluation of a cough. Which action by the nurse would be least appropriate in promoting atraumatic care for the child?

   a. Having the parents stay with the child during the examination

   b. Allowing the child to touch the stethoscope before listening to his heart

   c. Informing the child that the stethoscope might feel a bit cold but not hurt

   d. Wrapping the child tightly in a blanket to prevent him from moving around

Anatomy and Physiology of the Reproductive System

Upon completion of the chapter, you will be able to:

- Define the key terms used in this chapter.
- Contrast the structure and function of the major external and internal female genital organs.
- Outline the phases of the menstrual cycle, the dominant hormones involved, and the changes taking place in each phase.
- Classify external and internal male reproductive structures and the function of each in hormonal regulation.

SECTION I: ASSESSING YOUR UNDERSTANDING

Activity A FILL IN THE BLANKS

1. The vagina is a tubular, fibromuscular organ lined with a mucous membrane that lies in a series of transverse folds called _____.

2. _____ stimulates the production of milk within a few days after childbirth.

3. The _____, which lies against the testes, is a coiled tube almost 20 ft long that collects sperm from the testes and provides the space and environment for sperm to mature.

4. In the male, the _____ is the terminal duct of the reproductive and urinary systems, serving as a passageway for semen and urine.

5. The _____ is the mucosal layer that lines the uterine cavity in nonpregnant women.

6. _____ glands, located on either side of the female urethral opening, secrete a small amount of mucus to keep the opening moist and lubricated for the passage of urine.

7. The incision made into the perineal tissue to provide more space for the presenting part of the delivering fetus is called an _____.

8. In the male, the _____ gland lies just under the bladder in the pelvis and surrounds the middle portion of the urethra.

9. The _____ is a pear-shaped muscular organ at the top of the vagina.

10. The _____ is the thin-skinned sac that surrounds and protects the testes.

Activity B MATCHING

Match the hormones in Column A with their functions in Column B.

Column A

____ **1.** Gonadotropin-releasing hormone (GnRH)

____ **2.** Follicle-stimulating hormone (FSH)

____ **3.** Luteinizing hormone (LH)

____ **4.** Estrogen

____ **5.** Progesterone

Column B

a. It maintains the uterine decidual lining and reduces uterine contractions, allowing pregnancy to be maintained

b. It is required for the final maturation of preovulatory follicles and luteinization of the ruptured follicle

c. It is primarily responsible for the maturation of the ovarian follicle

d. It inhibits FSH production and stimulates LH production

e. It induces the release of FSH and LH to assist with ovulation

Activity C SEQUENCING

Put the activities in correct sequence by writing the letters in the boxes provided below.

1. Given below, in random order, are steps occurring during the endometrial cycle. Arrange them in the correct sequence.

   a. The endometrium becomes thickened and more vascular and glandular.

   b. Cervical mucus becomes thin, clear, stretchy, and more alkaline.

   c. The spiral arteries rupture, releasing blood into the uterus.

   d. The ischemia leads to shedding of the endometrium down to the basal layer.

   □ → □ → □ → □

2. Given below, in random order, are pubertal events. Arrange them in the correct sequence.

   a. Growth spurt

   b. Appearance of pubic and then axillary hair

   c. Development of breast buds

   d. Onset of menstruation

   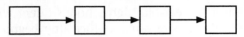

Activity D SHORT ANSWERS

Briefly answer the following.

1. What is vulva?

_____

_____

_____

2. What is colostrum?

_____

_____

_____

3. What are the physical changes observed in women during their perimenopausal years?

_____

_____

_____

4. What is the role of the nurse when caring for menopausal women?

_____

_____

_____

5. What is the function of the testes?

_____

_____

_____

6. What is the function of the bulbourethral, or Cowper, glands?

_____

_____

SECTION II: APPLYING YOUR KNOWLEDGE

Activity E CASE STUDY

Consider this scenario and answer the questions.

Susan is a 14-year-old high school student who came to the school nurse's office after beginning her first menstrual period. She has received health education information in class, but has many questions about her body. She asks the school nurse several questions.

1. Describe what a nurse should teach Susan about the changes in her body and menstruation.

   _____

   _____

   _____

2. Describe the nurse's response when Susan asks how long her cycles will last.

   _____

   _____

   _____

3. Susan reports that most of her close friends have not yet started their periods. What information can be provided about factors that influence the onset of menstruation?

   _____

   _____

   _____

SECTION III: PRACTICING FOR NCLEX

Activity F

Answer the following questions.

1. A client is trying to have a baby and wants to know the best time to have intercourse to increase the chances of pregnancy. Which of the following is the ideal time for intercourse, to help her chances of conceiving?
   a. A week after ovulation
   b. One or 2 days before ovulation
   c. Any time after ovulation
   d. Any time during the week before ovulation

2. Which of the following organs is responsible for providing lubrication during intercourse?
   a. Endocrine glands
   b. Pituitary glands
   c. Skene glands
   d. Bartholin glands

3. Which of the following is the mucosal layer that lines the uterine cavity in nonpregnant women?
   a. Endometrium
   b. Fundus
   c. Mons pubis
   d. Clitoris

4. A nurse is caring for a client who has given birth. The client reports that her breast milk is dark yellow. Which of the following information should the nurse give to the client regarding the situation?
   a. Modify diet to reduce excess fat intake.
   b. The yellow fluid is colostrum and is rich in maternal antibodies.
   c. Breastfeeding should be avoided until the breast milk becomes normal.
   d. Completely stop breastfeeding and use formula instead.

5. A client complains of pain on one side of the abdomen. On further questioning, the nurse discovers that the pain occurs regularly around 2 weeks before menstruation. The client has not missed a period, and she exercises regularly. Which of the following is the most likely cause of the pain?
   a. Early signs of pregnancy
   b. Irregular menstruation cycle
   c. Pain during ovulation
   d. Exercising regularly

6. A client asks the nurse how she would know if ovulation has occurred. Which of the following is a sign of ovulation that the nurse should inform the client about?
   a. Pain in the vaginal area
   b. Rise in temperature by 0.5° to 1° F
   c. Uneasiness or sickness
   d. Lack of sleep

7. A nurse is assessing a 45-year-old client. The client asks for information regarding the changes that are most likely to occur with menopause. Which of the following should the nurse tell the client?

   a. Uterus tilts backward

   b. Uterus shrinks and gradually atrophies

   c. Cervical muscle content increases

   d. Outer layer of the cervix becomes rough

8. Which of the following hormones is called the hormone of pregnancy because it reduces uterine contractions during pregnancy?

   a. LH

   b. Estrogen

   c. FSH

   d. Progesterone

9. During cold conditions, how does the body react to maintain scrotal temperature?

   a. Cremaster muscles relax

   b. Frequency of urination increases

   c. Scrotum is pulled closer to the body

   d. Increase in blood flow to genital area

10. A nurse is screening an elderly client for prostate cancer. What are the effects of aging on the prostate gland?

    a. Prostate gland enlarges with age.

    b. Production of semen stops.

    c. Prostate gland stops functioning.

    d. Prostate gland causes painful erection.

11. Which of the following organs provides the space and environment for sperm cells to mature?

    a. Vas deferens

    b. Epididymis

    c. Testes

    d. Cowper glands

12. A nurse is explaining the menstrual cycle to a 12-year-old client who has experienced menarche. Which of the following should the nurse tell the client?

    a. An average cycle length is about 15 to 20 days.

    b. Ovary contains 400,000 follicles at birth.

    c. Duration of the flow is about 3 to 7 days.

    d. Blood loss averages 120 to 150 mL.

13. A nurse is providing information regarding ovulation to a couple who want to have a baby. Which of the following should the nurse tell the clients?

    a. Ovulation takes place 10 days before menstruation.

    b. The lifespan of the ovum is only about 48 hours.

    c. At ovulation, a mature follicle ruptures, releasing an ovum.

    d. When ovulation occurs, there is a rise in estrogen.

14. Which of the following hormones is secreted from the hypothalamus in a pulsatile manner throughout the reproductive cycle?

    a. FSH

    b. GnRH

    c. LH

    d. Estrogen

15. Which of the following statements best expresses the role of the corpus luteum?

    a. The corpus luteum promotes the increased production of estrogen before ovulation.

    b. The corpus luteum secretes progesterone to promote the preparation of the endometrium for implantation.

    c. During the luteal phase, the corpus luteum secretes glycogen.

    d. Increasing amounts of cervical mucus are produced as a result of the LH produced by the corpus luteum.

Common Reproductive Issues

Upon completion of the chapter, you will be able to:

- Define the key terms used in this chapter.
- Examine common reproductive concerns in terms of symptoms, diagnostic tests, and appropriate interventions.
- Identify risk factors and outline appropriate client education needed in common reproductive disorders.
- Compare and contrast the various contraceptive methods available and their overall effectiveness.
- Analyze the physiologic and psychological aspects of menopausal transition.
- Delineate the nursing management needed for women experiencing common reproductive disorders.

SECTION I: ASSESSING YOUR UNDERSTANDING

Activity A FILL IN THE BLANKS

1. _____ involves the ingrowth of the endometrium into the uterine musculature.

2. Primary dysmenorrhea is caused by increased _____ production by the endometrium in an ovulatory cycle.

3. _____ is the direct visualization of the internal organs with a lighted instrument inserted through an abdominal incision.

4. During _____, the ovary begins to falter, producing irregular and missed periods and an occasional hot flash.

5. Male sterilization is accomplished with a surgical procedure known as a _____.

6. In a _____ abortion, the woman takes certain medications to induce a miscarriage to remove the products of conception.

7. _____ is a condition in which bone mass declines to such an extent that fractures occur with minimal trauma.

8. At the onset of ovulation, cervical mucus that is more abundant, clear, slippery, and smooth is known as _____ mucus.

9. The _____ body temperature refers to the lowest body temperature and is reached upon awakening.

10. Oral contraceptives (OC), called _____, contain only progestin and work primarily by thickening the cervical mucus to prevent penetration of the sperm and make the endometrium unfavorable for implantation.

Activity B MATCHING

Match the terms in Column A with the correct description in Column B.

Column A	Column B
____ **1.** Amenorrhea	**a.** Bleeding between periods
____ **2.** Dysmenorrhea	**b.** Bleeding occurring at intervals of more than 35 days
____ **3.** Metrorrhagia	
____ **4.** Menometrorrhagia	**c.** Absence of menses during the reproductive years
____ **5.** Oligomenorrhea	
	d. Difficult, painful, or abnormal menstruation
	e. Heavy bleeding occurring at irregular intervals with flow lasting more than 7 days

Activity C SEQUENCING

Put the steps in correct sequence by writing the letters in the boxes provided below.

1. Given below, in random order, are steps occurring during diaphragm insertion. Write the correct sequence.

   a. Hold the diaphragm between the thumb and fingers and compress it to form a "figure-eight" shape.

   b. Place a tablespoon of spermicidal jelly or cream in the dome and around the rim of the diaphragm.

   c. Select the position that is most comfortable for insertion.

   d. Tuck the front rim of the diaphragm behind the pubic bone so that the rubber hugs the front wall of the vagina.

   e. Insert the diaphragm into the vagina, directing it downward as far as it will go.

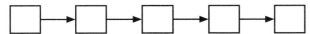

2. Given below, in random order, are steps occurring during cervical cap insertion. Write the correct sequence.

   a. Pinch the sides of the cervical cap together.

   b. Use one finger to feel around the entire circumference to make sure there are no gaps between the cap rim and the cervix.

   c. Pinch the cap dome and tug gently to check for evidence of suction.

   d. Insert the cervical cap into the vagina and place over the cervix.

   e. Compress the cervical cap dome.

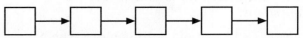

Activity D SHORT ANSWERS

Briefly answer the following.

1. What are the common laboratory tests ordered to determine the cause of amenorrhea?

   _____

   _____

   _____

2. What is menopause?

   _____

   _____

   _____

3. What are the risk factors associated with endometriosis?

   _____

   _____

   _____

4. Compare and contrast primary and secondary infertility.

   _____

   _____

   _____

5. What is the Two-Day Method for contraception?

   _____

   _____

   _____

6. What are intrauterine systems?

   _____

   _____

   _____

SECTION II: APPLYING YOUR KNOWLEDGE

Activity E CASE STUDY

Consider this scenario and answer the questions.

Alexa is a 14-year-old lacrosse player who has been training vigorously for selection on her high school team. Alexa comes to the health care provider's office to have her health forms for school completed. The office nurse takes her history, and the client describes that she has been experiencing amenorrhea.

a. How should the nurse describe "primary amenorrhea" to Alexa?

_____

_____

_____

b. State the causes of "primary amenorrhea" that may be related to Alexa.

_____

_____

_____

c. What treatments may be considered for Alexa?

_____

_____

_____

d. What counseling and education should the nurse provide for Alexa at this visit?

_____

_____

_____

SECTION III: PRACTICING FOR NCLEX

Activity F NCLEX-STYLE QUESTIONS

Answer the following questions.

1. The nurse is assessing a client for amenorrhea. Which of the following should the nurse document as evidence of androgen excess secondary to a tumor?

   a. Reduced subcutaneous fat
   b. Hypothermia
   c. Irregular heart rate and pulse
   d. Facial hair and acne

2. A nurse is teaching a female client about fertility awareness as a method of contraception. Which of the following should the nurse mention as an assumption for this method?

   a. Sperm can live up to 24 hours after intercourse.
   b. The "unsafe period" is approximately 6 days.
   c. The exact time of ovulation can be determined.
   d. The "safe period" is 3 days after ovulation.

3. The nurse is instructing a client with dysmenorrhea on how to manage her symptoms. Which of the following should the nurse include in the teaching plan? Select all that apply.

   a. Increase intake of salty foods.
   b. Increase water consumption.
   c. Avoid keeping legs elevated while lying down.
   d. Use heating pads or take warm baths.
   e. Increase exercise and physical activity.

4. A client is to be examined for the presence and extent of endometriosis. Which of the following tests should the nurse prepare the client for?

   a. Tissue biopsy
   b. Hysterosalpingogram
   c. Clomiphene citrate challenge test
   d. Laparoscopy

5. A couple is being assessed for infertility. The male partner is required to collect a semen sample for analysis. What instruction should the nurse give him?

   a. Abstain from sexual activity for 10 hours before collecting the sample.
   b. Avoid strenuous activity for 24 hours before collecting the sample.
   c. Collect a specimen by ejaculating into a condom or plastic bag.
   d. Deliver sample for analysis within 1 to 2 hours after ejaculation.

6. A client needs additional information about the cervical mucus ovulation method after

having read about it in a magazine. She asks the nurse about cervical changes during ovulation. Which of the following should the nurse inform the client about?

   a. Cervical os is slightly closed

   b. Cervical mucus is dry and thick

   c. Cervix is high or deep in the vagina

   d. Cervical mucus breaks when stretched

7. A client has been following the conventional 28-day regimen for contraception. She is now considering switching to an extended OC regimen. She is seeking information about specific safety precautions. Which of the following is true for the extended OC regimen?

   a. It is not as effective as the conventional regimen.

   b. It prevents pregnancy for 3 months at a time.

   c. It carries the same safety profile as the 28-day regimen.

   d. It does not ensure restoration of fertility if discontinued.

8. A 30-year-old client would like to try using basal body temperature (BBT) as a fertility awareness method. Which of the following instructions should the nurse provide the client?

   a. Avoid unprotected intercourse until BBT has been elevated for 6 days.

   b. Avoid using other fertility awareness methods along with BBT.

   c. Use the axillary method of taking the temperature.

   d. Take temperature before rising and record it on a chart.

9. The nurse is caring for a client at the ambulatory care clinic who questions the nurse for information about contraception. The client reports that she is not comfortable about using any barrier methods and would like the option of regaining fertility after a couple of years. Which of the following methods should the nurse suggest to this client?

   a. BBT

   b. Coitus interruptus

   c. Lactational amenorrhea method

   d. Cycle Beads or Depo-Provera

10. A client would like some information about the use of a cervical cap. Which of the following should the nurse include in the teaching plan of this client? Select all that apply.

   a. Inspect the cervical cap before insertion.

   b. Apply spermicide to the rim of the cervical cap.

   c. Wait for 30 minutes after insertion before engaging in intercourse.

   d. Remove the cervical cap immediately after intercourse.

   e. Do not use the cervical cap during menses.

11. A healthy 28-year-old female client who has a sedentary lifestyle and is a chain smoker is seeking information about contraception. The nurse informs this client of the various options available and the benefits and the risks of each. Which of the following should the nurse recognize as contraindicated in the case of this client?

   a. The Lunelle injection or Depo-Provera

   b. Combination OCs

   c. A copper intrauterine device

   d. Implantable contraceptives

12. A client in her second trimester of pregnancy asks the nurse for information regarding certain oral medications to induce a miscarriage. What information should this client be given about such medications?

   a. They are available only in the form of suppositories.

   b. They can be taken only in the first trimester.

   c. They present a high risk of respiratory failure.

   d. They are considered a permanent end to fertility.

13. A client reports that she has multiple sex partners and has a lengthy history of various pelvic infections. She would like to know if there is any temporary contraceptive method that would suit her condition. Which of the following should the nurse suggest for this client?

   a. Intrauterine device

   b. Condoms

   c. OCs

   d. Tubal ligation

14. When caring for a client with reproductive issues, the nurse is required to clear up misconceptions. This enables new learning to take hold and a better client response to whichever methods are explored and ultimately selected. Which of the following are misconceptions that the nurse needs to clear up? Select all that apply.

    a. Breastfeeding does not protect against pregnancy.

    b. Taking birth control pills protects against sexually transmitted infections (STIs).

    c. Douching after sex will prevent pregnancy.

    d. Pregnancy can occur during menses.

    e. Irregular menstruation prevents pregnancy.

15. A 52-year-old client is seeking treatment for menopause. She is not very active and has a history of cardiac problems. Which of the following therapy options should the nurse recognize as contraindicated for this client?

    a. Long-term hormone replacement therapy

    b. Selective estrogen receptor modulators

    c. Lipid-lowering agents

    d. Bisphosphonates

16. A 49-year-old client who is in the perimenopausal phase of life reports to the nurse a loss of lubrication during intercourse, which she feels is hampering her sex life. Which of the following responses is appropriate for the nurse?

    a. "Don't worry! This is a normal process of aging."

    b. "Have you considered contacting a support group for women your age?"

    c. "You can manage the condition by using over-the-counter (OTC) moisturizers or lubricants."

    d. "All you need is a positive outlook and a supportive partner."

17. A client has opted to use an intrauterine device for contraception. Which of the following effects of the device on monthly periods should the nurse inform the client about?

    a. Periods become lighter

    b. Periods become more painful

    c. Periods become longer

    d. Periods reduce in number

18. A 30-year-old client tells the nurse that she would like to use a contraceptive sponge but does not know enough about its use and whether it will protect her against STIs. Which of the following information should the nurse provide the client about using a contraceptive sponge? Select all that apply.

    a. Keep the sponge for more than 30 hours to prevent STIs.

    b. Wet the sponge with water before inserting it.

    c. Insert the sponge 24 hours before intercourse.

    d. Leave the sponge in place for at least 6 hours following intercourse.

    e. Replace sponge every 2 hours for the method to be effective.

CHAPTER 5

Sexually Transmitted Infections

Learning Objectives

Upon completion of the chapter, you will be able to:

- Define the key terms used in this chapter.
- Evaluate the spread and control of STIs.
- Identify risk factors and outline appropriate client education needed in common STIs.
- Describe how contraceptives can play a role in the prevention of STIs.
- Analyze the physiologic and psychological aspects of STIs.
- Outline the nursing management needed for women with STIs.

SECTION I: ASSESSING YOUR UNDERSTANDING

Activity A FILL IN THE BLANKS

1. _____ is a common vaginal infection characterized by a heavy yellow, green, or gray frothy discharge.

2. The _____ stage of syphilis is characterized by diseases affecting the heart, eyes, brain, central nervous system, and/or skin.

3. _____ are a common cause of skin rash and pruritus throughout the world.

4. _____ is an intense pruritic dermatitis caused by a mite.

5. Vulvovaginal candidiasis, if not treated effectively during pregnancy, can cause the newborn to contract an oral infection known as _____ during the birth process.

6. _____ is a complex, curable bacterial infection caused by the spirochete Treponema pallidum.

7. Hepatitis B virus (HBV) can result in serious, permanent damage to the _____.

8. Cervicitis, acute urethral syndrome, salpingitis, pelvic inflammatory disease (PID), and infertility are conditions associated with _____ infection.

9. A person is said to be in the last stage of AIDS when the _____ T-cell count is less than or equal to 200.

10. Any woman suspected of having gonorrhea should be tested for _____ also, because co-infection (45%) is extremely common.

Activity B LABELING

Consider the following figures.

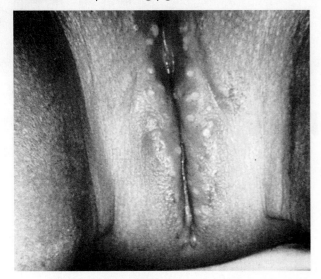

1. a. Identify this disease.

    _____

    _____

    b. What are the risk factors of this disease?

    _____

    _____

    c. What treatments are available to manage this disease?

    _____

    _____

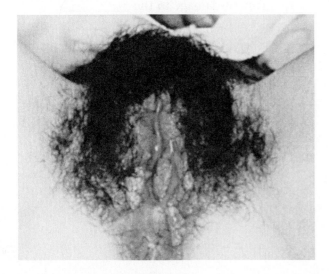

2. a. Identify this disease.

    _____

    _____

b. What are the clinical manifestations of this disease?

    _____

    _____

c. What medications may be prescribed to manage this condition?

    _____

    _____

Activity C MATCHING

Match the STIs in Column A with their related descriptions in Column B.

Column A

____ 1. HIV

____ 2. Vaginitis

____ 3. Hepatitis

____ 4. Gonorrhea

____ 5. Genital herpes

____ 6. Human papilloma virus (HPV)

Column B

a. Inflammation and infection of the vagina

b. Acute, systemic viral infection that can be transmitted sexually

c. Retrovirus causes breakdown in immune function, leading to AIDS

d. A recurrent, lifelong viral infection

e. Cause of essentially all cases of cervical cancer

f. Very severe bacterial infection in the columnar epithelium of the endocervix

Activity D SEQUENCING

Given below, in random order, are the manifestations of syphilis in its various stages. Arrange the stages in their correct order.

1. Flu-like symptoms; rash on trunk, palms, and soles

2. Life-threatening heart disease and neurologic disease that slowly destroys the heart, the eyes, the brain, the central nervous system, and the skin

3. Painless ulcer at site of bacterial entry that disappears in 1 to 6 weeks

4. No clinical manifestations even though serology is positive

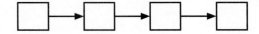

Activity E SHORT ANSWER

Briefly answer the following.

1. What are the predisposing factors for the occurrence of vulvovaginal candidiasis?

   _____

   _____

   _____

2. What are the symptoms of hepatitis A?

   _____

   _____

   _____

3. How is HIV transmitted?

   _____

   _____

   _____

4. What is AIDS?

   _____

   _____

   _____

5. What are the causes of vaginitis?

   _____

   _____

   _____

6. What are clinical manifestations of Chlamydia?

   _____

   _____

   _____

SECTION II: APPLYING YOUR KNOWLEDGE

Activity F CASE STUDY

Consider this scenario and answer the questions.

1. A nurse is caring for a 22-year-old pregnant client who has been diagnosed with gonorrhea. The client seems to be very apprehensive about seeking treatment and wants to know if her newborn would be at risk for the infection.

   a. What information should the nurse provide the client regarding the transmission of the infection to the newborn?

   _____

   _____

   _____

   b. What factors should a nurse be aware of when caring for the client with gonorrhea or any other STI?

   _____

   _____

   _____

   c. Which groups of clients are at a higher risk for developing gonorrhea?

   _____

   _____

   _____

SECTION III: PRACTICING FOR NCLEX

Activity G NCLEX-STYLE QUESTIONS

Answer the following questions.

1. A nurse is caring for a female client who has a history of recurring vulvovaginal candidiasis. Which of the following instructions should the nurse include in the teaching session with the client?
   a. Use superabsorbent tampons.
   b. Douche the affected area regularly.
   c. Wear white, 100% cotton underpants.
   d. Increase intake of carbonated drinks.

2. An HIV-positive client who is on antiretroviral therapy complains of anorexia, nausea, and vomiting. Which of the following suggestions should the nurse offer the client to cope with this condition?
   a. Use high-protein supplements.
   b. Eat dry crackers after meals.
   c. Limit number of meals to three a day.
   d. Constantly drink fluids while eating.

3. A client complaining of genital warts has been diagnosed with HPV. The genital warts have been treated, and they have disappeared. Which of the following should the

nurse include in the teaching plan when educating the client about the condition?

a. Applying steroid creams in affected area promotes comfort.

b. Even after warts are removed, HPV still remains.

c. All women above the age of 30 should get themselves vaccinated against HPV.

d. Use of latex condoms is associated with increased risk of cervical cancer.

4. A female client is prescribed metronidazole for the treatment of trichomoniasis. Which of the following instructions should the nurse give the client undergoing treatment?

a. Avoid extremes of temperature to the genital area.

b. Use condoms during sex.

c. Increase fluid intake.

d. Avoid alcohol.

5. A nurse is required to assess a client complaining of unusual vaginal discharge for bacterial vaginosis. Which of the following is a classic manifestation of this condition that the nurse should assess for?

a. Characteristic "stale fish" odor

b. Heavy yellow discharge

c. Dysfunctional uterine bleeding

d. Erythema in the vulvovaginal area

6. A nurse needs to assess a female client for primary stage herpes simplex virus (HSV) infection. Which of the following symptoms related to this condition should the nurse assess for?

a. Rashes on the face

b. Yellow-green vaginal discharge

c. Loss of hair or alopecia

d. Genital vesicular lesions

7. A nurse working in a community health education program is assigned to educate community members about STIs. Which of the following nursing strategies should be adopted to prevent the spread of STIs in the community?

a. Promote use of oral contraceptives.

b. Emphasize the importance of good body hygiene.

c. Discuss limiting the number of sex partners.

d. Emphasize not sharing personal items with others.

8. A nurse who is conducting sessions on preventing the spread of STIs in a particular community discovers that there is a very high incidence of hepatitis B in the community. Which of the following measures should she take to ensure the prevention of the disease?

a. Ensure that the drinking water is disease free.

b. Instruct people to get vaccinated for hepatitis B.

c. Educate about risks of injecting drugs.

d. Educate teenagers to delay onset of sexual activity.

9. A nurse is caring for a client undergoing treatment for bacterial vaginosis. Which of the following instructions should the nurse give the client to prevent recurrence of bacterial vaginosis? Select all that apply.

a. Practice monogamy

b. Use oral contraceptives

c. Avoid smoking

d. Undergo colposcopy tests frequently

e. Avoid foods containing excessive sugar

10. A pregnant client arrives at the community clinic complaining of fever blisters and cold sores on the lips, eyes, and face. The primary health care provider has diagnosed it as the primary episode of genital herpes simplex, for which antiviral therapy is recommended. Which of the following information should the nurse offer the client when educating her about managing the infection?

a. Antiviral drug therapy cures the infection completely.

b. Kissing during the primary episode does not transmit the virus.

c. Safety of antiviral therapy during pregnancy has not been established.

d. Recurrent HSV infection episodes are longer and more severe.

11. A 19-year-old female client has been diagnosed with pelvic inflammatory disease due to untreated gonorrhea. Which of the following instructions should the nurse offer when caring for the client? Select all that apply.

a. Use an intrauterine device (IUD).

b. Avoid douching vaginal area.

c. Complete the antibiotic therapy.

d. Increase fluid intake.

e. Limit the number of sex partners.

12. A client complaining of genital ulcers has been diagnosed with syphilis. Which of the following nursing interventions should the nurse implement when caring for the client? Select all that apply.

    a. Have the client urinate in water if urination is painful.

    b. Suggest the client apply ice packs to the genital area for comfort.

    c. Instruct the client to wash her hands with soap and water after touching lesions.

    d. Instruct the client to wear nonconstricting, comfortable clothes.

    e. Instruct the client to abstain from sex during the latency period.

13. A nurse is conducting an AIDS awareness program for women. Which of the following instructions should the nurse include in the teaching plan to empower women to develop control over their lives in a practical manner so that they can prevent becoming infected with HIV? Select the most appropriate responses.

    a. Give opportunities to practice negotiation techniques.

    b. Encourage women to develop refusal skills.

    c. Encourage women to use female condoms.

    d. Support youth-development activities to reduce sexual risk-taking.

    e. Encourage women to lead a healthy lifestyle.

14. A nurse is caring for an HIV-positive client who is on triple-combination highly active antiretroviral therapy (HAART). Which of the following should the nurse include in the teaching plan when educating the client about the treatment? Select all that apply.

    a. Exposure of fetus to antiretroviral agents is completely safe.

    b. Successful antiretroviral therapy may prevent AIDS.

    c. Unpleasant side effects such as nausea and diarrhea are common.

    d. Provide written materials describing diet, exercise, and medications.

    e. Ensure that the client understands the dosing regimen and schedule.

15. A nurse is caring for a female client who is undergoing treatment for genital warts due to HPV. Which of the following information should the nurse include when educating the client about the risk of cervical cancer? Select all that apply.

    a. Use of broad-spectrum antibiotics increases risk of cervical cancer.

    b. Obtaining Pap smears regularly helps early detection of cervical cancer.

    c. Abnormal vaginal discharge is a sign of cervical cancer.

    d. Recurrence of genital warts increases risk of cervical cancer.

    e. Use of latex condoms is associated with a lower rate of cervical cancer.

16. A nurse is caring for a client who has just delivered a baby. Which of the following information should the nurse give the client regarding hepatitis B vaccination for the baby?

    a. Vaccine may not be safe for underweight or premature babies.

    b. Vaccine consists of a series of three injections given within 6 months.

    c. Vaccine is administered only after the infant is at least 6 months old.

    d. Vaccine is required only if mother is identified as high-risk for hepatitis B.

17. A pregnant client has been diagnosed with gonorrhea. Which of the following nursing interventions should be performed to prevent gonococcal ophthalmia neonatorum in the baby?

    a. Administer cephalosporins to mother during pregnancy.

    b. Instill a prophylactic agent in the eyes of the newborn.

    c. Perform a cesarean operation to prevent infection.

    d. Administer an antiretroviral syrup to the newborn.

18. A pregnant client is diagnosed with AIDS. Which of the following interventions should the nurse undertake to minimize the risk of transmission of AIDS to the infant?

    a. Ensure that the baby is delivered via cesarean.

    b. Begin triple-combination HAART for the newborn.

    c. Ensure that the baby is breastfed instead of being given formula.

    d. Administer antiretroviral syrup to the infant within 12 hours after birth.

Disorders of the Breast

Learning Objectives

Upon completion of the chapter, you will be able to:

- Define the key terms used in this chapter.
- Identify the incidence, risk factors, screening methods, and treatment modalities for benign breast conditions.
- Outline preventive strategies for breast cancer through lifestyle changes and health screening.
- Analyze the incidence, risk factors, treatment modalities, and nursing considerations related to breast cancer.
- Develop an educational plan to teach breast self-examination to a group of high-risk women.

SECTION I: ASSESSING YOUR UNDERSTANDING

Activity A FILL IN THE BLANKS

1. _____ is a useful adjunct to mammography that produces images of the breasts by sending sound waves through a conductive gel applied to the breasts.

2. _____, an alternative to radiation therapy, involves the use of a catheter to implant radioactive seeds into the breast after a tumor has been removed surgically.

3. Hormone therapy is used to block or counter the effect of the hormone _____ while treating breast cancer.

4. _____ is contraindicated for women whose active connective tissue conditions make them especially sensitive to the side effects of radiation.

5. _____ involves taking x-ray pictures of the breasts while they are compressed between two plastic plates.

6. _____, a type of therapy for breast cancer, leads to side effects such as hair loss, weight loss, and fatigue.

7. The removal of all breast tissue, the nipple, and the areola for breast cancer treatment is known as _____.

8. When diagnosing a woman with intraductal papilloma, a _____ card is used to evaluate nipple discharge for the presence of occult blood.

9. _____ is used as an adjunct therapy for breast cancer.

10. _____ are common benign solid breast tumors that occur in about 10% of all women and account for up to half of all breast biopsies.

Activity B MATCHING

Match the benign breast disorders in Column A with their related descriptions in Column B.

Column A

____ 1. Fibrocystic breast changes

____ 2. Fibroadenomas

____ 3. Intraductal papilloma

____ 4. Mammary duct ectasia

____ 5. Mastitis

Column B

a. An infection of the connective tissue in the breast, occurring primarily in lactating women

b. Dilation and inflammation of the ducts behind the nipple

c. Benign, wart-like growths found in the mammary ducts, usually near the nipple

d. Firm, rubbery, well-circumscribed, freely mobile nodules that might or might not be tender when palpated

e. Lumpy, tender breasts; multiple, smooth, tiny "pebbles" or lumpy "oatmeal" under the skin in later stages

Activity C SEQUENCING

1. Listed below in random order are steps taken to diagnose a breast mass. Arrange the steps in order of typical occurrence.

   a. Core needle biopsy

   b. Clinical manual breast examination

c. Imaging studies

d. Advanced Breast Biopsy Instrument biopsy

☐ → ☐ → ☐ → ☐

Activity D SHORT ANSWERS

Briefly answer the following.

1. What are benign breast disorders?

_____

_____

_____

2. What are the three aspects on which breast cancers are classified?

_____

_____

_____

3. What is breast-conserving surgery?

_____

_____

_____

4. What is adjunct therapy?

_____

_____

_____

5. What are the side effects of chemotherapy?

_____

_____

_____

6. Why is the status of the axillary lymph nodes important in the diagnosis of breast cancer?

_____

_____

_____

SECTION II: APPLYING YOUR KNOWLEDGE

Activity E CASE STUDY

Consider this scenario and answer the questions.

Mrs. Taylor, age 54, presents to the women's health community clinic, where a nurse assesses her. She is very upset and crying. She tells the nurse that she found one large lump in her left breast and she knows that "it's cancer and I will die." When the nurse asks about her problem, she states that she does not routinely check her breasts and she hasn't had a mammogram for years because "they're too expensive." She also describes the intermittent pain she experiences in her breast.

1. What specific questions should the nurse include in her assessment of Mrs. Taylor?

   _____

   _____

   _____

2. What education does Mrs. Taylor need regarding breast health?

   _____

   _____

   _____

3. Explain what treatment modalities are available if Mrs. Taylor does have a malignancy.

   _____

   _____

   _____

4. What community referrals are needed to meet Mrs. Taylor's future needs?

   _____

   _____

   _____

SECTION III: PRACTICING FOR NCLEX

Activity F NCLEX-STYLE QUESTIONS

Answer the following questions.

1. A client complains of lumpy, tender breasts, particularly during the week before menses. She complains of pain that often dissipates after the onset of menses. The nurse has to examine the client's breasts to confirm fibrocystic breast changes. Which of the following is the best time in the client's menstrual cycle to perform a breast examination?

   a. When the client is ovulating

   b. During the second phase of the client's menstrual cycle

   c. A week after the client has completed her menses

   d. Immediately after the client's menses

2. A client arrives at the health care facility complaining of a lump that she felt during her breast self-examination. Upon diagnosis, the physician suspects fibroadenomas. Which of the following questions should the nurse ask when assessing the client?

   a. "Do you consume foods high in fat?"

   b. "Are you lactating?"

   c. "Are you taking oral contraceptives?"

   d. "Do you smoke regularly?"

3. A female client who has a 2-month-old baby arrives at a health care facility complaining of flulike symptoms with fever and chills. When examining the breast, the nurse observes an increase in warmth, tenderness, and swelling with abraded nipples. The diagnosis indicates mastitis. Which of the following instructions should the nurse provide the client to help her cope with the condition?

   a. Increase fluid intake.

   b. Avoid breastfeeding for a month.

   c. Avoid changing positions while nursing.

   d. Apply cold compresses to the affected breast.

4. Mammography is recommended for a client diagnosed with intraductal papilloma. Which of the following factors should the nurse ensure when preparing the client for a mammography?
   a. Client has not consumed fluids an hour before testing.
   b. Client has not applied deodorant on the day of testing.
   c. Client is just going to start her menses.
   d. Client has taken an aspirin before the testing.

5. A female client with a malignant tumor of the breast has to undergo chemotherapy for a period of 6 months. Which of the following side effects should the nurse monitor for when caring for this client?
   a. Vaginal discharge
   b. Headache
   c. Chills
   d. Constipation

6. A client diagnosed with fibroadenoma is worried about her chances of developing breast cancer. She also asks the nurse about various breast disorders and their risks. Which of the following benign breast disorders should the nurse include as having the greatest risk for the development of breast cancer?
   a. Fibroadenomas
   b. Mastitis
   c. Mammary duct ectasia
   d. Intraductal papilloma

7. It is recommended that a 48-year-old female client with breast cancer undergo a sentinel lymph node biopsy before lumpectomy. The client is anxious to know the reason for removing the sentinel lymph node. Which of the following information should the nurse offer the client?
   a. It will prevent lymphedema, which is a common side effect.
   b. It will reveal the hormone receptor status of the cancer.
   c. It will lessen the aggressiveness of the subsequent chemotherapy.
   d. It will allow the degree of human epidermal growth factor receptor 2 (HER-2)/neu oncoprotein to be revealed.

8. A client has undergone a mastectomy for breast cancer. Which of the following instructions should the nurse include in the postsurgery client-teaching plan?
   a. Breathe rapidly for an hour
   b. Elevate the affected arm on a pillow
   c. Avoid moving the affected arm in any way
   d. Restrict intake of medication

9. A 62-year-old female client arrives at a health care facility complaining of skin redness in the breast area, along with skin edema. The physician suspects inflammatory breast cancer. Which of the following is a symptom of inflammatory breast cancer that the nurse should assess for?
   a. Palpable mobile cysts
   b. Palpable papilloma
   c. Increased warmth of the breast
   d. Induced nipple discharge

10. A 41-year-old female client arrives at a health care setting complaining of dull nipple pain with a burning sensation, accompanied by pruritus around the nipple. The physician suspects mammary duct ectasia. Which of the following is a manifestation of mammary duct ectasia that the nurse should assess for?
    a. Torturous tubular swellings in the upper half of the breast
    b. Increased warmth of the breasts, along with redness
    c. Skin retractions on the breast when the skin is pulled
    d. Green-colored nipple discharge with consistency of toothpaste

11. A 52-year-old female client with an estrogen receptors positive (ER+) breast cancer has to undergo hormonal therapy after her initial treatment. The client has to be administered selective estrogen receptor modulator (SERM). Which of the following side effects of SERM should the nurse monitor for when caring for the client?
    a. Fever
    b. Weight loss
    c. Hot flashes
    d. Chills

12. A nurse is assigned to educate a group of women on cancer awareness. Which of the following are the modifiable risk factors for breast cancer? Select all that apply.

    a. Failing to breastfeed for up to a year after pregnancy

    b. Early menarche or late menopause

    c. Postmenopausal use of estrogen and progestins

    d. Not having children until after age 30

    e. Previous abnormal breast biopsy

13. A nurse is educating a client on the technique for performing breast self-examination. Which of the following instructions should the nurse include in the teaching plan with regard to the different degrees of pressure that need to be applied on the breast?

    a. Light pressure midway into the tissue

    b. Medium pressure around the areolar area

    c. Medium pressure on the skin throughout

    d. Hard pressure applied down to the ribs

14. A female client with metastatic breast disease is prescribed trastuzumab as part of her immunotherapy. Which of the following is the adverse effect of trastuzumab that a nurse should monitor for with the first infusion of the antibody?

    a. Stroke

    b. Hepatic failure

    c. Myelosuppression

    d. Dyspnea

15. A nurse is caring for a female client undergoing radiation therapy after her breast surgery. Which of the following is the side effect of radiation therapy that the client is likely to experience?

    a. Anorexia

    b. Infection

    c. Fever

    d. Nausea

16. A nurse is caring for a client who has just had her intraductal papilloma removed through a surgical procedure. What instructions should the nurse give this client as part of her care?

    a. Apply warm compresses to the affected breast.

    b. Continue monthly breast self-examinations.

    c. Wear a supportive bra 24 hours a day.

    d. Refrain from consuming salt in diet.

17. Lumpectomy is a treatment option for clients diagnosed with breast cancer with tumors smaller than 5 cm. For which of the following clients is lumpectomy contraindicated? Select all that apply.

    a. Client who has had an early menarche or late onset of menopause

    b. Client who has had previous radiation to the affected breast

    c. Client who has failed to breastfeed for up to a year after pregnancy

    d. Client whose connective tissue is reported to be sensitive to radiation

    e. Client whose surgery will not result in a clean margin of tissue

18. A 38-year-old female client has to undergo lymph node surgery in conjunction with mastectomy. The client is likely to experience lymphedema due to the surgery. Post-surgery, which of the following factors will make the client more susceptible to lymphedema? Select all that apply.

    a. Use of the affected arm for drawing blood or measuring blood pressure

    b. Engaging in activities like gardening without using gloves

    c. Not consuming foods that are rich in phytochemicals

    d. Not wearing a well-fitted compression sleeve

    e. Not consuming a diet high in fiber and protein

19. A 33-year-old female client complains of yellow nipple discharge and a pain in her breasts a week before menses that dissipates on the onset of menses. Diagnosis reveals that the client is experiencing fibrocystic breast changes. Which of the following instructions should the nurse offer the client to help alleviate the condition? Select all that apply.

   a. Increase fluid intake steadily.

   b. Avoid caffeine.

   c. Practice good hand-washing techniques.

   d. Maintain a low-fat diet.

   e. Take diuretics as recommended.

20. A nurse is educating a 43-year-old female client about required lifestyle changes to help avoid breast cancer. Which of the following instructions regarding diet and food habits should the nurse include in the teaching plan? Select all that apply.

   a. Restrict intake of salted foods.

   b. Limit intake of processed foods.

   c. Consume seven or more portions of complex carbohydrates daily.

   d. Increase liquid intake to 3 L daily.

   e. Consume at least five servings of proteins daily.

CHAPTER 7

Benign Disorders of the Female Reproductive Tract

Learning Objectives

Upon completion of the chapter, you will be able to:

- Define the key terms.
- Identify the major pelvic relaxation disorders in terms of etiology, management, and nursing interventions.
- Outline the nursing management needed for the most common benign reproductive disorders in women.
- Evaluate urinary incontinence in terms of pathology, clinical manifestations, treatment options, and effect on quality of life.
- Compare the various benign growths in terms of their symptoms and management.
- Analyze the emotional impact of polycystic ovarian syndrome and the nurse's role as a counselor, educator, and advocate.

SECTION I: ASSESSING YOUR UNDERSTANDING

Activity A FILL IN THE BLANKS

1. _____ occurs when the posterior bladder wall protrudes downward through the anterior vaginal wall.

2. Uterine _____ occurs when the uterus descends through the pelvic floor and into the vaginal canal.

3. A _____ is a silicone or plastic device that is placed into the vagina to support the uterus, bladder, and rectum as a space-filling device.

4. _____ are small benign growths that may be associated with chronic inflammation, an abnormal local response to increased levels of estrogen, or local congestion of the cervical vasculature.

5. Uterine fibroids, or _____, are benign proliferations composed of smooth muscle and fibrous connective tissue in the uterus.

6. _____ exercises strengthen the pelvic floor muscles to support the inner organs and prevent further prolapse.

7. Rectocele occurs when the _____ relaxes and pushes against or into the posterior vaginal wall.

8. Weakened pelvic floor musculature also prevents complete closure of the _____, resulting in urine leakage during moments of physical activity.

9. _____, or irregular, acyclic uterine bleeding, is the most frequent clinical manifestation of women with endometrial polyps.

10. _____ ultrasound is used to distinguish fluid-filled ovarian cysts from a solid mass.

Activity B MATCHING

Match the benign disorders of the female reproductive tract in Column A with their correct definitions in Column B.

Column A

_____ **1.** Pelvic organ prolapsed

_____ **2.** Stress incontinence

_____ **3.** Uterine fibroids

_____ **4.** Polycystic ovarian syndrome

_____ **5.** Urge incontinence

Column B

a. Abnormal descent or herniation of the pelvic organs from their original attachment sites or their normal positions in the pelvis

b. Benign tumors composed of muscular and fibrous tissue in the uterus

c. Presence of multiple inactive follicle cysts within the ovary that interfere with ovarian function

d. Precipitous loss of urine, preceded by a strong urge to void, with increased bladder pressure and detrusor contraction

e. Accidental leakage of urine that occurs with increased pressure on the bladder from coughing, sneezing, laughing, or physical exertion

Activity C SHORT ANSWERS

Briefly answer the following.

1. What are the causes of pelvic organ prolapse?

_____

_____

_____

2. What are Kegel exercises?

_____

_____

_____

3. What are the causes of urinary incontinence?

_____

_____

_____

4. What is the Colpexin Sphere?

_____

_____

_____

5. What is uterine artery embolization (UAE)?

_____

_____

_____

6. What are Bartholin cysts?

_____

_____

_____

SECTION II: APPLYING YOUR KNOWLEDGE

Activity D CASE STUDY

Consider this scenario and answer the questions.

Mrs. Scott, age 57, comes in for a gynecologic examination and reports to the nurse that she "feels like something is coming down in her vagina." She has chronic smoker's cough. Upon completion of a pelvic exam, uterine prolapse is diagnosed.

1. What factors may contribute to the development of this disorder?

_____

_____

_____

2. What are the symptoms of uterine prolapse that may affect Mrs. Scott's daily activities?

_____

_____

_____

3. What are the nonsurgical and surgical interventions available to Mrs. Scott?

_____

_____

_____

SECTION III: PRACTICING FOR NCLEX

Activity E **NCLEX-STYLE QUESTIONS**

Answer the following questions.

1. A 40-year-old client arrives at the community health center experiencing a strange dragging feeling in the vagina. She stated that "at times it feels as if there is a lump" there as well. Which of the following conditions may be an indication of these symptoms?
   a. Urinary incontinence
   b. Endocervical polyps
   c. Pelvic organ prolapse
   d. Uterine fibroids

2. A nurse is caring for a client for whom estrogen replacement therapy has been recommended for pelvic organ prolapse. Which of the following is the most appropriate nursing intervention the nurse should implement before the start of the therapy?
   a. Discuss the effective dose of estrogen required to treat the client.
   b. Evaluate the client to validate her risk for complications.
   c. Discuss the dietary modifications following therapy.
   d. Discuss the cost of estrogen replacement therapy.

3. A nurse is caring for a female client with symptoms of first-degree pelvic organ prolapse. Which of the following instructions related to dietary and lifestyle modifications should the nurse provide to the client to help prevent pelvic relaxation and chronic problems later in life?
   a. Increase dietary fiber
   b. Avoid caffeine products
   c. Avoid excess intake of fluids
   d. Increase high-impact aerobics

4. Myomectomy is recommended to a client for removal of uterine fibroids. The client is concerned about the surgery and wants to know if there are any disadvantages associated with it. Which of the following is a disadvantage of myomectomy?
   a. Fertility is jeopardized.
   b. Uterus is scarred and adhesions may form.
   c. Uterine walls are weakened.
   d. Fibroids may grow back.

5. Kegel exercises are recommended for a client with pelvic organ prolapse. Which of the following should the nurse inform the client about the exercises?
   a. They should be performed after food intake.
   b. They alleviate mild prolapse symptoms.
   c. They are not recommended after surgery.
   d. They increase blood pressure.

6. A nurse is assessing a 45-year-old client for uterine fibroids. Which of the following are the predisposing factors for uterine fibroids? Select all that apply.
   a. Age
   b. Nulliparity
   c. Smoking
   d. Obesity
   e. Hyperinsulinemia

7. A nurse is caring for a client who has been prescribed GnRH medication for uterine fibroids. Which of the following is a side effect of GnRH medications that the nurse should monitor the client for?
   a. Increased vaginal discharge
   b. Vaginal dryness
   c. Urinary tract infections
   d. Vaginitis

8. A nurse is caring for a 32-year-old client for whom pessary usage is recommended for uterine prolapse. Which of the following instructions should the nurse include in the teaching plan for the client concerning the pessary?
   a. Avoid jogging and jumping.
   b. Wear a girdle or abdominal support.
   c. Report any discomfort with urination and defecation.
   d. Avoid lifting heavy objects.

9. A nurse is caring for a 45-year-old client using a pessary to help decrease leakage of urine and support a prolapsed vagina. Which of the following is the most common recommendation a nurse should provide to the client regarding pessary care?

    a. Douche vaginal area with diluted vinegar or hydrogen peroxide.

    b. Remove the pessary twice weekly, and clean it with soap and water.

    c. Use estrogen cream to make the vaginal mucosa more resistant to erosion.

    d. Remove the pessary before sleeping or intercourse.

10. A client with abnormal uterine bleeding is diagnosed with small ovarian cysts. The nurse has to educate the client on the importance of routine check-ups. Which of the following is the most appropriate assessment for this client's condition?

    a. Monitor gonadotropin level every month.

    b. Monitor blood sugar level every 15 days.

    c. Schedule periodic Pap smears.

    d. Schedule ultrasound every 3 to 6 months.

11. A client with large uterine fibroids is scheduled to undergo a hysterectomy. Which of the following interventions should the nurse perform as a part of the preoperative care for the client?

    a. Teach turning, deep breathing, and coughing.

    b. Instruct the client to reduce activity level.

    c. Educate the client on the need for pelvic rest.

    d. Instruct the client to avoid a high-fat diet.

12. A 40-year-old client complains of low back pain after standing for a long time. The primary care provider has diagnosed the client with pelvic organ prolapse. The nurse correctly recognizes that which of the following clients is likely not a candidate for corrective surgery for pelvic organ prolapsed. Select all that apply.

    a. Clients with low back pain and pelvic pressure

    b. Clients at high risk of recurrent prolapse after surgery

    c. Client who is morbidly obese before surgery

    d. Client who has severe pelvic organ prolapse

    e. Client who has chronic obstructive pulmonary disease

13. A nurse is caring for a female client with urinary incontinence. Which of the following instructions should the nurse include in the client's teaching plan to reduce the incidence or severity of incontinence? Select all that apply.

    a. Continue pelvic floor exercises.

    b. Increase fiber in the diet.

    c. Increase intake of orange juice.

    d. Control blood glucose levels.

    e. Wipe from back to front.

14. A client has undergone an abdominal hysterectomy to remove uterine fibroids. Which of the followings interventions should a nurse perform as a part of the postoperative care for the client? Select all that apply.

    a. Administer analgesics promptly and use a patient-controlled analgesia (PCA) pump

    b. Avoid pillows and changing positions frequently

    c. Avoid intake of excess carbonated beverages in the diet

    d. Frequent ambulation

    e. Administer antiemetics to control nausea and vomiting

15. A client with complaints of changes in her normal voiding patterns and altered bowel habits is diagnosed with polycystic ovarian syndrome. Which of the following is the most appropriate instruction the nurse should provide to the client to help alleviate her condition?

    a. Adhere to follow-up care.

    b. Increase intake of fiber-rich foods.

    c. Increase fluid intake.

    d. Perform Kegel exercises.

CHAPTER 8

Cancers of the Female Reproductive Tract

Learning Objectives

Upon completion of the chapter, you will be able to:

- Define the key terms in the chapter.
- Evaluate the major modifiable risk factors for reproductive tract cancers.
- Analyze the screening methods and treatment modalities for cancers of the female reproductive tract.
- Outline the nursing management needed for the most common malignant reproductive tract cancers in women.
- Examine lifestyle changes and health screenings that can reduce the risk of or prevent reproductive tract cancers.
- Assess at least three website resources available for a woman diagnosed with cancer of the reproductive tract.
- Appraise the psychological distress felt by women diagnosed with cancer, and outline information that can help them to cope.

SECTION I: ASSESSING YOUR UNDERSTANDING

Activity A FILL IN THE BLANKS

1. High-grade _____ can progress to invasive cervical cancer; the progression takes up to 2 years.

2. _____ is a microscopic examination of the lower genital tract with use of a magnifying instrument.

3. _____ is the use of liquid nitrogen to freeze abnormal cervical tissue.

4. _____ or uterine cancer is a malignant neoplastic growth of the uterine lining.

5. Pap smear results are classified by the _____ system.

6. _____ refers to the surgical removal of the uterus.

7. _____ is a biologic tumor marker associated with ovarian cancer.

8. The two major types of vulvar intraepithelial neoplasia (VIN) are classic (undifferentiated) and _____ (differentiated).

9. Ovarian cancer usually originates in the ovarian _____.

10. _____ cell carcinomas that begin in the epithelial lining of the vagina tend to spread early by directly invading the bladder and rectal walls.

Activity B MATCHING

Match the stages of endometrial cancer in Column A with the relevant organs affected during that stage in Column B.

Column A	Column B
____ 1. Stage I	a. Cervix
____ 2. Stage II	b. Muscle wall of the uterus
____ 3. Stage III	
____ 4. Stage IV	

c. Bladder mucosa, with distant metastases to the lungs, the liver, and bone

d. Bowel or vagina, with metastases to pelvic lymph nodes

Given below, in random order, are some of the steps performed by a nurse while assisting with the collection of a Pap smear. Choose the most likely sequence in which they would have occurred.

1. Provide support to the client as the practitioner obtains a sample.

2. Drape the client with a sheet, leaving the perineal area exposed.

3. Wash hands thoroughly.

4. Transfer the specimen to a container or a slide.

5. Position the client in stirrups or foot pedals so that her knees fall outward.

6. Assemble the equipment.

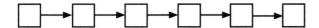

Briefly answer the following.

1. What are the risk factors associated with cervical cancer?

_____

_____

_____

2. What are the treatment options for endometrial cancer?

_____

_____

_____

3. What are the risk factors for ovarian cancer?

_____

_____

_____

4. What is a transvaginal ultrasound used for?

_____

_____

_____

5. What are the nursing interventions when caring for clients with cancers of the female reproductive tract?

_____

_____

_____

6. What are the diagnostic options for endometrial cancer?

_____

_____

_____

SECTION II: APPLYING YOUR KNOWLEDGE

Consider this scenario and answer the questions.

Amy, age 60, has been diagnosed with ovarian cancer. Because this cancer develops slowly, remains silent, and is without symptoms until the cancer is far advanced, it is considered one of the worst gynecologic malignancies.

1. What are the most common symptoms of ovarian cancer?

_____

_____

_____

2. There is still no adequate screening test to identify early cancer of the ovary. What suggestions should a nurse give a client to facilitate early detection of this type of cancer?

_____

_____

_____

3. State the nursing diagnoses related to malignancies of the reproductive tract.

_____

_____

_____

4. Explain the four stages of ovarian cancer.

_____

_____

_____

SECTION III: PRACTICING FOR NCLEX

Activity F **NCLEX-STYLE QUESTIONS**

Answer the following questions.

1. A nurse is educating a 25-year-old client with a family history of cervical cancer. Which of the following tests should the nurse inform the client about to detect cervical cancer at an early stage?
   a. Papanicolaou test
   b. Blood tests for mutations in the BRCA genes
   c. CA-125 blood test
   d. Transvaginal ultrasound

2. A client presents for her annual Pap test. She wants to know about the risk factors that are associated with cervical cancer. Which of the following should the nurse inform the client is a risk factor for cervical cancer?
   a. Early age at first intercourse
   b. Obesity (at least 50 lb overweight)
   c. Hypertension
   d. Infertility

3. A client is waiting for the results of an endometrial biopsy for suspected endometrial cancer. She wants to know more about endometrial cancer and asks the nurse about the available treatment options. Which of the following treatment information should the nurse give the client?
   a. Surgery involves removal of the uterus only.
   b. In advanced cancers, radiation and chemotherapy are used instead of surgery.
   c. Surgery involves removal of the uterus, fallopian tubes, and ovaries; adjuvant therapy is used if relevant.
   d. Follow-up care after the relevant treatment should last for at least 6 months after the treatment.

4. A 65-year-old client presents at a local community health care center for a routine check-up. While obtaining her medical history, the nurse learns that the client had her menarche when she was 13 years old. She experienced menopause at 51. She is between 5 and 10 lb underweight but is otherwise in good physical condition. The nurse should inform the client of which of the following factors that increase the client's risk of getting ovarian cancer?
   a. The client's age at menarche
   b. The client's present age
   c. The client's age at menopause
   d. The client's weight

5. A client presents at a community health care center for a routine check-up. The client wants to know about any tests that can effectively detect ovarian cancer early. About which of the following tests that can aid in the detection of ovarian cancer should the nurse inform the client?
   a. Pap smears
   b. Serum CA-125
   c. Yearly bimanual pelvic examinations
   d. Regular x-rays of the pelvic area

6. A client presents for a routine check-up at a local health care center. One of the client's distant relatives died of ovarian cancer, and the client wants to know about measures that can reduce the risk of ovarian cancer. About which of the following measures to reduce the risk of ovarian cancer should the nurse inform the client?
   a. Provide genetic counseling and thorough assessment.
   b. Instruct the client to avoid use of oral contraceptives.
   c. Instruct the client to avoid breastfeeding.
   d. Instruct the client to use perineal talc or hygiene sprays.

7. A nurse is caring for a client who has been diagnosed with genital warts due to HPV. The nurse explains to the client that HPV increases the risk of vulvar cancer. Which of the following preventive measures to reduce the risk of vulvar cancer should the nurse explain to the client?
   a. Genital examination should be done only by the primary health care provider.
   b. Genital examination should be done by the client.
   c. The client should avoid tight undergarments.
   d. The client should use OTC drugs for self-medication of suspicious lesions.

8. When working in a local community health care center, a nurse is frequently asked about cervical cancer and ways to prevent it. Which of the following should be included in the information provided by the nurse? Select all that apply.
   a. Encourage the use of an IUD for contraception.
   b. Encourage cessation of smoking and drinking.
   c. Encourage prevention of STIs to reduce risk factors.
   d. Avoid stress and high blood pressure.
   e. Counsel teenagers to avoid early sexual activity.

9. The endometrial biopsy of a client reveals cancerous cells, and the primary health care provider has diagnosed it as endometrial cancer. Which of the following are responsibilities of the nurse as part of the treatment of the client? Select all that apply.
   a. Make sure the client understands all the available treatment options.
   b. Inform the client that changes in sexuality are normal and need not be reported.
   c. Inform the client about the possible advantages of a support group.
   d. Offer the family explanations and emotional support throughout the treatment.
   e. Inform the client that follow-up care is not required unless something unusual occurs.

10. A nurse is conducting a session on education about cancers of the reproductive tract and is explaining the importance of visiting a health care professional if certain unusual symptoms appear. Which of the following should the nurse include in her list of symptoms that merit a visit to a health care professional for further evaluation? Select all that apply.
    a. Irregular bowel movements
    b. Irregular vaginal bleeding
    c. Increase in urinary frequency
    d. Persistent low backache not related to standing
    e. Elevated or discolored vulvar lesions

11. A client has been referred for a colposcopy by the physician. The client wants to know more about the examination. Which of the following information regarding a colposcopy should the nurse give to the client?
    a. Client may feel pain in the vaginal area during the examination.
    b. The test is conducted because of abnormal results in Pap smears.
    c. Intercourse should be avoided for at least a week afterward.
    d. Client may experience pain during urination for a week following the test.

12. The results of a Pap smear test have been classified as atypical squamous cells with possible HSIL (ASC-H) as per the 2001 Bethesda system. Which of the following is the correct interpretation of the result?
    a. Repeat the Pap smear in 4 to 6 months, or refer for a colposcopy.
    b. Refer for a colposcopy without HPV testing.
    c. Immediate colposcopy; follow-up is based on the results of findings.
    d. No need for any further Pap smear screenings.

13. Which of the following is the major initial symptom of endometrial cancer?
    a. Abnormal and painless vaginal bleeding
    b. Diabetes mellitus
    c. Liver disease
    d. Severe back pain

14. Which of the following risk factors are associated with vaginal cancer? Select all that apply.

  a. Advancing age

  b. HIV infection

  c. Persistent ovulation over time

  d. Smoking

  e. Hormone replacement therapy for more than 10 years

15. Which of the following risk factors has been linked to the development of vulvar cancer?

  a. Lichen sclerosus

  b. Previous pelvic radiation

  c. Exposure to diethylstilbestrol (DES) in utero

  d. Tamoxifen use

CHAPTER 9

Violence and Abuse

Learning Objectives

After completion of the chapter, you should be able to:

- Define the key terms.
- Examine the incidence of violence in women.
- Characterize the cycle of violence and appropriate interventions.
- Evaluate the various myths and facts about violence.
- Analyze the dynamics of rape and sexual abuse.
- Select the resources available to women experiencing abuse.
- Outline the role of the nurse who cares for abused women.

SECTION I: ASSESSING YOUR UNDERSTANDING

Activity A FILL IN THE BLANKS

1. A victim of _____ woman syndrome has experienced deliberate and repeated physical or sexual assault at the hands of an intimate partner.

2. _____ is any type of sexual exploitation between blood relatives or surrogate relatives before the victim reaches 18 years of age.

3. _____ rape is sexual activity between an adult and a person below the age of 18 and is considered to have occurred despite the willingness of the underage person.

4. _____, also known as roofies, forget pills, and the drop drug, is a common date rape drug.

5. Female genital mutilation, also known as female _____, refers to procedures involving injury, or partial or total removal of the female genital organs.

6. _____ rape involves someone being forced to have sex by a person he or she knows.

7. Forcing objects into a woman's vagina against her will constitutes _____ abuse.

8. Increased emotional arousal, exaggerated startle response, and irritability are some of the symptoms of _____ during post-traumatic stress disorder (PTSD).

9. To assess for the presence of _____ reactions during PTSD, the nurse should find out if the client feels numb emotionally or tries to avoid thinking of the trauma.

10. During the _____ phase, the abuser is sorry for the abuse inflicted.

Activity B MATCHING

Match the four phases of rape recovery in Column A with the survivor's response in Column B.

Column A	Column B
___ 1. Acute phase (disorganization)	a. The survivor attempts to make life adjustments by moving or changing jobs and using emotional distancing to cope
___ 2. Outward adjustment phase (denial)	

_____ **3.** Reorganization

_____ **4.** Integration and recovery

b. The survivor appears outwardly composed, refuses to discuss the assault, and denies need for counseling

c. The survivor begins to feel safe, starts to trust others, and may become an advocate for other rape victims

d. The survivor experiences shock, fear, disbelief, anger, shame, guilt, and feelings of being unclean

Activity C **SEQUENCING**

Given below are the interventions that a nurse performs when caring for a client who has been physically or sexually abused. Choose the order in which the interventions would have occurred.

1. Document and report findings.

2. Screen for abuse during every health care visit.

3. Isolate the client from her partner immediately.

4. Ask direct and indirect questions about abuse.

☐ → ☐ → ☐ → ☐

Activity D **SHORT ANSWERS**

Briefly answer the following.

1. What is the cycle of violence?

_____

_____

_____

2. What is financial abuse?

_____

_____

_____

3. What are the potential nursing diagnoses related to violence against women?

_____

_____

_____

4. What is PTSD? What are its symptoms?

_____

_____

_____

5. What signs should the nurse assess the client for, to find out if she is a victim of abuse?

_____

_____

_____

6. What are the effects of physical abuse on the pregnant woman?

_____

_____

_____

SECTION II: APPLYING YOUR KNOWLEDGE

Activity E **CASE STUDY**

Consider this scenario and answer the questions.

A visit to a health care agency is an ideal time for women to be assessed for violence. Suzanne, a married 24-year-old, presents to the Women's Center with complaints of pelvic pain, headaches, and sleep disruption. The triage nurse in the center recognizes that Suzanne became uncomfortable when discussing her marital relationship.

1. What are common symptoms of suspected physical abuse?

_____

_____

2. Explain why Suzanne may not seek help when she is in an abusive relationship.

_____

_____

_____

3. What appropriate strategies should the nurse suggest that might help Suzanne to manage the situation?

_____

_____

_____

SECTION III: PRACTICING FOR NCLEX

Activity F NCLEX-STYLE QUESTIONS

Answer the following questions.

1. A nurse is caring for a client who is being hospitalized for physical injuries. She later confides to the nurse that the injuries are a result of a physical assault by her partner when he was drunk. The client feels degraded and ashamed but realizes that her partner was under the influence of alcohol. How should the nurse respond to this client?

  a. "Violent tendencies have gone on for generations; you need to accept it as part of life."

  b. "Try to avoid provoking your partner in any way that might lead to abuse."

  c. "Being drunk is not an excuse for physically assaulting an intimate partner."

  d. "Violence occurs to only a small percentage of women who deserve it."

2. A client is receiving treatment for injuries sustained during a fight with her partner. The nurse observes that the partner visits her daily in the hospital and appears very solicitous and contrite. When questioned, she tries to convince the nurse that her partner always apologizes and brings gifts after a fight. Which of the following information should the nurse give to the client?

  a. "No one deserves to be a victim of physical abuse."

  b. "Your partner seems to be genuinely contrite."

  c. "You should try not to upset your partner in the future."

  d. "Don't worry; this is a normal part of any relationship."

3. A nurse is caring for a client who has been admitted with an ear infection. While discussing her partner with the nurse, the client says that her lover's behavior is "threatening" and "intimidating" at times, even though he has not physically harmed her. She wants to know what emotional abuse is. Which of the following should the nurse include as an example of emotional abuse while educating the client?

  a. Being overly watchful of the client's every move

  b. Throwing objects at the client

  c. Destroying valued possessions or attacking pets

  d. Forcing the client to have intercourse

4. A nurse is conducting an awareness session on sexual abuse, and she is explaining the psychological profile of an average abuser. Which of the following traits is displayed by abusers?

  a. They have parents who are divorced.

  b. They exhibit antisocial behaviors.

  c. They belong to the low-income group.

  d. They are usually physically imposing.

5. A nurse is working in a community hospital situated in an area with a history of grievous assaults on women, including rape. The nurse discovers that most rape victims come to the hospital but leave without seeking medical treatment. Which of the following interventions should the nurse perform to ensure that rape victims get legal and medical aid?

  a. Let them wait in waiting rooms to collect their thoughts before approaching them.

  b. Treat them as any other client to make them feel more comfortable.

  c. Focus on treating them rather than on collecting evidence.

  d. Ensure that the appropriate law enforcement agencies are apprised of the incident.

6. A client comes to a local community health care facility for a routine check-up. While talking to the nurse, the client happens to mention that every time she has a serious fight with her husband, he forces her to have intercourse with him. The client seems to be very disturbed when revealing this to the nurse. Which of the following is an appropriate response by the nurse?

    a. "Your husband is just trying to reconcile using intimacy."

    b. "It's okay in cases of fights where you're really at fault."

    c. "This behavior is considered sexual abuse."

    d. "Such behavior is considered normal in a married couple."

7. A 13-year-old immigrant from Asia is admitted to the health care facility with vaginal bleeding. An examination reveals unhealed circumcision wounds. The client can understand English but cannot speak the language fluently. Hence, the service of an interpreter is employed. What are the points the nurse should keep in mind when interacting with this client?

    a. Convey important information in precise medical terms.

    b. Allow the interpreter to question the client directly.

    c. Use pictures and diagrams to assist the client's understanding.

    d. Condemn the cultural practice and explain why it is wrong.

8. A woman comes to a local community health care facility with her partner. She has a broken arm and bruises on the face that she claims were caused by a fall. The nature of the injuries, however, causes the nurse to be convinced that this is a case of physical abuse. Which of the following interventions should the nurse perform?

    a. Ask the partner directly if he was responsible.

    b. Attempt to interview the woman in private.

    c. Tell the partner to leave the room immediately.

    d. Question the client about the injury in front of the partner.

9. A nurse is caring for a client who was raped at gunpoint. The client does not want any photos taken of her injuries. The client also does not want the police to be informed about the incident even though state laws require reporting life-threatening injuries. Which of the following interventions should the nurse perform to document and report the findings of the case?

    a. Use direct quotes and specific language when documenting.

    b. Obtain photos to substantiate the client's case in a court of law.

    c. Document only descriptions of medical interventions taken.

    d. Respect the client's opinion and avoid informing the police.

10. A nurse observes telltale signs of injuries from physical abuse on the face and neck of a female client. When questioned, the client tells the nurse that the injuries are the result of a physical attack by her partner and that she has developed palpitations thereafter. Which of the following should the nurse do to gain the trust of the client and enhance the nurse–client relationship?

    a. Offer referrals to the client so she can get help that will allow her to heal.

    b. Tell the client to forget about the incident to avoid the trauma.

    c. Inform the client that there is no connection between the violence and palpitations.

    d. Confirm with the partner whether the client's story is true.

11. A nurse is caring for a rape victim who has just arrived at the local health care facility. Which of the following interventions should the nurse perform to minimize risk of pregnancy in this client?

    a. Administer prescribed double dose of emergency contraceptive pills.

    b. Wait for first signs of pregnancy before taking action.

    c. Apply spermicidal cream or gel near the vaginal area.

    d. Administer regular oral contraceptive pills.

12. A nurse is caring for a pregnant client and discovers signs of bruises near her neck. On questioning, the nurse learns that the bruises were caused by her husband. The client tells the nurse that her husband had stopped abusing her some time ago, but this was the first time during the pregnancy that she was assaulted. She blames herself because she admits to not paying enough attention to her husband. Which of the following facts about abuse during pregnancy should the nurse tell the client to convince her that the abuse was not her fault? Select all that apply.

    a. Abuse is a result of concern for the unborn child when the mother doesn't fulfill her responsibilities toward the newborn.

    b. Abuse is a result of resentment toward the interference of the growing fetus and change in the woman's shape.

    c. Abuse is a result of the perception of the partner that the baby will be a competitor after he or she is born.

    d. Abuse is a result of insecurity and jealousy of the pregnancy and the responsibilities it brings.

    e. Most men exhibit violent reactions during pregnancy as a way of coping with the stress.

13. A nurse is caring for a 16-year-old female immigrant. Which of the following questions must she ask the client to assess if she is a victim of human trafficking? Select all that apply.

    a. "Can you leave your job or situation if you wish?"

    b. "Can you come and go as you please?"

    c. "What is your education level?"

    d. "What do your parents and siblings do?"

    e. "Is there a lock on your door so you cannot get out?"

14. A nurse is working in a local community health care facility where she frequently encounters victims of abuse. Which of the following signs should the nurse assess for to find out if a client is a victim of abuse? Select all that apply.

    a. Client is affected by STIs frequently.

    b. Client has mental health problems such as depression, anxiety, or substance abuse.

    c. Client has injuries on the face, head, and neck.

    d. Partner of the suspected victim seems relaxed and not overly worried.

    e. The reported history of the injury is inconsistent with the actual presenting problem.

15. A nurse is caring for a rape victim. Which of the following questions should the nurse ask the client to know the extent of physical symptoms of PTSD? Select all that apply.

    a. "Are you having trouble sleeping?"

    b. "Have you felt irritable or experienced outbursts of anger?"

    c. "Do you have heart palpitations or sweating?"

    d. "Do you feel numb emotionally?"

    e. "Do you get upset?"

CHAPTER 10

Fetal Development and Genetics

Learning Objectives

Upon completion of the chapter, you will be able to:

- Characterize the process of fertilization, implantation, and cell differentiation.
- Examine the functions of the placenta, umbilical cord, and amniotic fluid.
- Outline normal fetal development from conception through birth.
- Compare the various inheritance patterns, including nontraditional patterns of inheritance.
- Analyze examples of ethical and legal issues surrounding genetic testing.
- Research the role of the nurse in genetic counseling and genetic-related activities.

SECTION I: ASSESSING YOUR UNDERSTANDING

Activity A FILL IN THE BLANKS

1. _____ is one of two or more alternative versions of a gene at a given position or locus on a chromosome that imparts the same characteristic of that gene.

2. Any change in gene structure or location leads to a _____, which may alter the type and amount of protein produced.

3. Human beings typically have 22 pairs of nonsex chromosomes or _____ and 1 pair of sex chromosomes.

4. The _____ originates from the ectoderm germ layer during the early stages of embryonic development; it is a thin protective membrane that contains the amniotic fluid.

5. _____ are long, continuous strands of DNA that carry genetic information.

6. The _____ reaches the uterine cavity about 72 hours after fertilization.

7. The pictorial analysis of the number, form, and size of an individual's chromosomes is termed _____.

8. _____ causes an increase in the number of haploid sets (23) of chromosomes in a cell.

9. A genetic disorder is a disease caused by an abnormality in an individual's genetic material or _____.

10. The genotype, together with environmental variation that influences the individual, determines the _____, or the observed, outward characteristics of an individual.

Activity B LABELING

Consider the following figure and identify the structural abnormality depicted.

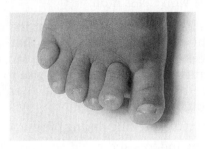

_____

_____

_____

Activity C MATCHING

Match the terms related to genetics in Column A with their descriptions in Column B.

Column A	Column B
____ **1.** Monosomies	**a.** Both alleles for a trait are the same in the individual
____ **2.** Trisomies	
____ **3.** Triploidy	**b.** Chromosomal abnormalities that do not show up in every cell
____ **4.** Mosaicism	
____ **5.** Homozygous	**c.** Three whole sets of chromosomes in a single cell
	d. There is only one copy of a particular chromosome instead of the usual pair
	e. There are three copies of a particular chromosome instead of the usual two

Activity D SEQUENCING

Write the correct sequence of events in human development after fertilization in the boxes provided below.

1. Formation of the placenta

2. Development of the fluid-filled blastocyst

3. Development of the morula

4. Formation of the amnion

5. Development of the trophoblast

☐ → ☐ → ☐ → ☐ → ☐

Activity E SHORT ANSWERS

Briefly answer the following.

1. How does conception occur?

_____

_____

2. What are the different stages of fetal development?

_____

_____

_____

3. What determines the sex of a zygote?

_____

_____

_____

4. What happens during differentiation of the zygote?

_____

_____

_____

5. What is amniotic fluid?

_____

_____

_____

6. What are the hormones produced by the placenta?

_____

_____

_____

SECTION II: APPLYING YOUR KNOWLEDGE

Activity F CASE STUDY

Consider the scenario and answer the questions.

Shana is 16 weeks pregnant and comes into the prenatal clinic for a routine check-up. She tells the nurse she is worried because she feels the baby moving a lot and has concerns "it might get tangled in its cord." She wants to know if this could be true and, if so, why. Shana also wants to know about the functions of amniotic fluid, the placenta, and the umbilical cord.

1. Describe how the nurse should respond to Shana's concerns about the baby's movements and potentially getting "tangled in the umbilical cord."

   _____

   _____

   _____

2. What information should the nurse provide to Shana concerning the function of the amniotic fluid, the placenta, and the umbilical cord?

   _____

   _____

   _____

SECTION III: PRACTICING FOR NCLEX

Activity G NCLEX-STYLE QUESTIONS

Answer the following questions.

1. The nurse is counseling a couple who are concerned that the woman has achondroplasia in her family. The woman is not affected. Which of the following statements by the couple indicates the need for more teaching?
   a. "If the mother has the gene, then there is a 50% chance of passing it on."
   b. "If the father doesn't have the gene, then his son won't have achondroplasia."
   c. "If the father has the gene, then there is a 50% chance of passing it on."
   d. "Since neither one of us has the disorder, we won't pass it on."

2. A client has been informed that the result of the pregnancy test indicates that she is 3 weeks pregnant. Which of the following instructions should the nurse give to the client that is most appropriate given her condition?
   a. Avoid exercising during pregnancy.
   b. Stay indoors and avoid going out for the duration of pregnancy.
   c. Instruct client to stop using drugs, alcohol, and tobacco.
   d. Wear comfortable clothes that are not tight or restrictive.

3. A nurse is obtaining the genetic history of a pregnant client by questioning family members. Which of the following questions is most appropriate for the nurse to ask?
   a. Were there any instances of premature birth in the family?
   b. Is there a family history of drinking or drug abuse?
   c. What was the cause and age of death for deceased family members?
   d. Were there any instances of depression during pregnancy?

4. A nurse is caring for a 37-year-old pregnant client who is expecting twins, both boys. The client used to smoke but has stopped during pregnancy. A relative of the client has Klinefelter syndrome, and the client wants to find out more about the disorder. Which of the following information will the nurse give to the client during genetic counseling?
   a. There is a greater risk of Klinefelter syndrome due to the client's age.
   b. Klinefelter syndrome occurs only in girls and not boys.
   c. Having twins increases the risk of Klinefelter syndrome.
   d. The client's previous smoking habit will increase the risk of a genetic disorder.

5. A 25-year-old client wants to know if her baby boy is at risk for Down syndrome, as one of her distant relatives was born with it. Which of the following will the nurse tell the client while counseling her about Down syndrome?

a. Instances of Down syndrome in the family increase the risk for the baby.

b. Children with Down syndrome have 47 chromosomes instead of 46.

c. Down syndrome occurs only in females, and there is no risk as the baby is male.

d. Children with Down syndrome are intellectually normal.

6. A nurse is questioning the family members of a pregnant client to obtain a genetic history. While asking questions, which of the following should the nurse keep in mind?

a. Inquire about the socioeconomic status of the family members.

b. Avoid questions about race or ethnic background.

c. Ask questions regarding physical characteristics of family members.

d. Find out if couples are related to each other or have blood ties.

7. A pregnant client and her husband have had a session with a genetic specialist. What is the role of the nurse after the client has seen a specialist?

a. Identify the best decision to be taken for the client.

b. Refer the client to another specialist for a second opinion.

c. Review what has been discussed with the specialist.

d. Refer the client for further diagnostic and screening tests.

8. A nurse is caring for a client who is pregnant with a female baby. The client and her husband are both Jewish. The client is in her early 30s. They are not directly related by blood. There has been an instance of Tay–Sachs disease occurring in the family.

Which of the following information does the nurse need to give the client regarding Tay–Sachs disease?

a. Tay–Sachs disease affects both male and female babies.

b. The age of the client increases the susceptibility of the baby to Tay–Sachs disease.

c. There is no risk of Tay–Sachs disease because the parents are not related by blood.

d. There is no risk of the baby developing Tay–Sachs disease because both parents are healthy.

9. A pregnant client arrives at the community health center for a routine check-up. She informs the nurse that a relative on her mother's side has hemophilia, and she wants to know the chances of her child acquiring hemophilia. Which of the following characteristics of hemophilia should the nurse explain to the client to help her understand the odds of acquiring the disease? Select all that apply.

a. Affected individuals will have affected parents.

b. Affected individuals are usually males.

c. Daughters of an affected male are unaffected and are not carriers.

d. Female carriers have a 50% chance of transmitting the disorder to their sons.

e. Females are affected by the condition if it is a dominant X-linked disorder.

10. A nurse is providing genetic counseling to a pregnant client. Which of the following are the nursing responsibilities related to counseling the client? Select all that apply.

a. Explaining basic concepts of probability and disorder susceptibility

b. Ensuring complete informed consent to facilitate decisions about genetic testing

c. Instructing the client on the appropriate decision to be taken

d. Knowing basic genetic terminology and inheritance patterns

e. Avoiding explaining ethical or legal issues and concentrating on genetic issues

11. The nurse is caring for a client at the prenatal care clinic. The client reports to the nurse that she heard her baby referred to as an embryo. The client questions what this means. What statement by the nurse is most appropriate?

    a. "The embryo is the name given to the baby when the lungs are still immature to survive outside of the womb."

    b. "The embryonic period is that time from conception till approximately 4 weeks of gestation."

    c. "The embryo refers to the products of conception from until the placenta begins to fully function."

    d. "The products of conception become an embryo around 2 weeks after conception and until it becomes a fetus."

12. A client has just been told she is pregnant with twins. The ultrasound reveals that the babies are monozygotic. She has several questions about her babies. What information should be shared with the client by the nurse?

    a. "Your babies likely will share the same placenta."

    b. "We will need to wait for a few more weeks to determine if you have a boy and a girl or if both are the same gender."

    c. "Your babies have developed from a single fertilized egg."

    d. "Your babies will be very similar in appearance."

    e. "Your babies will share a single amniotic sac."

13. A pregnant client asks the nurse about the relationship between her circulation and that of the unborn child. What response by the nurse is most appropriate?

    a. "The shared circulation between mother and unborn child begins at the time of conception."

    b. "There is no actual shared blood circulation but the substances in the mother's blood stream may be filtered to the fetus through the placenta."

    c. "Shared circulation is greatest during the second trimester."

    d. "The sharing of circulation begins once the products of conception begin the embryonic stage of development."

14. The nurse is caring for a client and her partner who are considering a future pregnancy. The client reports her last two pregnancies ended in stillbirth related to an underlying genetic disorder. What response by the nurse is most appropriate?

    a. "You should contact a geneticist after you become pregnant to closely watch your condition."

    b. "Your risk of repeated occurrences likely increases with future pregnancies."

    c. "You are strong to consider such an undertaking."

    d. "Consultation with a genetic counselor before you become pregnant would likely be beneficial."

15. The physician has ordered a karyotype for a newborn. The mother questions what the type of information that will be provided by the test. What information should be included in the nurse's response?

    a. The karyotype will provide information about the severity of your baby's condition.

    b. A karyotype is useful in determining the potential complications the baby may face as a result of its condition.

    c. The karyotype will assess the baby's chromosomal makeup.

    d. The karyotype will determine the treatment needed for the infant.

Maternal Adaptation During Pregnancy

Learning Objectives

Upon completion of the chapter, you will be able to:

■ Define the key terms used in this chapter.
■ Differentiate between subjective (presumptive), objective (probable), and diagnostic (positive) signs of pregnancy.
■ Appraise maternal physiologic changes that occur during pregnancy.
■ Summarize the nutritional needs of the pregnant woman and her fetus.
■ Characterize the emotional and psychological changes that occur during pregnancy.

SECTION I: ASSESSING YOUR UNDERSTANDING

Activity A FILL IN THE BLANKS

1. During the stress of pregnancy, _____, secreted by the adrenal glands, helps keep up the level of glucose in the plasma by breaking down noncarbohydrate sources.

2. _____, or having conflicting feelings at the same time, is an emotion expressed by most women upon learning they are pregnant.

3. _____, released by the posterior pituitary gland, is responsible for milk ejection during breastfeeding.

4. At birth, as soon as the _____ is expelled, and there is a drop in progesterone, lactogenesis can begin.

5. Palmar erythema, a well-delineated pinkish area on the palmar surface of the hands, is caused by elevated _____ levels.

6. The postural changes of pregnancy coupled with the loosening of the _____ joints may result in lower back pain.

7. Constipation, increased venous pressure, and pressure from the gravid uterus can lead to the formation of _____ during pregnancy.

8. During pregnancy, elevated _____ levels cause smooth-muscle relaxation, which results in delayed gastric emptying and decreased peristalsis.

9. _____ is the creamy, yellowish breast fluid that provides nourishment for the newborn during the first few days of life.

10. Most women experience an increase in a whitish vaginal discharge, called _____, during pregnancy.

Activity B LABELING

Consider the following figure.

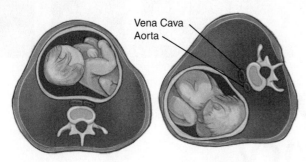

Supine position   Side-lying position

1. What condition is illustrated in the figure above?

   _____

   _____

   _____

2. What causes this condition to occur?

   _____

   _____

   _____

3. What symptoms are associated with this condition?

   _____

   _____

   _____

Activity C MATCHING

Match the parts of the female reproductive tract in Column A with the physiologic changes that occur in them during pregnancy, in Column B.

Column A

_____ **1.** Uterus

_____ **2.** Cervix

_____ **3.** Vagina

_____ **4.** Ovaries

_____ **5.** Ureters

Column B

a. Between weeks 6 and 8 of gestation, softens due to vaso-congestion

b. Elongate, widen, and curve above pelvic rim by 10th gestational week

c. Connective tissue loosens and smooth muscle begins hypertrophy

d. Produce more hormones until weeks 6 to 7 of gestation

e. Weighs 2 lb at full term

Activity D SEQUENCING

Given in random order are the changes in the uterus as pregnancy progresses. Arrange the items in sequence.

1. Uterus progressively ascends into the abdomen.

2. Fundal height drops as fetus begins to descend and engage into the pelvis.

3. Fundus reaches its highest level at the xiphoid process.

4. Softening and compressibility of the lower uterine segment are noted.

5. Fundus is at the level of the umbilicus and measures 20 cm.

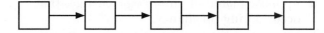

Activity E SHORT ANSWERS

Briefly answer the following.

1. What are stretch marks?

   _____

   _____

   _____

2. Why does hypertrophy of the heart occur in pregnant women?

   _____

   _____

   _____

3. Why do iron requirements increase during pregnancy?

   _____

   _____

   _____

4. What is pica?

_____

_____

_____

5. What is the role of oxytocin?

_____

_____

_____

6. Why do pregnant women develop varicose veins?

_____

_____

_____

SECTION II: APPLYING YOUR KNOWLEDGE

Activity F CASE STUDY

Consider this scenario and answer the questions.

A nurse working in a private doctor's office has been assigned to be the primary nurse for Maggie, age 40, who is in her first trimester of pregnancy. Maggie states that she is very nervous about the pregnancy and is concerned because "she is not very excited." She adds that she is also worried about her baby, avoids travel, stays indoors because she feels nauseous most of the time, and has little interaction with the outside world. She asks the nurse if it is normal to feel this way.

1. Describe how the nurse should respond to the client about her lack of excitement.

_____

_____

_____

2. How should the nurse explain to the client how introversion, or focusing on oneself, may be common in early pregnancy?

_____

_____

_____

3. How should the nurse describe to the client how she may feel in the second trimester?

_____

_____

_____

4. How should the nurse reassure Maggie about her mood swings?

_____

_____

_____

SECTION III: PRACTICING FOR NCLEX

Activity G NCLEX-STYLE QUESTIONS

Answer the following questions.

1. A 28-year-old client complains of skipping her menses and suspects she is pregnant. When assessing this client, which of the following would the nurse identify as a presumptive sign of pregnancy?

a. Positive home pregnancy test

b. Urinary frequency

c. Abdominal enlargement

d. Softening of the cervix

2. A pregnant client complains of an increase in a thick, whitish vaginal discharge. Which of the following information should a nurse provide to this client?

a. Refrain from any sexual activity.

b. Consult physician for fungal infection.

c. Such discharge is normal during pregnancy.

d. Use local antifungal agents regularly.

3. When teaching a client about hormones, which of the following should the nurse identify as responsible in developing the ductal system of the breasts in preparation for lactation during pregnancy?

a. Estrogen

b. Prolactin

c. Progesterone

d. Oxytocin

4. A 28-year-old client in her first trimester of pregnancy complains of conflicting feelings. She expresses feeling proud and excited about her pregnancy while at the same time feeling fearful and anxious of its implications. Which of the following maternal emotional responses is the client experiencing?

   a. Introversion

   b. Mood swings

   c. Acceptance

   d. Ambivalence

5. A pregnant client arrives at the maternity clinic complaining of constipation. Which of the following factors could be the cause of constipation during pregnancy? Select all that apply.

   a. Decreased activity level

   b. Increase in estrogen levels

   c. Use of iron supplements

   d. Reduced stomach acidity

   e. Intestinal displacement

6. A client in her 10th week of gestation arrives at the maternity clinic complaining of morning sickness. The nurse needs to inform the client about the body system adaptations during pregnancy. Which of the following factors corresponds to the morning sickness period during pregnancy?

   a. Reduced stomach acidity

   b. Elevation of human chorionic gonadotropin (hCG)

   c. Increase in red blood cell (RBC) production

   d. Increase in estrogen level

   e. Elevation of human placental lactogen (hPL)

7. A pregnant client in her first trimester of pregnancy complains of spontaneous, irregular, painless contractions. What does this indicate?

   a. Preterm labor

   b. Infection of the gastrointestinal (GI) tract

   c. Braxton Hicks contractions

   d. Acid indigestion

8. A client in her 29th week of gestation complains of dizziness and clamminess when assuming a supine position. During the assessment, the nurse observes there is a marked decrease in the client's blood pressure. Which of the following interventions should the nurse implement to help alleviate this client's condition?

   a. Keep the client's legs slightly elevated.

   b. Place the client in an orthopneic position.

   c. Keep the head of the client's bed slightly elevated.

   d. Place the client in the left lateral position.

9. A client in her 20th week of gestation expresses concern about her 5-year-old son, who is behaving strangely by not approaching her anymore. He does not seem to be taking the news of a new family member very well. Which of the following strategies can a nurse discuss with the mother to deal with the situation?

   a. Provide constant reinforcement of love and care to the child.

   b. Avoid talking to the child about the new arrival.

   c. Pay less attention to the child to prepare him for the future.

   d. Consult a child psychologist about the situation.

10. When caring for a newborn, the nurse observes that the neonate has developed white patches on the mucus membranes of the mouth. Which of the following conditions is the newborn most likely to be experiencing?

    a. Rubella

    b. Thrush

    c. Cytomegalovirus infection

    d. Toxoplasmosis

11. A client in her 39th week of gestation arrives at the maternity clinic stating that earlier in her pregnancy, she experienced shortness of breath. However, for the past few days, she's been able to breathe easily, but she has also begun to experience increased urinary frequency. A nurse is assigned to perform the

physical examination of the client. Which of the following is the nurse most likely to observe?

a. Fundal height has dropped since the last recording.

b. Fundal height is at its highest level at the xiphoid process.

c. The fundus is at the level of the umbilicus and measures 20 cm.

d. The lower uterine segment and cervix have softened.

12. A client in her second trimester of pregnancy is anxious about the blotchy, brown pigmentation appearing on her forehead and cheeks. She also complains of increased pigmentation on her breasts and genitalia. When educating the client, which of the following would the nurse identify as the condition experienced by the client?

a. Linea nigra

b. Striae gravidarum

c. Facial melisma (chloasma)

d. Vascular spiders

13. A client in her 39th week of gestation complains of swelling in the legs after standing for long periods of time. The nurse recognizes that these factors increase the client's risk for which of the following conditions?

a. Hemorrhoids

b. Embolism

c. Venous thrombosis

d. Supine hypotension syndrome

14. A nurse is assigned to educate a pregnant client regarding the changes in the structures of the respiratory system taking place during pregnancy. Which of the following conditions are associated with such changes? Select all that apply.

a. Nasal and sinus stuffiness

b. Persistent cough

c. Nosebleed

d. Kussmaul's respirations

e. Thoracic rather than abdominal breathing

15. During a prenatal visit, a client in her second trimester of pregnancy verbalizes positive feelings about the pregnancy and conceptualizes the fetus. Which of the following is the most appropriate nursing intervention when the client expresses such feelings?

a. Encourage the client to focus on herself, not on the fetus.

b. Inform the primary health care provider about the client's feeling.

c. Inform the client that it is too early to conceptualize the fetus.

d. Offer support and validation about the client's feelings.

16. A client in her second trimester of pregnancy complains of discomfort during sexual activity. Which of the following instructions should a nurse provide?

a. Perform frequent douching, and use lubricants.

b. Modify sexual positions to increase comfort.

c. Restrict contact to alternative, noncoital modes of sexual expression.

d. Perform stress-relieving and relaxing exercises.

17. A nurse is educating a client about the various psychological feelings experienced by a woman and her partner during pregnancy. Which of the following is the feeling experienced by the expectant partner during the second trimester of pregnancy?

a. Ambivalence along with extremes of emotions

b. Confusion when dealing with the partner's mood swings

c. Preparation for the new role as a parent and negotiating his or her role during labor

d. Sympathetic response to the partner's pregnancy

CHAPTER 12

Nursing Management During Pregnancy

Learning Objectives

Upon completion of the chapter, you will be able to:

- Define the key terms used in this chapter.
- Relate the information typically collected at the initial prenatal visit.
- Select the assessments completed at follow-up prenatal visits.
- Evaluate the tests used to assess maternal and fetal well-being, including nursing management for each.
- Outline appropriate nursing management to promote maternal self-care and to minimize the common discomforts of pregnancy.
- Examine the key components of perinatal education.

SECTION I: ASSESSING YOUR UNDERSTANDING

Activity A FILL IN THE BLANKS

1. A _____ is a laywoman trained to provide women and their families with encouragement, emotional and physical support, and information through late pregnancy, labor, and birth.

2. A _____ is a woman who has given birth once after a pregnancy of at least 20 weeks.

3. _____ height is the distance (in cm) measured with a tape measure from the top of the pubic bone to the top of the uterus while the client is lying on her back with her knees slightly flexed.

4. In a pregnant woman, darker pigmentation of the nipple and areola develops, along with enlargement of _____ glands in the breast.

5. Bluish coloration of the cervix and vaginal mucosa is known as _____ sign.

6. _____ is the craving for nonfood substances such as clay, cornstarch, laundry detergent, baking soda, soap, paint chips, dirt, ice, or wax.

7. _____ involves a transabdominal perforation of the amniotic sac to obtain a sample of amniotic fluid for analysis.

8. Alpha-fetoprotein is a substance produced by the fetal _____ between weeks 13 and 20 of gestation.

9. The basis for the _____ test is that the normal fetus produces characteristic fetal heart rate patterns in response to fetal movements.

10. _____ are varicosities of the rectum which occur as a result of progesterone-induced vasodilation and from pressure of the enlarged uterus on the lower intestine and rectum.

Activity B MATCHING

Match the different types of assessment tests conducted to determine fetal well-being in Column A with their uses in Column B.

Column A

____ **1.** Ultrasonography

____ **2.** Doppler flow studies

____ **3.** Nuchal translucency screening (ultrasound)

____ **4.** Percutaneous umbilical blood sampling

____ **5.** Contraction stress test

Column B

a. Allows for earlier detection and diagnosis of some fetal chromosomes and structural abnormalities

b. Permits the collection of a blood specimen directly from the fetal circulation for rapid chromosomal analysis

c. Determines the fetal heart rate response under stress, such as during contractions

d. Acts as a guide for the need for invasive intrauterine tests and used to monitor fetal growth and placental location

e. Help to identify abnormalities in diastolic flow within the umbilical vessels

Activity C SEQUENCING

Pregnant women are at an increased risk for epistaxis (nosebleeds). Given below, in random order, are steps that should be followed when caring for the client who experiences an epistaxis. Rearrange in the correct sequence.

1. Pinch her nostrils with her thumb and forefinger for 10 to 15 minutes.

2. Loosen the clothing around her neck.

3. Apply an ice pack to the bridge of her nose.

4. Sit with her head tilted forward.

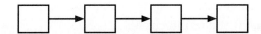

Activity D SHORT ANSWERS

Briefly answer the following.

1. What are the key areas which the nurse should include in preconception care?

_____

_____

_____

2. What is the role of a nurse in preconception care to ensure a positive impact on the pregnancy?

_____

_____

_____

3. Discuss the priority assessment by the nurse during a client's initial prenatal visit.

_____

_____

_____

4. What are the roles of a nurse with regard to providing counseling and education to the client at a prenatal visit?

_____

_____

_____

5. What assessments should a nurse perform when conducting a chest examination for a pregnant client on her first prenatal visit?

_____

_____

_____

6. What assessments should the nurse perform during follow-up visits?

_____

_____

_____

SECTION II: APPLYING YOUR KNOWLEDGE

Activity E CASE STUDY

Consider this scenario and answer the questions.

A pregnant client and her husband are preparing for the birth of their first baby. The couple wants to ensure that they are well prepared for the baby's birth and homecoming and seek guidance from the nurse. The pregnant client also wants to know the importance of breastfeeding and wants to prepare for it.

1. What are the items in the checklist used by the nurse to ensure that the client is well prepared for the newborn's birth and homecoming?

   _____

   _____

   _____

2. What interventions should the nurse perform in preparing the client for breastfeeding?

   _____

   _____

   _____

3. What advantages of breastfeeding should the nurse educate the pregnant client about?

   _____

   _____

   _____

SECTION III: PRACTICING FOR NCLEX

Activity F NCLEX-STYLE QUESTIONS

Answer the following questions.

1. A 28-year-old client who has just conceived arrives at a health care facility for her first prenatal visit to undergo a physical examination. Which of the following interventions should the nurse perform to prepare the client for the physical examination?

   a. Ensure that the client is lying down.

   b. Ensure that the client's family is present.

   c. Instruct the client to empty her bladder.

   d. Instruct the client to keep taking deep breaths.

2. A client in her third month of pregnancy arrives at the health care facility for a regular follow-up visit. The client complains of discomfort due to increased urinary frequency. Which of the following instructions should the nurse offer the client to reduce the client's discomfort?

   a. Avoid consumption of caffeinated drinks.

   b. Drink fluids with meals rather than between meals.

   c. Avoid an empty stomach at all times.

   d. Munch on dry crackers and toast in the early morning.

3. A pregnant client has come to a health care provider for her first prenatal visit. The nurse needs to document useful information about the past health history. What are goals of the nurse in the history-taking process? Select all that apply.

   a. To prepare a plan of care that suits the client's lifestyle

   b. To develop a trusting relationship with the client

   c. To prepare a plan of care for the pregnancy

   d. To assess the client's partner's sexual health

   e. To urge the client to achieve an optimal body weight

4. A pregnant client has come to a health care facility for a physical examination. Which of the following assessments should a nurse perform when doing a physical examination of the head and neck? Select all that apply.

   a. Assess for previous injuries and sequelae.

   b. Check the eye movements.

   c. Check for levels of estrogen.

   d. Evaluate for limitations in range of motion.

   e. Palpate the thyroid gland for enlargement.

5. A pregnant client in her 12th week of gestation has come to a health care center for a physical examination of her abdomen. Where should the nurse palpate for the fundus in this client?

   a. At the umbilicus

   b. Below the ensiform cartilage

c. Midway between the symphysis and umbilicus

d. At the symphysis pubis

6. A pregnant client has come to a clinic for a pelvic examination. What assessments should a nurse perform when examining external genitalia?

a. Ensure that the cervix is smooth, long, thick, and closed.

b. Assess for bluish coloration of cervix and vaginal mucosa.

c. Assess for any infection due to hematomas, varicosities, and inflammation.

d. Assess for hemorrhoids, masses, prolapse, and lesions.

7. Which of the following nursing interventions should the nurse perform when assessing fetal well-being through abdominal ultrasonography in a client?

a. Inform the client that she may feel hot initially.

b. Instruct the client to refrain from emptying her bladder.

c. Instruct the client to report the occurrence of fever.

d. Obtain and record vital signs of the client.

8. A pregnant client wishes to know if sexual intercourse would be safe during her pregnancy. Which of the following should the nurse confirm before educating the client regarding sexual behavior during pregnancy?

a. Client does not have an incompetent cervix.

b. Client does not have anxieties and worries.

c. Client does not have anemia.

d. Client does not experience facial and hand edema.

9. A client in her second trimester arrives at a health care facility for a follow-up visit. During the exam, the client complains of constipation. Which of the following instructions should the nurse offer to help alleviate constipation?

a. Ensure adequate hydration and bulk in the diet.

b. Avoid spicy or greasy foods in meals.

c. Practice Kegel exercises.

d. Avoid lying down for 2 hours after meals.

10. A client in the third trimester of pregnancy has to travel a long distance by car. The client is anxious about the effect the travel may have on her pregnancy. Which of the following instructions should the nurse provide to promote easy and safe travel for the client?

a. Activate the air bag in the car.

b. Use a lap belt that crosses over the uterus.

c. Apply a padded shoulder strap properly.

d. Always wear a three-point seat belt.

11. A pregnant client's last menstrual period was March 10. Using Naegele's rule, the nurse knows that which of the following dates should be the child's estimated date of birth?

a. January 7

b. December 17

c. February 21

d. January 30

12. A nurse who has been caring for a pregnant client understands that the client has pica and has been regularly consuming soil. Which of the following conditions should the nurse monitor for in the client as a manifestation of consuming soil?

a. Iron-deficiency anemia

b. Constipation

c. Tooth fracture

d. Inefficient protein metabolism

13. A client who is in her 6th week of gestation is being seen for a routine prenatal care visit. The client asks the nurse about changes in her eating habits that she should make during her pregnancy. The client informs the nurse that she is a vegetarian. The nurse knows that she has to monitor the client for which of the following risks arising from her vegetarian diet? Select all that apply.

a. Risk of epistaxis

b. Iron-deficiency anemia

c. Decreased mineral absorption

d. Increased risk of constipation

e. Low gestational weight gain

14. A nurse is caring for a pregnant client in her second trimester of pregnancy. The nurse educates the client to look for which of the following danger signs of pregnancy needing immediate attention by the physician.

    a. Vaginal bleeding

    b. Painful urination

    c. Severe, persistent vomiting

    d. Lower abdominal and shoulder pain

15. A client in her third trimester of pregnancy wishes to use the method of feeding formula to her infant. Which of the following instructions should the nurse provide to assist the client in feeding her baby?

    a. Mix one scoop of powder with an ounce of water.

    b. Feed the infant every 8 hours.

    c. Serve the formula at room temperature.

    d. Refrigerate any leftover formula.

16. A nurse caring for a client in labor has asked her to perform Lamaze breathing techniques to avoid pain. Which of the following should the nurse keep in mind to promote effective Lamaze-method breathing?

    a. Ensure deep abdominopelvic breathing.

    b. Ensure abdominal breathing during contractions.

    c. Ensure client's concentration on pleasurable sensations.

    d. Remain quiet during client's period of imagery.

17. A nurse is caring for a client in her second trimester of pregnancy. During a regular follow-up visit, the client complains of varicosities of the legs. Which of the following instructions should the nurse provide to help the client alleviate varicosities of the legs?

    a. Avoid sitting in one position for long.

    b. Refrain from crossing legs when sitting for long periods.

    c. Apply heating pads on the extremities.

    d. Refrain from wearing any kind of stockings.

18. A nurse is assigned to care for a pregnant client as she undergoes a nonstress test. Given below are the steps involved in conducting the nonstress test. Arrange the steps in correct order.

    a. Client is handed an event marker

    b. Client consumes a meal

    c. External electronic fetal-monitoring device applied

    d. Fetal monitor strip marked for fetal movement

    e. Client placed in left lateral recumbent position

Labor and Birth Process

Upon completion of the chapter, you will be able to:

- Relate premonitory signs of labor.
- Compare and contrast true versus false labor.
- Categorize the critical factors affecting labor and birth.
- Analyze the cardinal movements of labor.
- Evaluate the maternal and fetal responses to labor and birth.
- Classify the stages of labor and the critical events in each stage.
- Characterize the normal physiologic/psychological changes occurring during all four stages of labor.
- Formulate the concept of pain as it relates to the woman in labor.

SECTION I: ASSESSING YOUR UNDERSTANDING

Activity A FILL IN THE BLANKS

1. Vaginal birth is most favorable with a _____ type of pelvis because the inlet is round and the outlet is roomy.

2. The thinning out process of the cervix during labor is termed _____.

3. The _____ suture is located between the parietal bones and divides the skull into the right and left halves.

4. _____ station is designated when the presenting part is at the level of the maternal ischial spines.

5. _____ occurs when the fetal presenting part begins to descend into the maternal pelvis.

6. An increase in prostaglandins leads to myometrial _____ and to a reduction in cervical resistance.

7. Oxytocin aids in stimulating prostaglandin synthesis through receptors in the _____.

8. The birth _____ is the route through which the fetus must travel to be birthed vaginally.

9. A sudden increase in energy on the part of the expectant woman 24 to 48 hours before the onset of labor is sometimes referred to as _____.

10. The elongated shape of the fetal skull at birth as a result of overlapping of the cranial bones is known as _____.

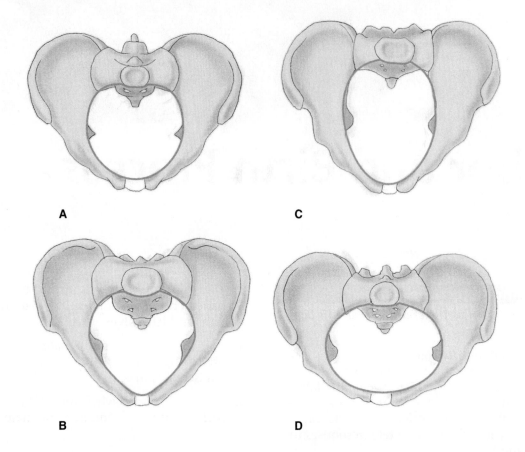

A

C

B

D

Activity B LABELING

Consider the following figures.

1. Identify the four types of pelvic shapes shown in the image. Which one of the four images is most favorable for a vaginal birth?

_____

_____

_____

2. Identify the different types of breeched positions shown in the figure. In which clients are such cases observed?

_____

_____

_____

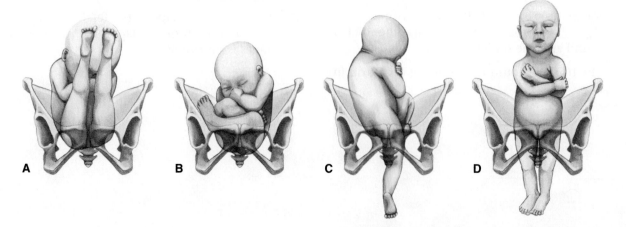

A   B   C   D

Activity C MATCHING

Match the cardinal movements of labor in Column A with the corresponding fetal movements observed in Column B.

Column A

____ **1.** Engagement

____ **2.** Descent

____ **3.** Flexion

____ **4.** Extension

____ **5.** External rotation

Column B

a. Occurs when the greatest transverse diameter of the head in vertex passes through the pelvic inlet

b. Downward movement of the fetal head until it is within the pelvic inlet

c. Allows the shoulders to rotate internally to fit the maternal pelvis

d. The head emerges through extension under the symphysis pubis, along with the shoulders

e. Occurs as the vertex meets resistance from the cervix, walls of the pelvis, or the pelvic floor

Activity D SEQUENCING

Given below, in random order, are the phases of labor. Arrange them in the order of their occurrence. Put the items in correct sequence by writing the letters in the boxes provided below.

1. Pelvic phase

2. Perineal phase

3. Placental expulsion

4. Latent phase

5. Active phase

6. Placental separation

7. Transition phase

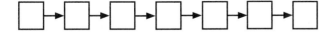

Activity E SHORT ANSWERS

Briefly answer the following.

1. What are the reasons that cause women to adopt back-lying positions during labor?

_____

_____

_____

2. Why should the nurse encourage the pregnant client experiencing contractions to adopt the upright or lateral position?

_____

_____

_____

3. What are the maternal physiologic responses that occur as a woman progresses through childbirth?

_____

_____

_____

4. What are the factors influencing the ability of a woman to cope with labor stress?

_____

_____

_____

5. What are the signs of separation that indicate the placenta is ready to deliver?

_____

_____

_____

6. What are the factors that ensure a positive birth experience for the pregnant client?

_____

_____

_____

SECTION II: APPLYING YOUR KNOWLEDGE

Activity F CASE STUDY

Consider this scenario and answer the questions.

Becca is a primigravida at 36 weeks' gestation. During her prenatal visit, she asks the nurse the following questions about labor. Describe how the nurse should respond.

1. "How will I know I am in labor?"

   _____

   _____

   _____

2. "When should I come to the hospital?"

   _____

   _____

   _____

3. "My sister just had a baby and she told me that the nurse midwife encouraged her to change positions and to walk to help her labor; will this help me in labor?"

   _____

   _____

   _____

4. "How do we determine that it's time to push?"

   _____

   _____

   _____

SECTION III: PRACTICING FOR NCLEX

Activity G

Answer the following questions.

1. A client in her third trimester of pregnancy arrives at a health care facility complaining of cramping and low back pain; she also notes that she is urinating more frequently and that her breathing has become easier the past few days. Physical examination conducted by the nurse indicates that the client has edema of the lower extremities, along with an increase in vaginal discharge. The nurse knows that the client is experiencing which of the following conditions?

   a. Nesting
   b. Lightening
   c. Braxton Hicks contractions
   d. Bloody show

2. The assessment of a pregnant client, who is toward the end of her third trimester, reveals that she has increased prostaglandin levels. Which of the following factors should the nurse assess for in the client? Select all that apply.

   a. Reduction in cervical resistance
   b. Myometrial contractions
   c. Boggy appearance of the uterus
   d. Softening and thinning of the cervix
   e. Hypotonic character of the bladder

3. A client experiencing contractions presents at a health care facility. Assessment conducted by the nurse reveals that the client has been experiencing Braxton Hicks contractions. The nurse has to educate the client on the usefulness of Braxton Hicks contractions. Which of the following is the role of Braxton Hicks contractions in aiding labor?

   a. These contractions help in softening and ripening the cervix.
   b. These contractions increase the release of prostaglandins.
   c. These contractions increase oxytocin sensitivity.
   d. These contractions make maternal breathing easier.

4. A pregnant client wants to know why the labor of a first-time-pregnant woman usually lasts longer than that of a woman who has already delivered once and is pregnant a second time. What explanation should the nurse offer the client?

   a. Braxton Hicks contractions are not strong enough during first pregnancy.
   b. Contractions are stronger during the first pregnancy than the second.
   c. The cervix takes around 12 to 16 hours to dilate during first pregnancy.
   d. Spontaneous rupture of membranes occurs during first pregnancy.

5. A pregnant client is admitted to a maternity clinic for childbirth. The client wishes to adopt the kneeling position during labor. The nurse knows that which of the following is the advantage of adopting a kneeling position during labor?

   a. It helps the woman in labor to save energy.

   b. It facilitates vaginal examinations.

   c. It facilitates external belt adjustment.

   d. It helps to rotate fetus in a posterior position.

6. A nurse is caring for a pregnant client who is in labor. Which of the following maternal physiologic responses should the nurse monitor for in the client as the client progresses through childbirth? Select all that apply.

   a. Increase in heart rate

   b. Increase in blood pressure

   c. Increase in respiratory rate

   d. Slight decrease in body temperature

   e. Increase in gastric emptying and pH

7. A nurse is caring for a client in labor who is delivering. Which of the following fetal responses should the nurse monitor for in the client's baby?

   a. Decrease in arterial carbon dioxide pressure

   b. Increase in fetal breathing movements

   c. Increase in fetal oxygen pressure

   d. Decrease in circulation and perfusion to the fetus

8. A client in the third stage of labor has experienced placental separation and expulsion. Why is it necessary for a nurse to massage the woman's uterus briefly until it is firm?

   a. To reduce boggy nature of the uterus

   b. To remove pieces left attached to uterine wall

   c. To constrict the uterine blood vessels

   d. To lessen the chances of conducting an episiotomy

9. A nurse is caring for a pregnant client in labor in a health care facility. The nurse knows that which of the following marks the termination of the first stage of labor in the client?

   a. Diffuse abdominal cramping

   b. Rupturing of fetal membranes

   c. Start of regular contractions

   d. Dilation of cervix diameter to 10 cm

10. A nurse is caring for a client who is in the first stage of labor. The client is experiencing extreme pain due to the labor. The nurse understands that which of the following is causing the extreme pain in the client? Select all that apply.

    a. Lower uterine segment distention

    b. Fetus moving along the birth canal

    c. Stretching and tearing of structures

    d. Spontaneous placental expulsion

    e. Dilation of the cervix

11. A pregnant client in labor has to undergo a sonogram to confirm the fetal position of a shoulder presentation. The nurse should assess for which of the following conditions associated with shoulder presentation during a vaginal birth?

    a. Uterine abnormalities

    b. Fetal anomalies

    c. Congenital anomalies

    d. Prematurity

12. A nurse is assigned the task of educating a pregnant client about childbirth. Which of the following nursing interventions should the nurse perform as a part of prenatal education for the client to ensure a positive childbirth experience? Select all that apply.

    a. Provide the client clear information on procedures involved.

    b. Encourage the client to have a sense of mastery and self-control.

    c. Encourage the client to have a positive reaction to pregnancy.

    d. Instruct the client to spend some time alone each day.

    e. Instruct the client to begin changing the home environment.

13. A pregnant client is admitted to a maternity clinic for childbirth. Which assessment finding indicates that the client's fetus is in the transverse lie position?

   a. Long axis of fetus is at 60° to that of client.

   b. Long axis of fetus is parallel to that of client.

   c. Long axis of fetus is perpendicular to that of client.

   d. Long axis of fetus is at 45° to that of client.

14. A pregnant client is admitted to a maternity clinic after experiencing contractions. The assigned nurse observes that the client experiences pauses between contractions. The nurse knows that which of the following marks the importance of the pauses between contractions during labor?

   a. Effacement and dilation of the cervix

   b. Shortening of the upper uterine segment

   c. Reduction in length of the cervical canal

   d. Restoration of blood flow to uterus and placenta

15. A nurse is caring for a pregnant client during labor. Which of the following methods should the nurse use to provide comfort to the pregnant client? Select all that apply.

   a. Hand holding

   b. Chewing gum

   c. Massaging

   d. Acupressure

   e. Prescribed pain killers

CHAPTER 14

Nursing Management During Labor and Birth

Learning Objectives

Upon completion of the chapter, you will be able to:

- Define the key terms related to the labor and birth process.
- Examine the measures used to evaluate maternal status during labor and birth.
- Differentiate the advantages and disadvantages of external and internal fetal monitoring, including the appropriate use for each.
- Choose appropriate nursing interventions to address nonreassuring fetal heart rate patterns.
- Outline the nurse's role in fetal assessment.
- Appraise the various comfort-promotion and pain-relief strategies used during labor and birth.
- Summarize the assessment data collected on admission to the perinatal unit.
- Relate the ongoing assessments involved in each stage of labor and birth.
- Analyze the nurse's role throughout the labor and birth process.

SECTION I: ASSESSING YOUR UNDERSTANDING

Activity A FILL IN THE BLANKS

1. _____ comfort measures are usually simple, safe, effective, and inexpensive to use.

2. If the woman is a diabetic, it is critical to alert the newborn nursery of potential _____ in the newborn.

3. If the nitrazine test is inconclusive, an additional test, called the _____ test, can be used to confirm rupture of membranes.

4. The nurse reviews the prenatal record to identify risk factors that may contribute to a decrease in _____ circulation during pregnancy and/or labor.

5. The _____ spines serve as landmarks for estimating the descent of the fetal presenting part and have been designated as zero station.

6. The primary power of labor is _____ contractions, which are involuntary.

7. The _____ is placed over the uterine fundus in the area of greatest contractility to electronically monitor uterine contractions.

8. _____ describes the irregular variations or absence of fetal heart rate (FHR) due to erroneous causes on the fetal monitor record.

9. Baseline variability represents the interplay between the _____ and sympathetic nervous systems.

10. Fetal _____ are transitory increases in the FHR above the baseline that are associated with sympathetic nervous stimulation.

Activity B MATCHING

Match the extent of the lacerations in Column A with their depths in Column B.

Column A

_____ **1.** First-degree laceration

_____ **2.** Second-degree laceration

_____ **3.** Third-degree laceration

_____ **4.** Fourth-degree laceration

Column B

a. Through the anal sphincter muscle

b. Through the muscles of the perineal body

c. Through the skin

d. Through the anterior rectal wall

Activity C SEQUENCING

Put the items in correct sequence by writing the letters in the boxes provided below.

1. Given below, in random order, are nursing interventions during various stages of labor and birth. Arrange them in the correct order.

a. Check the fundus to ensure that it is firm (size and consistency of a grapefruit), located in the midline and below the umbilicus.

b. Ascertain whether the woman is in true or false labor.

c. Position the woman and cleanse the vulva and perineal areas.

d. Check for lengthening of the umbilical cord protruding from the vagina.

e. Check for crowning, low grunting sounds from the woman, and increase in blood-tinged show.

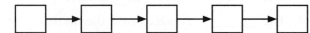

Activity D SHORT ANSWERS

Briefly answer the following.

1. What information should a nurse include when taking the maternal health history?

_____

_____

_____

2. What does the Apgar score assess?

_____

_____

_____

3. What is the purpose of vaginal examination during maternal assessment?

_____

_____

_____

4. What are the advantages and disadvantages of continuous electronic fetal monitoring?

_____

_____

_____

5. What are the typical signs of the second stage of labor?

_____

_____

_____

6. What positions are used for the second stage of labor?

_____

_____

_____

SECTION II: APPLYING YOUR KNOWLEDGE

Activity E CASE STUDY

Consider this scenario and answer the questions.

Susan, a pregnant client, has been admitted to the health care facility because she is in labor. The nurse is prepared to do maternal assessment during labor and delivery. Susan informs the nurse that there is no vaginal bleeding.

1. What nursing intervention should the nurse perform?

_____

_____

_____

2. What is the purpose of vaginal examination during maternal assessment?

   _____

   _____

   _____

3. What is the procedure for conducting vaginal examination?

   _____

   _____

   _____

SECTION III: PRACTICING FOR NCLEX

Activity F NCLEX-STYLE QUESTIONS

Answer the following questions.

1. It is the nurse's first meeting with a pregnant client. What is the first point that the nurse needs to ascertain as part of the admission assessment to check whether the client needs to be admitted?
   a. Whether the client is in true or false labor
   b. Whether the client is pregnant for the first time
   c. Whether the client is addicted to drugs
   d. Whether the client has a history of drug allergy

2. A nurse is assigned to conduct an admission assessment on the phone for a pregnant client. Which of the following information should the nurse obtain from the client? Select all that apply.
   a. Estimated due date
   b. History of drug abuse
   c. Characteristics of contractions
   d. Appearance of vaginal blood
   e. History of drug allergy

3. A nurse is caring for a pregnant client who is in the active phase of labor. At what intervals should the nurse monitor the client's vital signs?
   a. Every 15 to 30 minutes
   b. Every 30 minutes
   c. Every 30 to 60 minutes
   d. Every 4 hours

4. A nurse is required to obtain the FHR for a pregnant client. If the presentation is cephalic, which maternal site should the nurse monitor to hear the FHR clearly?
   a. Lower quadrant of the maternal abdomen
   b. At the level of the maternal umbilicus
   c. Above the level of the maternal umbilicus
   d. Just below the maternal umbilicus

5. The nurse is assessing the laboring client to determine fetal oxygenation status. What indirect assessment method will the nurse likely use?
   a. External electronic fetal monitoring
   b. Fetal blood pH
   c. Fetal oxygen saturation
   d. Fetal position

6. A client in labor is administered lorazepam to help her relax enough so that she can participate effectively during her labor process rather than fighting against it. Which of the following is an adverse effect of the drug that the nurse should monitor for?
   a. Increased sedation
   b. Newborn respiratory depression
   c. Nervous system depression
   d. Decreased alertness

7. A pregnant client with a history of spinal injury is being prepared for a cesarean birth. Which of the following methods of anesthesia is to be administered to the client?
   a. Local infiltration
   b. Epidural block
   c. Regional anesthesia
   d. General anesthesia

8. The nurse is monitoring a pregnant client admitted to a health care center who is in the latent phase of labor. The nurse demonstrates appropriate nursing care by monitoring the FHR with the Doppler at least how often?
   a. Every 30 minutes
   b. Every hour
   c. Every 15 to 30 minutes
   d. Continuously

9. During an admission assessment of a client in labor, the nurse observes that there is no vaginal bleeding yet. What nursing intervention is appropriate in the absence of vaginal

bleeding when the client is in the early stage of labor?

a. Monitor vital signs.

b. Assess amount of cervical dilation.

c. Obtain urine specimen for urinalysis.

d. Monitor hydration status.

10. A pregnant client is admitted with vaginal bleeding. The nurse performs a nitrazine test to confirm that the membranes have ruptured. The nitrazine tape remains yellow to olive green, with pH between 5 and 6. What does this indicate?

a. Membranes have ruptured

b. Presence of amniotic fluid

c. Presence of vaginal fluid

d. Presence of excess blood

11. A nurse assisting a pregnant client during pregnancy is to monitor uterine contractions. Which of the following factors should the nurse assess to monitor uterine contraction? Select all that apply.

a. Uterine resting tone

b. Frequency of contractions

c. Change in temperature

d. Change in blood pressure

e. Intensity of contractions

12. The nurse performing Leopold's maneuvers for a pregnant client explains to the client the purpose of the maneuvers. Which of the following is the purpose of the maneuvers? Select all that apply.

a. Determining the presentation of the fetus

b. Determining the position of the fetus

c. Determining the lie of the fetus

d. Determining the weight of the fetus

e. Determining the size of the fetus

13. A nurse caring for a pregnant client in labor observes that the FHR is below 110. Which of the following interventions should the nurse perform? Select all that apply.

a. Turn the client on her left side.

b. Reduce intravenous (IV) fluid rate.

c. Administer oxygen by mask.

d. Assess client for underlying causes.

e. Ignore questions from the client.

14. The nurse caring for a client in preterm labor observes nonreassuring FHR patterns. Which of the following nursing interventions should the nurse perform?

a. Application of vibroacoustic stimulation

b. Tactile stimulation

c. Administration of oxygen by mask

d. Fetal scalp stimulation

15. A nurse is caring for a client who has been administered an epidural block. Which of the following symptoms must the nurse monitor the client for?

a. Respiratory depression

b. Accidental intrathecal blockade

c. Inadequate or failed block

d. Postdural puncture headache

16. A client administered combined spinal–epidural analgesia is showing signs of hypotension and associated FHR changes. What interventions should the nurse perform to manage the changes?

a. Assist client to a supine position.

b. Provide supplemental oxygen.

c. Discontinue IV fluid.

d. Turn client to her left side.

17. A nurse is caring for a client administered general anesthesia for an emergency cesarean birth. What complications associated with general anesthesia should the nurse monitor for?

a. Pruritus

b. Uterine relaxation

c. Inadequate or failed block

d. Maternal hypotension

18. A pregnant client has opted for hydrotherapy for pain management during labor. Which of the following should the nurse consider when assisting the client during the birthing process?

a. Initiate the technique only when the client is in active labor.

b. Do not allow the client to stay in the bath for long.

c. Ensure that the water temperature exceeds body temperature.

d. Allow the client into the water only if her membranes have ruptured.

19. A nurse is teaching a couple about patterned breathing during their childbirth education. Which of the following techniques should the nurse suggest for slow-paced breathing?

   a. Inhale and exhale through the mouth at a rate of 4 breaths every 5 seconds.

   b. Inhale slowly through nose and exhale through pursed lips.

   c. Punctuated breathing by a forceful exhalation through pursed lips every few breaths.

   d. Hold breath for 5 seconds after every 3 breaths.

20. A pregnant client requires administration of an epidural block for management of pain during labor. Which of the following conditions should the nurse check for in the client before administering the epidural block? Select all that apply.

   a. Spinal abnormality

   b. Hypovolemia

   c. Varicose veins

   d. Coagulation defects

   e. Skin rashes or bruises

15

Postpartum Adaptations

Learning Objectives

Upon completion of the chapter, you will be able to:

- Define the key terms used in this chapter.
- Examine the systemic physiologic changes occurring in the woman after childbirth.
- Assess the phases of maternal role adjustment and accompanying behaviors.
- Analyze the psychological adaptations occurring in the mother's partner after childbirth.

SECTION I: ASSESSING YOUR UNDERSTANDING

Activity A FILL IN THE BLANKS

1. Within 10 days of birth, the fundus of the uterus usually cannot be palpated because it has descended into the true _____.

2. If retrogressive changes do not occur as a result of retained placental fragments or infection, _____ results.

3. _____ are the painful uterine contractions some women experience during the early postpartum period.

4. Increased prolactin levels and abundant milk supply, combined with inadequate emptying of the breast, may cause breast _____.

5. During pregnancy, stretching of the abdominal wall muscles occurs to accommodate the enlarging _____.

6. _____ elicits the milk letdown reflex so that milk can be ejected from the alveoli to the nipple.

7. For _____ women, menstruation usually resumes 7 to 9 weeks after giving birth.

8. _____ is the secretion of milk by the breasts.

9. _____ from the anterior pituitary gland, secreted in increasing levels throughout pregnancy, triggers synthesis and secretion of milk after giving birth.

10. The profuse _____ that is common during the early postpartum period is one of the most noticeable adaptations in the integumentary system and is a way of eliminating excess body fluids retained during pregnancy.

Activity B MATCHING

Match the terms in Column A with their descriptions in Column B.

Column A

____ 1. Engrossment

____ 2. Involution

____ 3. Lochia

____ 4. Puerperium

____ 5. Uterine atony

Column B

a. The discharge that occurs after birth

b. Encompasses the time after delivery as the woman's body begins to return to the pre-pregnant state

c. Allows excessive bleeding

d. The father's developing a bond with his newborn, which is a time of intense absorption, preoccupation, and interest

e. Involves three retrogressive processes, which are contraction of muscle fibers, catabolism, and regeneration of uterine epithelium

Activity C SEQUENCING

Put the items in correct sequence by writing the letters in the boxes provided below.

1. Lochia refers to the discharge that occurs after birth. Given below, in random order, are the three stages of lochia. Choose the correct sequence in which they appear after birth.

   a. Lochia alba

   b. Lochia rubra

   c. Lochia serosa

   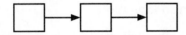

2. Given below, in random order, are the three stages a woman goes through immediately after she gives birth to a child. Choose the correct sequence in which they occur.

   a. Letting-go phase

   b. Taking-hold phase

   c. Taking-in phase

   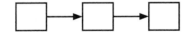

Activity D SHORT ANSWERS

Briefly answer the following.

1. Explain why breastfeeding is not a reliable method of contraception?

   _____

   _____

   _____

2. Why are afterpains more acute in multiparous women?

   _____

   _____

   _____

3. What are the factors that facilitate uterine involution?

   _____

   _____

   _____

4. What are the factors that inhibit uterine involution?

   _____

   _____

   _____

5. Why do women who have had cesarean births tend to have less flow of lochial discharge?

   _____

   _____

   _____

6. Why are afterpains usually stronger during breastfeeding? What can be done to reduce this discomfort?

   _____

   _____

   _____

SECTION II: APPLYING YOUR KNOWLEDGE

Activity E CASE STUDY

Consider this scenario and answer the questions.

A nurse is caring for two clients, one who is breastfeeding and has developed breast engorgement and another who is not breastfeeding and has developed breast engorgement.

1. What relief measures should the nurse suggest to resolve engorgement in the client who is breastfeeding?

   _____

   _____

   _____

2. What relief measures should a nurse suggest for nonbreastfeeding engorgement?

_____

_____

_____

SECTION III: PRACTICING FOR NCLEX

Activity F NCLEX-STYLE QUESTIONS

Answer the following questions.

1. A nurse is caring for a client in the postpartum period. Which of the following processes should the nurse identify as retrogressive processes involved in involution? Select all that apply.

a. Contraction of muscle fibers

b. Return of breasts to their prepregnancy size

c. Catabolism, which reduces individual myometrial cells

d. Regeneration of uterine epithelium

e. Retention of urine

2. A client who gave birth about 12 hours ago informs the nurse that she has been voiding small amounts of urine frequently. The nurse examines the client and notes the displacement of the uterus from the midline to the right. What intervention will help the client most?

a. A warm shower

b. Practicing good body mechanics

c. A warm compress

d. Urinary catheterization

3. A client who has given birth a week ago complains to the nurse of discomfort when defecating and ambulating. The birth involved an episiotomy. Which of the following should the nurse suggest to the client to provide local comfort? Select all that apply.

a. Maintain correct posture

b. Use of warm sitz baths

c. Use of anesthetic sprays

d. Use of witch hazel pads

e. Use good body mechanics

4. A nurse is caring for a client who has had a vaginal birth. The nurse understands that pelvic relaxation can occur in any woman experiencing a vaginal birth. Which of the following should the nurse recommend to the client to improve pelvic floor tone?

a. Kegel exercises

b. Urinating immediately when the urge is felt

c. Abdominal crunches

d. Sitz baths

5. The nurse is caring for a client who had been administered an anesthetic block during labor. Which of the following are risks that the nurse should watch for in the client? Select all that apply.

a. Incomplete emptying of bladder

b. Bladder distention

c. Ambulation difficulty

d. Urinary retention

e. Perineal laceration

6. A client who delivered a baby 36 hours ago informs the nurse that she has been passing unusually large volumes of urine very often. How should the nurse explain this to the client?

a. "Bruising and swelling of the perineum often causes excessive urination."

b. "Larger than normal amounts of urine frequently occurs due to swelling of tissues surrounding the urinary meatus."

c. "Your body usually retains extra fluids during pregnancy, so this is one way it rids itself of the excess fluid."

d. "Anesthesia causes decreased bladder tone, which causes you to urinate more frequently."

7. A client complains to the nurse of pain in the lower back, hips, and joints 10 days after the birth of her baby. What instruction should the nurse give the client after birth to prevent low back pain and injury to the joints?

a. Try to avoid carrying the baby for a few days.

b. Maintain correct posture and positioning.

c. Soak in a warm bath several times a day.

d. Apply ice to the sore joints.

8. A concerned client tells the nurse that her husband, who was very excited about the baby before its birth, is apparently happy but seems to be afraid of caring for the baby. What suggestions should the nurse give to the client's husband to resolve the issue?

    a. Suggest that her husband begin by holding the baby frequently.

    b. Encourage the husband to speak to his friends who have children.

    c. Advise that her husband read up on parental care.

    d. Recommend that she speak to the physician on her husband's behalf.

9. A client who gave birth 5 days ago complains to the nurse of profuse sweating during the night. What should the nurse recommend to the client in this regard?

    a. "I would suggest that you speak with your physician about this."

    b. "Drink plenty of cold fluids before you go to bed."

    c. "Be sure to change your pajamas to prevent you from chilling."

    d. "I'm not sure why this is occurring since this usually doesn't occur until much later in the postpartum period."

10. A client is undergoing a routine check-up 2 months after the birth of her child. The nurse understands that the client is not practicing Kegel exercises. Which of the following should the nurse tell the client is caused by poor perineal muscular tone?

    a. Pain in the joints

    b. Pain in the lower back

    c. Urinary incontinence

    d. Postpartum diuresis

11. A breastfeeding client informs the nurse that she is unable to maintain her milk supply. What instructions should the nurse give to the client to improve milk supply?

    a. Take cold baths.

    b. Apply ice to the breasts.

    c. Empty the breasts frequently.

    d. Perform Kegel exercises.

12. A nurse is examining a client who underwent a vaginal birth 24 hours ago. The client asks the nurse why her discharge is such a deep red color. What explanation is most accurate for the nurse to give to the client?

    a. "The discharge consists of mucus, tissue debris, and blood; this gives it the deep red color."

    b. "It is normal for the discharge to be deep red since it consists of leukocytes, decidual tissue, RBCs, and serous fluid."

    c. "The discharge at this point in the postpartum period consists of RBCs and leukocytes."

    d. "This discharge is called lochia, and it consists of leukocytes and decidual tissue."

13. A nurse is caring for a client who gave birth a week ago. The client informs the nurse that she experiences painful uterine contractions when breastfeeding the baby. The nurse would be accurate in identifying which hormone as the cause of these afterpains?

    a. Relaxin

    b. Progesterone

    c. Prolactin

    d. Oxytocin

14. A client who had a vaginal delivery 2 days ago asks the nurse when she will be able to breathe normally again. Which response by the nurse is accurate?

    a. "You should notice a change in your respiratory status within the next 24 hours."

    b. "Everyone is different, so it is difficult to say when your respirations will be back to normal."

    c. "It usually takes about 3 months before all of your abdominal organs return to normal, allowing you to breathe normally."

    d. "Within 1 to 3 weeks, your diaphragm should return to normal and your breathing will feel like it did before your pregnancy."

15. The nurse is caring for a client of Asian descent 1 day after she has given birth. Which foods will the client most likely refuse to eat when her meal tray is delivered? Select all that apply.

a. Ice cream

b. Hot soup

c. Raw carrots and celery

d. Orange slices

e. Mashed potatoes with gravy

16. While caring for a client following a lengthy labor and delivery, the nurse notes that the client repeatedly reviews her labor and delivery and is very dependent on her family for care. The nurse is correct in identifying the client to be in which phase of maternal role adjustment?

a. Letting-go

b. Taking-hold

c. Taking-in

d. Acquaintance/attachment

Nursing Management During the Postpartum Period

Learning Objectives

Upon completion of the chapter, you will be able to:

- Define the key terms.
- Characterize the normal physiologic and psychological adaptations to the postpartum period.
- Determine the parameters that need to be assessed during the postpartum period.
- Compare the bonding and attachment process.
- Select behaviors that enhance or inhibit the attachment process.
- Outline nursing management for the woman and her family during the postpartum period.
- Examine the role of the nurse in promoting successful breastfeeding.
- Plan areas of health education needed for discharge planning, home care, and follow-up.

SECTION I: ASSESSING YOUR UNDERSTANDING

Activity A FILL IN THE BLANKS

1. The _____ is a plastic squeeze bottle filled with warm tap water that is sprayed over the perineal area after each voiding and before applying a new perineal pad.

2. Palpate the breasts for any nodules, masses, or areas of warmth, which may indicate a plugged duct that may progress to _____ if not treated promptly.

3. Elevations in blood pressure from the woman's baseline might suggest pregnancy-induced _____.

4. _____ is considered the fifth vital sign.

5. _____ hypotension can occur when the woman changes rapidly from a lying or sitting position to a standing one.

6. The top portion of the uterus, known as the _____, is assessed to determine uterine involution.

7. Women who experience _____ births will have less lochia discharge than those having a vaginal birth.

8. _____ is the process by which the infant's capabilities and behavioral characteristics elicit parental response.

9. _____ refers to the enduring nature of the attachment relationship.

10. Any discharge from the nipple should be described and documented if it is not _____ or foremilk.

Activity B MATCHING

Match the terms in Column A with their descriptions in Column B.

Column A

_____ **1.** Bonding

_____ **2.** Proximity

_____ **3.** Process of attachment

_____ **4.** Postpartum blues

_____ **5.** Contact

Column B

a. Physical and psychological experience of the parents being close to their infant

b. Transient emotional disturbances

c. Development of a close emotional attachment to a newborn by the parents during the first 30 to 60 minutes after birth

d. Development of strong affectional ties between an infant and a significant other (e.g., mother, father, sibling, caretaker)

e. Sensory experiences such as touching, holding, and gazing at the newborn

Activity C SHORT ANSWERS

Briefly answer the following.

1. What does the postpartum assessment of the mother include?

_____

_____

_____

2. What nutritional recommendations can a nurse provide to a client during the postpartum period?

_____

_____

_____

3. What are the causes of postpartum stress?

_____

_____

_____

4. What are the postpartum physiologic danger signs?

_____

_____

_____

5. Discuss ways a nurse can model behavior to facilitate parental role adaptation and attachment during the postpartum period.

_____

_____

_____

6. What suggestions can a nurse provide to the parents to minimize sibling rivalry during the postpartum period?

_____

_____

_____

SECTION II: APPLYING YOUR KNOWLEDGE

Activity D CASE STUDY

Consider this scenario and answer the questions.

A nurse is caring for a client who has just delivered a healthy baby girl. The client is aware of the benefits of breastfeeding. She expresses her desire to breastfeed her newborn.

1. What assessments should the nurse perform in this regard?

_____

_____

_____

2. How often should the client breastfeed her infant during the postpartum period?

_____

_____

_____

SECTION III: PRACTICING FOR NCLEX

Activity E NCLEX-STYLE QUESTIONS

Answer the following questions.

1. A nurse has been assigned to the care of a client who has just given birth. How frequently should the nurse perform the assessments during the first hour after delivery?

    a. Every 30 minutes

    b. Every 15 minutes

    c. After 60 minutes

    d. After 45 minutes

2. A nurse, assigned to check the pulse, discerns tachycardia in a postpartum client. Which of the following does it suggest?

    a. Pulmonary edema

    b. Atelectasis

    c. Excessive blood loss

    d. Pulmonary embolism

3. During assessment of the mother during the postpartum period, what would alert the nurse that the client is likely experiencing uterine atony?

    a. Fundus feels firm

    b. Foul-smelling urine

    c. Purulent vaginal drainage

    d. Boggy or relaxed uterus

4. The nurse observes a 2-in lochia stain on the perineal pad of a postpartum client. Which of the following terms should the nurse use to describe the amount of lochia present?

    a. Light

    b. Scant

    c. Moderate

    d. Large

5. A nurse is caring for a client who has just received an episiotomy. The nurse observes that the laceration extends through the perineal area and continues through the anterior rectal wall. Which of the following classifications will the nurse use to describe the laceration?

    a. First-degree laceration

    b. Second-degree laceration

    c. Third-degree laceration

    d. Fourth-degree laceration

6. A nurse is applying ice packs to the perineal area of a client who has had a vaginal delivery. Which of the following interventions should the nurse perform to ensure that the client gets the optimum benefits of the procedure?

    a. Apply ice packs directly to the perineal area.

    b. Apply ice packs for 40 minutes continuously.

    c. Ensure ice pack is changed frequently.

    d. Use ice packs for a week after delivery.

7. Which of the following exercises should a nurse suggest to the client during the first day of postpartum?

    a. Abdominal exercises

    b. Buttock exercises

    c. Thigh-toning exercises

    d. Kegel exercises

8. A first-time mother is nervous about breastfeeding. Which of the following interventions should the nurse perform to reduce maternal anxiety about breastfeeding?

    a. Reassure the mother that some newborns "latch on and catch on" right away, and some newborns take more time and patience.

    b. Explain that breastfeeding comes naturally to all mothers.

    c. Tell her that breastfeeding is a mechanical procedure that involves burping once in a while and that she should try finishing it quickly.

    d. Ensure that the mother breastfeeds the newborn using the cradle method.

9. A client who has a breastfeeding newborn complains of sore nipples. Which of the following interventions can the nurse suggest to alleviate the client's condition?

    a. Recommend a moisturizing soap to clean the nipples.

    b. Encourage use of breast pads with plastic liners.

    c. Offer suggestions based on observation to correct positioning or latching.

    d. Fasten nursing bra flaps immediately after feeding.

10. A client who has given birth is being discharged from the health care facility. She wants to know how safe it would be for her to have intercourse. Which of the following instructions should the nurse provide to the client regarding intercourse after childbirth?

    a. Avoid use of water-based gel lubricants.

    b. Resume intercourse if bright-red bleeding stops.

    c. Avoid performing pelvic floor exercises.

    d. Use oral contraceptives for contraception.

11. A client has been discharged from the hospital after a cesarean birth. Which of the following is the most appropriate time for scheduling a follow-up appointment for the client?

    a. Within 3 weeks of hospital discharge

    b. Between 4 and 6 weeks after hospital discharge

    c. Within 2 weeks of hospital discharge

    d. Within 1 week of hospital discharge

12. A client is Rh-negative and has given birth to a newborn who is Rh-positive. Within how many hours should Rh immunoglobulin be injected in the mother?

    a. 72

    b. 75

    c. 78

    d. 80

13. A nurse is to care for a client during the postpartum period. The client complains of pain and discomfort in her breasts. What signs should a nurse look for to find out if the client has engorged breasts? Select all that apply.

    a. Breasts are hard.

    b. Breasts are tender.

    c. Nipples are fissured.

    d. Nipples are cracked.

    e. Breasts are soft.

14. A nurse is assessing a client during the postpartum period. Which of the following indicate normal postpartum adjustment? Select all that apply.

    a. Abdominal pain

    b. Active bowel sounds

    c. Tender abdomen

    d. Passing gas

    e. Nondistended abdomen

15. When teaching the new mother about breastfeeding, the nurse is correct when providing what instructions? Select all that apply.

    a. Give newborns water and other foods to balance nutritional needs.

    b. Show mothers how to initiate breastfeeding within 30 minutes of birth.

    c. Encourage breastfeeding of the newborn infant on demand.

    d. Provide breastfeeding newborns with pacifiers.

    e. Place baby in uninterrupted skin-to-skin contact with the mother.

Newborn Transitioning

Learning Objectives

Upon completion of the chapter, you will be able to:

- Define the key terms used in this chapter.
- Examine the major physiologic changes that occur as the newborn transitions to extrauterine life.
- Determine the primary challenges faced by the newborn during transition to extrauterine life.
- Differentiate the three behavioral patterns that newborns progress through after birth.
- Assess the five typical behavioral responses triggered by external stimuli of the newborn.

SECTION I: ASSESSING YOUR UNDERSTANDING

Activity A FILL IN THE BLANKS

1. _____ is the newborn's ability to process and respond to visual and auditory stimuli.

2. A _____ is an involuntary muscular response to a sensory stimulus.

3. The immune system's responses may be natural or _____.

4. _____ is the first stool passed by the newborn, which is composed of amniotic fluid, shed mucosal cells, intestinal secretions, and blood.

5. Human breast milk provides a passive mechanism to protect the newborn against the dangers of a deficient _____ defense system.

6. At birth, the pH of the stomach contents is mildly acidic, reflecting the pH of the _____ fluid.

7. _____ refers to the yellowing of the skin, sclera, and mucous membranes as a result of increased bilirubin blood levels.

8. The source of bilirubin in the newborn is the _____ of erythrocytes.

9. Newborn iron stores are determined by total body _____ content and length of gestation.

10. The primary body temperature regulators are located in the _____ and the central nervous system.

Activity B LABELING

Consider the following figures. Identify figures A, B, C, and D by the mechanisms of heat loss for the newborn.

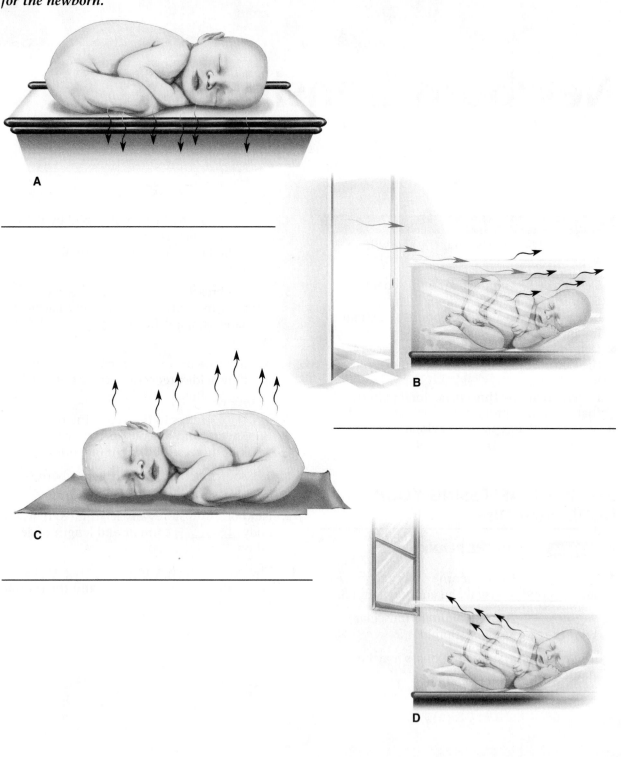

A

_____

B

_____

C

_____

D

_____

Activity C MATCHING

Match the blood-supplying structures in Column A with their corresponding functions in Column B.

Column A

___ **1.** Umbilical vein

___ **2.** Ductus venosus

___ **3.** Foramen ovale

___ **4.** Ductus arteriosus

___ **5.** Placenta

Column B

a. Allows majority of the umbilical vein blood to bypass liver and merge with blood moving through the vena cava, bringing it to the heart sooner

b. Connects pulmonary artery to the aorta, which allows bypassing of the pulmonary circuit

c. Allows more than half the blood entering the right atrium to cross immediately to the left atrium

d. Carries oxygenated blood from placenta to the fetus

e. Provides oxygen and nutrients to the fetus and removes waste products

Activity D SHORT ANSWERS

Briefly answer the following.

1. What is a newborn's response to auditory and visual stimuli?

2. What are the expected neurobehavioral responses of the newborn?

3. What events must occur before a newborn's lungs can maintain respiratory function?

4. How is the amniotic fluid removed from the lungs of a newborn?

5. What signs of abnormality should a nurse observe in a newborn's respiration?

6. What are the nursing interventions that may help minimize regurgitation?

SECTION II: APPLYING YOUR KNOWLEDGE

Activity E CASE STUDY

Consider this scenario and answer the questions.

A newborn is under the observation of a nurse in a health care facility. The child is crying, and its heartbeat has increased. Usually, heartbeats are highest after birth and reach a plateau within a week after birth. During the first few minutes after birth, a newborn's heart rate is approximately 120 to 180 bpm. Thereafter, the heart rate begins to decrease to somewhere between 120 and 130 bpm.

1. What are the factors that increase the heart rate and blood pressure in a newborn?

2. What are the factors that affect the hematologic values of a newborn?

3. What are the benefits of delayed cord clamping after birth?

_____

_____

_____

SECTION III: PRACTICING FOR NCLEX

Activity F **NCLEX-STYLE QUESTIONS**

Answer the following questions.

1. A client delivers a newborn in a local health care facility. What guidance should the nurse give to the client before discharge regarding care of the newborn at home?

   a. Ensure cool air is circulating over the newborn to prevent excess heat.

   b. Keep the newborn wrapped in a blanket, with a cap on its head.

   c. Hold the newborn close to the body after taking a shower.

   d. Refrain from using clothing and blankets in the crib.

2. A nurse is explaining the benefits of breastfeeding to a client who has just delivered. Which of the following immunoglobulins does breast milk contain that boost a newborn's immune system as opposed to formula?

   a. IgA

   b. IgD

   c. IgE

   d. IgM

3. Which of the following are factors that increase the risk of overheating in a newborn? Select all that apply.

   a. Limited sweating ability

   b. Underdeveloped lungs

   c. Too-warm crib

   d. Limited insulation

   e. Lack of brown fat

4. A 2-month-old infant is admitted to a local health care facility after experiencing heat loss. Which of the following manifestations should the nurse observe in the infant in order to confirm the occurrence of cold stress?

   a. Change in color of the urine

   b. Increase in the body temperature

   c. Lethargy and hypotonia

   d. Change in the color of the skin

5. Which of the following is a risk factor for the development of jaundice in a newborn?

   a. Formula feeding

   b. Oxytocin usage in the mother

   c. Female gender

   d. Hepatitis A vaccine

6. Which of the following complications should a nurse keep in mind while administering IV therapy to a newborn?

   a. Heart rate increase

   b. Lower blood pressure

   c. Decrease in alertness

   d. Fluid overload

7. A client is worried that her newborn's stools are greenish, with an unpleasant odor. The newborn is being formula-fed. What instruction should the nurse give this client?

   a. Switch to breast milk

   b. Greenish stools with an unpleasant odor are normal

   c. Increase newborn's fluid intake

   d. Administer Vitamin K supplements

8. A mother wants to know the caloric intake for her 2-week-old newborn. Which of the following should the nurse suggest as the ideal caloric intake for a term newborn to regain lost weight?

   a. 85 kcal/kg/day

   b. 108 kcal/kg/day

   c. 156 kcal/kg/day

   d. 212 kcal/kg/day

9. Which of the following newborns are at a greater risk for cold stress?

a. Preterm newborns

b. Newborns being fed formula

c. Postterm newborns

d. Larger-than-average newborns

10. A client delivers a baby in the maternity unit of a local health care facility. Which of the following behaviors of the newborn should the nurse identify as the self-quieting ability of a newborn?

a. Hand-to-mouth movements

b. Movement of head and eyes

c. Hyperactivity

d. Movements of the legs

11. A nurse needs to check the blood glucose levels of a newborn under observation at a health care facility. When should the nurse check the newborn's initial glucose level?

a. After the newborn has been fed

b. 24 hours after admission to the nursery

c. On admission to the nursery

d. 5 hours after admission to the nursery

12. Which of the following interventions can a nurse perform to maintain a neutral thermal environment?

a. Promote early breastfeeding

b. Avoid skin-to-skin contact with the mother

c. Keep the infant transporter cool

d. Avoid bathing the newborn

13. A nurse is required to assess the temperature of a newborn using a skin temperature probe. Which of the following points should the nurse keep in mind while taking the newborn's temperature?

a. Ensure that the newborn is lying on its abdomen

b. Place the temperature probe on the forehead

c. Place the temperature probe over the liver

d. Place the temperature probe on the buttocks

14. A nurse is assigned to care for a newborn with high bilirubin levels. Which of the following symptoms should the nurse monitor the newborn for?

a. Yellow mucous membranes

b. Pinkish appearance of tongue

c. Heart rate of 130 bpm

d. Bluish skin discoloration

15. The nurse is providing teaching to a new mother who is breastfeeding. The mother demonstrates understanding of teaching when she identifies which characteristics as being true of the stool of a breastfed newborn? Select all that apply.

a. Formed in consistency

b. Completely odorless

c. Firm in shape

d. Yellowish gold color

e. Stringy to pasty consistency

CHAPTER 18

Nursing Management of the Newborn

Learning Objectives

Upon completion of the chapter, you will be able to:

- Define the key terms.
- Relate the assessments performed during the immediate newborn period.
- Employ appropriate interventions that meet the immediate needs of the term newborn.
- Demonstrate the components of a typical physical examination of a newborn.
- Distinguish common variations that can be noted during a newborn's physical examination.
- Characterize common concerns in the newborn and appropriate interventions.
- Compare the importance of the newborn screening tests.
- Plan for common interventions that are appropriate during the early newborn period.
- Analyze the nurse's role in meeting the newborn's nutritional needs.
- Outline discharge planning content and education needed for the family with a newborn.

SECTION I: ASSESSING YOUR UNDERSTANDING

Activity A FILL IN THE BLANKS

1. The _____ score is used to evaluate newborns at 1 minute and 5 minutes after birth.

2. _____ refers to the soft, downy hair on the newborn's body.

3. _____ babies are babies with placental aging who are born after 42 weeks.

4. Babies weighing more than the 90th percentile on standard growth charts are referred to as _____ for gestational age.

5. Vitamin K, a fat-soluble vitamin, promotes blood clotting by increasing the synthesis of _____ by the liver.

6. Persistent cyanosis of fingers, hands, toes, and feet with mottled blue or red discoloration and coldness is called _____.

7. _____ are unopened sebaceous glands frequently found on a newborn's nose.

8. _____ sign refers to the dilation of blood vessels on only one side of the body, giving the newborn the appearance of paleness on one side of the body and ruddiness on the other.

9. The _____ fontanel of the baby is diamond shaped and closes by age 18 to 24 months.

10. _____ is a localized effusion of blood beneath the periosteum of the skull of the newborn.

Activity B LABELING

Consider the following figure. What is being depicted?

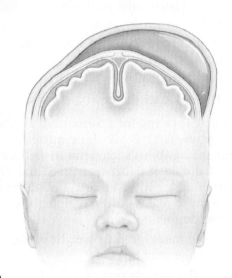

A

_____

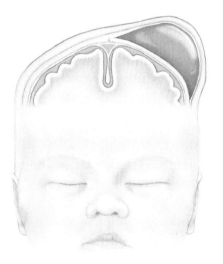

B

_____

Activity C MATCHING

Match the following anthropometric measurements of a term newborn in Column A with their appropriate value in Column B.

Column A	Column B
___ 1. Head circumference	a. 32–38 cm
___ 2. Chest circumference	b. 33–37 cm
___ 3. Weight	c. 2,500–4,000 g
___ 4. Length	d. 45–55 cm

Activity D SEQUENCING

Arrange the following reflexes in the correct order of their disappearance into adulthood.

1. Stepping

2. Babinski sign

3. Grasp

4. Rooting

5. Gag reflex

☐ → ☐ → ☐ → ☐ → ☐

Activity E SHORT ANSWERS

Briefly answer the following.

1. How can a mother achieve the football-hold position for breastfeeding?

_____

_____

_____

2. What is colostrum?

_____

_____

_____

3. What is the use of fiber optic pads in treatment of physiologic jaundice?

_____

_____

_____

4. How can a nurse test Moro reflex?

_____

_____

_____

5. What is caput succedaneum?

_____

_____

_____

6. What is erythema toxicum?

_____

_____

_____

SECTION II: APPLYING YOUR KNOWLEDGE

Activity F   CASE STUDY

Consider this scenario and answer the questions.

Karen, a first-time mother, is worried that her baby does not sleep properly and wakes up every 2 hours. Karen informs the nurse that she often brings the baby to her bed to nurse and falls asleep with the baby in her bed.

1. What information should the nurse offer regarding the sleeping habits of newborns?

_____

_____

_____

2. What safety precautions should the mother take when putting the baby to sleep?

_____

_____

_____

3. What education should the nurse impart to Karen to discourage bed-sharing?

_____

_____

_____

SECTION III: PRACTICING FOR NCLEX

Activity G   NCLEX-STYLE QUESTIONS

Answer the following questions.

1. The nurse caring for a newborn has to perform assessment at various intervals. When should the nurse complete the second assessment for the newborn?

a. Immediately after birth, in the birthing area

b. Within the first 2 to 4 hours, when the newborn is in the nursery

c. Before the newborn is discharged

d. The day after the newborn's birth

2. A nurse is caring for a 5-hour-old newborn. The physician has asked the nurse to maintain the newborn's temperature between 97.7° and 99.5° F (between 36.5° and 37.5° C). What nursing intervention should the nurse perform to maintain the temperature within the recommended range?

a. Avoid measuring the weight of the infant, as scales may be cold.

b. Use the stethoscope over the baby's garment.

c. Place the newborn close to the outer wall in the room.

d. Place the newborn skin-to-skin with the mother.

3. As a part of the newborn assessment, the nurse determines the skin turgor. Which of the following nursing interventions is relevant when observing the turgor of the newborn's skin?

a. Pinch skin and note return to original position.

b. Examine for stork bites or salmon patches.

c. Check for unopened sebaceous glands.

d. Inspect for blue or purple splotches on buttocks.

4. Which of the following information should the nurse give to a client who is breastfeeding her newborn regarding the nutritional requirements of newborns, as per the recommendations of the American Academy of Pediatrics (AAP)?

a. Feed the infant at least 10 mL per kg of water daily.

b. Give iron supplements to the newborn daily.

c. Give vitamin D supplements daily for the first 2 months.

d. Ensure adequate fluoride supplementation.

5. A first-time mother informs the nurse that she is unable to breastfeed her baby through the day as she is usually away at work. She adds that she wants to express her breast milk and store it for her baby. What instruction should the nurse offer the woman to ensure the safety of stored expressed breast milk?

a. Use sealed and chilled milk within 24 hours

b. Use frozen milk within 6 months of obtaining it

c. Use microwave ovens to warm chilled milk

d. Refreeze any unused milk for later use

6. A nurse is educating the mother of a newborn about feeding and burping. Which of the following strategies should the nurse offer to the mother regarding burping?

a. Hold the baby upright with the baby's head on her mother's shoulder.

b. Lay the baby on its back on its mother's lap.

c. Gently rub the baby's abdomen while the baby is in a sitting position.

d. Lay the baby on its mother's lap and give it frequent sips of warm water.

7. The mother of a formula-fed newborn asks how she will know if her newborn is receiving enough formula during feedings. Which response by the nurse is correct?

a. "Your newborn should finish a bottle in less than 15 minutes."

b. "A sign of good nutrition is when your newborn seems satisfied and is gaining sufficient weight."

c. "If your newborn is wetting three to four diapers and producing several stools a day, enough formula is likely being consumed."

d. "Your newborn should be taking about 2 oz of formula for every pound of body weight during each feeding."

8. A nurse, while examining a newborn, observes salmon patches on the nape and on the eyelids. Which of the following is the most likely cause of the salmon patches?

a. Concentration of pigmented cells

b. Eosinophils reacting to environment

c. Immature autoregulation of blood flow

d. Concentration of immature blood vessels

9. A nurse is required to obtain the temperature of a healthy newborn who is placed in an ordinary crib. Which of the following is the most appropriate method for measuring a newborn's temperature?

a. Tape electronic thermistor probe to the abdominal skin.

b. Obtain temperature orally.

c. Place electronic temperature probe in the midaxillary area.

d. Obtain temperature rectally.

10. A nurse observes that a newborn has a 1-minute Apgar score of 5 points. What should the nurse conclude from the observed Apgar score?

a. Severe distress in adjusting to extrauterine life

b. Better condition of the newborn

c. Moderate difficulty in adjusting to extrauterine life

d. Abnormal central nervous system status

11. The mother of a newborn observes a diaper rash on her baby's skin. Which of the following should the nurse instruct the parent to prevent diaper rash?

a. Expose the newborn's bottom to air several times a day.

b. Use plastic pants while bathing the newborn.

c. Use products such as powder and items with fragrance.

d. Place the newborn's buttocks in warm water often.

12. A nurse is caring for a newborn with transient tachypnea. What nursing interventions should the nurse perform while providing supportive care to the newborn? Select all that apply.

a. Provide warm water to drink.

b. Provide oxygen supplement.

c. Massage the newborn's back.

d. Ensure the newborn's warmth.

e. Observe respiratory status frequently.

13. A nurse is caring for a newborn with hypo-glycemia. What symptoms of hypoglycemia should the nurse monitor the newborn for? Select all that apply.

    a. Lethargy

    b. Low-pitched cry

    c. Cyanosis

    d. Skin rashes

    e. Jitteriness

14. A mother who is 4 days postpartum, and is breastfeeding, expresses to the nurse that her breast seems to be tender and engorged. What education should the nurse give to the mother to relieve breast engorgement? Select all that apply.

    a. Take warm-to-hot showers to encourage milk release.

    b. Feed the newborn in the sitting position only.

    c. Express some milk manually before breastfeeding.

    d. Massage the breasts from the nipple toward the axillary area.

    e. Apply warm compresses to the breasts prior to nursing.

15. A nurse is performing a detailed newborn assessment of a female baby. Which of the following observations indicate a normal finding? Select all that apply.

    a. Mongolian spots

    b. Enlarged fontanelles

    c. Swollen genitals

    d. Low-set ears

    e. Short, creased neck

CHAPTER 19

Nursing Management of Pregnancy at Risk: Pregnancy-Related Complications

Learning Objectives

Upon completion of the chapter, you will be able to:

- Evaluate the term "high-risk pregnancy."
- Determine the common factors that might place a pregnancy at high risk.
- Detect the causes of vaginal bleeding during early and late pregnancy.
- Outline nursing assessment and management for the pregnant woman experiencing vaginal bleeding.
- Develop a plan of care for the woman experiencing preeclampsia, eclampsia, and HELLP syndrome.
- Examine the pathophysiology of polyhydramnios and subsequent management.
- Evaluate factors in a woman's prenatal history that place her at risk for premature rupture of membranes (PROM).
- Formulate a teaching plan for maintaining the health of pregnant women experiencing a high-risk pregnancy.

SECTION I: ASSESSING YOUR UNDERSTANDING

Activity A FILL IN THE BLANKS

1. _____ is a decreased amount of amniotic fluid (<500 mL) between 32 and 36 weeks' gestation.

2. _____ is the presence of rhythmic involuntary contractions, most often at the foot or ankle.

3. The time interval from rupture of membranes to the onset of regular contractions is termed the _____ period.

4. Brisk reflexes, or _____, are a common presenting symptom of preeclampsia and are the result of an irritable cortex.

5. Rh _____ is a condition that develops when a woman with Rh-negative blood type is exposed to Rh-positive blood cells and subsequently develops circulating titers of Rh antibodies.

6. _____ twins develop when a single, fertilized ovum splits during the first 2 weeks after conception.

7. A foul odor of amniotic fluid indicates
   _____.

8. A _____ abortion refers to the loss of a
   fetus resulting from natural causes—that is,
   not elective or therapeutically induced by a
   procedure.

9. The most common cause for _____
   trimester abortions is fetal genetic abnormalities, usually unrelated to the mother.

10. _____ hypertension is characterized by
    hypertension without proteinuria after 20
    weeks of gestation and a return of the blood
    pressure to normal postpartum.

Activity B **MATCHING**

*Match the following conditions commonly
associated with pregnancy-related
complications in Column A with their
definitions in Column B.*

Column A

_____ **1.** Spontaneous
      abortion

_____ **2.** Ectopic
      pregnancy

_____ **3.** Gestational
      trophoblastic
      disease

_____ **4.** Cervical
      insufficiency

_____ **5.** Placenta previa

Column B

a. Spectrum of neo-
   plastic disorders
   that originate in the
   human placenta

b. Weak, structur-
   ally defective cervix
   that spontane-
   ously dilates in the
   absence of contrac-
   tions in the second
   trimester, resulting
   in the loss of the
   pregnancy

c. Loss of an early
   pregnancy, usu-
   ally before the 20th
   week of gestation

d. Painless bleed-
   ing condition that
   occurs in the last
   two trimesters of
   pregnancy

e. Pregnancy in which
   the fertilized ovum
   implants outside
   the uterine cavity

Activity C **SEQUENCING**

*Put the terms in correct sequence by writing the
letters in the boxes provided below.*

1. Given below, in random order, are the steps
   for assessing the patellar reflex. Write the correct sequence.

   a. Using a reflex hammer or the side of the
      hand, strike the area of the patellar ten-
      don firmly and quickly.

   b. Have the woman flex her knee slightly.

   c. Place the woman in the supine position.

   d. Repeat the procedure on the opposite leg.

   e. Note the movement of the leg and foot.

   f. Place a hand under the knee to support
      the leg and locate the patellar tendon.

□→□→□→□→□→□

Activity D **SHORT ANSWERS**

Briefly answer the following.

1. What are some possible complications of
   hyperemesis gravidarum?

   _____

   _____

2. What are the conditions associated with early
   bleeding during pregnancy?

   _____

   _____

   _____

3. What are the causes of ectopic pregnancies?

   _____

   _____

   _____

4. What are the risk factors for hyperemesis
   gravidarum?

   _____

   _____

   _____

5. What should a nurse include in prevention education for ectopic pregnancies?

_____

_____

_____

6. What is the Kleihauer–Betke test?

_____

_____

_____

SECTION II: APPLYING YOUR KNOWLEDGE

Activity E CASE STUDY

Consider this scenario and answer the questions.

The labor and birth triage nurse is admitting Jenna. By completing Jenna's history, the nurse learns that she is a single, 17-year-old African American, G-3 P-0020, who registered for prenatal care at the local clinic at 16 weeks of gestation. Her prenatal course has been unremarkable except for a urinary tract infection at 22 weeks that was treated with antibiotics. She did not return to the clinic for a follow-up urine culture after treatment. She is presenting at the hospital now, at 26 weeks, complaining of lower backache, cramping, and malaise. She reports to the nurse that she feels normal fetal movement and denies vaginal bleeding or discharge. She states that she feels her uterus "balling up" every 5 to 10 minutes. This has been going on all day, even after she came home from school and rested. The external fetal monitor, tocodynamometer, and ultrasound are applied to Jenna. The nurse's initial assessment indicates the client having contractions every 4 to 5 minutes that last 30 to 40 seconds, and the nurse palpates the contractions as mild.

1. Name the symptoms that indicate preterm labor and birth.

_____

_____

_____

2. The nurse caring for Jenna must ensure that she receives basic information about preterm labor, including information about harmful lifestyles, the signs of genitourinary infections, and preterm labor. What information should the nurse provide to the client to help better educate her in prevention strategies?

_____

_____

_____

SECTION III: PRACTICING FOR NCLEX

Activity F NCLEX-STYLE QUESTIONS

Answer the following questions.

1. A pregnant client with hyperemesis gravidarum needs advice on how to minimize nausea and vomiting. Which of the following instructions should a nurse give this client?

a. Lie down or recline for at least 2 hours after eating.

b. Avoid dry crackers, toast, and soda.

c. Eat small, frequent meals throughout the day.

d. Decrease intake of carbonated beverages.

2. When caring for a client with PROM, the nurse observes an increase in the client's pulse. What does this increase in pulse indicate?

a. Infection

b. Preterm labor

c. Cord compression

d. Respiratory distress syndrome

3. A nurse is caring for a client who has just undergone delivery. What is the best method for the nurse to assess this client for postpartum hemorrhage?

a. By assessing skin turgor

b. By assessing blood pressure

c. By frequently assessing uterine involution

d. By monitoring hCG titers

4. A nurse is monitoring a client with PROM who is in labor and observes meconium in the amniotic fluid. What does this indicate?

   a. Cord compression

   b. Fetal distress related to hypoxia

   c. Infection

   d. Central nervous system (CNS) involvement

5. The nurse is caring for a pregnant client with severe preeclampsia. Which of the following nursing interventions should a nurse perform to institute and maintain seizure precautions in this client?

   a. Provide a well-lit room.

   b. Keep head of bed slightly elevated.

   c. Place the client in a supine position.

   d. Keep the suction equipment readily available.

6. A client with preeclampsia is receiving magnesium sulfate to suppress or control seizures. Which of the following nursing interventions should a nurse perform to determine the effectiveness of therapy?

   a. Assess deep tendon reflexes.

   b. Monitor intake and output.

   c. Assess client's mucous membrane.

   d. Assess client's skin turgor.

7. A nurse is assessing pregnant clients for the risk of placenta previa. Which of the following clients faces the greatest risk for this condition?

   a. A 23-year-old client

   b. A client with a history of alcohol ingestion

   c. A client with a structurally defective cervix

   d. A client who had undergone a myomectomy to remove fibroids

8. A client is seeking advice for his pregnant wife, who is experiencing mild elevations in blood pressure. In which of the following positions should a nurse recommend the pregnant client rest?

   a. Supine position

   b. Lateral recumbent position

   c. Left lateral lying position

   d. Head of the bed slightly elevated

9. A nurse is caring for a client with hyperemesis gravidarum. Which of the following should be the first choice for fluid replacement for this client?

   a. Total parenteral nutrition

   b. IV fluids and antiemetics

   c. Percutaneous endoscopic gastrostomy

   d. 5% dextrose in lactated Ringer solution with vitamins and electrolytes

10. A nurse has been assigned to assess a pregnant client for abruptio placenta. Which of the following is a classic manifestation of this condition that the nurse should assess for?

    a. Painless bright red vaginal bleeding

    b. Increased fetal movement

    c. "Knife-like" abdominal pain with vaginal bleeding

    d. Generalized vasospasm

11. A nurse is caring for a client undergoing treatment for ectopic pregnancy. Which of the following symptoms is observed in a client if rupture or hemorrhaging occurs before the ectopic pregnancy is successfully treated?

    a. Phrenic nerve irritation

    b. Painless bright red vaginal bleeding

    c. Fetal distress

    d. Tetanic contractions

12. The nurse is required to assess a pregnant client who is complaining of vaginal bleeding. Which of the following assessments should be considered as a priority by the nurse?

    a. Monitoring uterine contractility

    b. Assessing signs of shock

    c. Determining the amount of funneling

    d. Assessing the amount and color of the bleeding

13. The nurse is required to monitor a pregnant client with fallopian tube rupture. Which of the following interventions should a nurse perform to identify development of hypovolemic shock in this client?

    a. Monitor the client's beta-hCG level.

    b. Monitor the mass with transvaginal ultrasound.

    c. Monitor the client's vital signs, bleeding.

    d. Monitor the fetal heart rate.

14. Which of the following instructions should a nurse give an Rh-negative nonimmunized client in her early weeks of pregnancy to prevent complications of blood incompatibility?

    a. Obtain RhoGAM at 28 weeks' gestation.

    b. Consume a well-balanced, nutritional diet.

    c. Avoid sexual activity until after 28 weeks.

    d. Undergo periodic transvaginal ultrasound.

15. A nurse is caring for a pregnant client with eclamptic seizure. Which of the following should the nurse know as a characteristic of eclampsia?

    a. Muscle rigidity is followed by facial twitching.

    b. Respirations are rapid during the seizure.

    c. Coma occurs after seizure.

    d. Respiration fails after the seizure.

16. A nurse is assessing a pregnant client with preeclampsia for suspected dependent edema. Which of the following is the most accurate description of dependent edema?

    a. Dependent edema leaves a small depression or pit after finger pressure is applied to a swollen area.

    b. Dependent edema occurs only in clients on bed rest.

    c. Dependent edema can be measured when pressure is applied.

    d. Dependent edema may be seen in the sacral area if the client is on bed rest.

17. The nurse is assessing a client who is in her 24th week of pregnancy. The nurse knows that which of the client's presenting symptoms should be further assessed as a possible sign of preterm labor? Select all that apply.

    a. Increase in vaginal discharge

    b. Phrenic nerve irritation

    c. Rupture of membranes

    d. Uterine contractions

    e. Hypovolemic shock

18. A pregnant client is brought to the health care facility with signs of PROM. Which of the following are the associated conditions and complications of premature rupture of the membranes? Select all that apply.

    a. Prolapsed cord

    b. Abruptio placenta

    c. Spontaneous abortion

    d. Placenta previa

    e. Preterm labor

19. The nurse is required to assess a client for HELLP syndrome. Which of the following are the signs and symptoms of this condition? Select all that apply.

    a. Blood pressure higher than 160/110

    b. Epigastric pain

    c. Oliguria

    d. Upper right quadrant pain

    e. Hyperbilirubinemia

20. A nurse is monitoring a client with spontaneous abortion who has been prescribed misoprostol. The nurse knows that which of the following symptoms are common adverse effects associated with misoprostol? Select all that apply.

    a. Constipation

    b. Dyspepsia

    c. Headache

    d. Hypotension

    e. Tachycardia

Nursing Management of the Pregnancy at Risk: Selected Health Conditions and Vulnerable Populations

Learning Objectives

Upon completion of the chapter, you will be able to:

- Select at least two conditions present before pregnancy that can have a negative effect on a pregnancy.
- Examine how a condition present before pregnancy can affect the woman physiologically and psychologically when she becomes pregnant.
- Evaluate the nursing assessment and management for a pregnant woman with diabetes from that of a pregnant woman without diabetes.
- Explore how congenital and acquired heart conditions can affect a woman's pregnancy.
- Design the nursing assessment and management of a pregnant woman with cardiovascular disorders and respiratory conditions.
- Differentiate among the types of anemia affecting pregnant women in terms of prevention and management.
- Relate the nursing care needed for the pregnant woman with an autoimmune disorder.

- Compare the most common infections that can jeopardize a pregnancy and propose possible preventive strategies.
- Develop a plan of care for the pregnant woman who is HIV-positive.
- Outline the nurse's role in the prevention and management of adolescent pregnancy.
- Determine the impact of pregnancy for a woman over the age of 35.
- Analyze the effects of substance abuse during pregnancy.

SECTION I: ASSESSING YOUR UNDERSTANDING

Activity A FILL IN THE BLANKS

1. Human placental lactogen and growth hormone _____ increase in direct correlation with the growth of placental tissue, causing insulin resistance.

2. _____ diabetes of any severity increases the risk of fetal macrosomia.

3. Asthma is known as reactive _____ disease.

4. The _____ is the major site of involvement in the client with tuberculosis.

5. _____ results in reduced capacity of the blood to carry oxygen to the vital organs of the mother and fetus as a result of reduced quantities of RBCs or hemoglobin.

6. Vaginal and rectal specimens of pregnant women may be cultured for the presence of _____ bacterium.

7. _____ is a widespread parasitic infection caused by a one-celled protozoan that may result from contact with cat feces.

8. _____ spans the time frame from the onset of puberty to the cessation of physical growth, roughly from 11 to 19 years of age.

9. _____ found in cigarettes causes vasoconstriction, transfers across the placenta, and reduces blood flow to the fetus, contributing to fetal hypoxia.

10. Maternal use of _____ early in a pregnancy often results in fetal neural tube defects and microencephaly.

Activity B MATCHING

Match the substances in Column A with their effect on pregnancy in Column B.

Column A

____ 1. Alcohol

____ 2. Caffeine

____ 3. Nicotine

____ 4. Cocaine

____ 5. Narcotics

____ 6. Sedatives

Column B

a. Respiratory problems, feeding difficulties, disturbed sleep

b. Neonatal abstinence syndrome, preterm labor, intrauterine growth restriction (IUGR), and pre-eclampsia

c. Vasoconstriction, tachycardia, hypertension, abruptio placenta, abortion, prune belly syndrome, IUGR

d. Reduced uteroplacental blood flow, decreased birth weight, abortion, prematurity, abruptio placenta

e. Decreased iron absorption; increased risk of anemia

f. Growth deficiencies, facial abnormalities, CNS impairment, behavioral disorders, and abnormal intellectual development

Activity C SHORT ANSWERS

Briefly answer the following.

1. What are the complications in a pregnant client with hypertension?

_____

_____

_____

2. What elements should be included during the physical examination of pregnant clients with asthma?

_____

_____

_____

3. What are the factors the nurse should include in the teaching plan for a pregnant client with asthma?

_____

_____

_____

4. What is the procedure involved in the assessment of tuberculosis in pregnant clients?

_____

_____

_____

5. What are the developmental tasks associated with adolescent behavior?

_____

_____

_____

6. What are the effects of abuse of sedatives by the mother on her infant?

_____

_____

_____

SECTION II: APPLYING YOUR KNOWLEDGE

Activity D CASE STUDY

Consider this scenario and answer the questions.

A nurse is caring for a pregnant client with asthma. During pregnancy, the respiratory system of the client is affected by hormonal changes, mechanical changes, and prior respiratory conditions.

1. When is a pregnant client likely to suffer an increase in asthma attacks?

_____

_____

_____

2. What does successful management of asthma in pregnancy involve?

_____

_____

_____

3. What are the nursing interventions involved for a client with asthma during labor?

_____

_____

_____

SECTION III: PRACTICING FOR NCLEX

Activity E NCLEX-STYLE QUESTIONS

Answer the following questions.

1. A nurse is caring for a pregnant client. The nurse learns from the report that the client is diabetic. Which of the following should the nurse identify as the effect of insulin resistance in the client?

a. Hypertension

b. Postprandial hyperglycemia

c. Hypercholesterolemia

d. Myocardial infarction

2. During the assessment of a pregnant client, the nurse learns that the client has CVD. Which of the following should the nurse identify as a major risk that can be faced by the newborn of the client?

a. Respiratory distress syndrome

b. Congenital varicella syndrome

c. SIDS

d. Prune belly syndrome

3. What is the role of the nurse during the preconception counseling of a pregnant client with chronic hypertension?

a. Stressing the avoidance of dairy products

b. Stressing the positive benefits of a healthy lifestyle

c. Stressing the increased use of Vitamin D supplements

d. Stressing regular walks and exercise

4. The nurse is caring for a pregnant client who is in her 30th week of gestation and has congenital heart disease. Which of the following should the nurse recognize as a symptom of cardiac decompensation with this client?

a. Swelling of the face

b. Dry, rasping cough

c. Slow, labored respiration

d. Elevated temperature

5. A nurse is caring for a pregnant client with heart disease in a labor unit. Which of the following is the most important intervention for this client in the first 48 hours postpartum?

a. Limiting sodium intake

b. Inspecting the extremities for edema

c. Ensuring that the client consumes a high-fiber diet

d. Assessing for cardiac decompensation

6. A nurse is caring for a pregnant client with asthma. Which of the following interventions should the nurse include during physical examination of this client?

a. Monitoring temperature frequently

b. Assessing for signs of fatigue

c. Monitoring frequency of headache

d. Assessing for feeling nauseated

7. What important instruction should the nurse give a pregnant client with tuberculosis?

a. Maintain adequate hydration.

b. Avoid direct sunlight.

c. Avoid red meat.

d. Wear light, cotton clothes.

8. Which of the following should the nurse identify as a risk associated with anemia during pregnancy?

a. Newborn with heart problems

b. Fetal asphyxia

c. Preterm birth

d. Newborn with an enlarged liver

9. A nurse is caring for a client with CVD who has just delivered. What nursing intervention should the nurse perform when caring for this client? Select all that apply.

a. Assess for shortness of breath.

b. Assess for a moist cough.

c. Assess for edema and note any pitting.

d. Auscultate heart sounds for abnormalities.

e. Monitor the client's hemoglobin and hematocrit.

10. A nurse is caring for a pregnant client who works at a daycare center and is in regular contact with children. What instructions should the nurse give this client in order to minimize risk of transmission of cytomegalovirus to the fetus?

a. Ensure thorough hand-washing.

b. Seek consultation for antibiotics.

c. Avoid interacting with children.

d. Drink plenty of fluids.

11. A nurse is caring for a pregnant adolescent client, who is in her first trimester, during a visit to the maternal child clinic. Which of the following is an important area that the nurse should address during assessment of the client?

a. Sexual development of the client

b. Whether sex was consensual

c. Options for birth control in the future

d. Knowledge of child development

12. A nurse is caring for a 45-year-old pregnant client with a cardiac disorder, who has been instructed by her physician to follow Class I functional activity recommendations. The nurse correctly instructs the client to follow which limitations?

a. "You will need to be on bedrest for the remainder of your pregnancy."

b. "It is important for you to rest after any physical activity in order to prevent any cardiac complications."

c. "It will be beneficial if you plan rest periods throughout your day."

d. "You do not need to limit your physical activity unless you experience any problems such as fatigue, chest pain, or shortness of breath."

13. A nurse is caring for a pregnant client who is HIV-positive. What is a priority issue that the nurse should discuss with the client?

a. The client's relationship with the spouse

b. The amount of physical contact that should occur with the infant

c. The client's plan for future pregnancies

d. The need for the client to avoid breast-feeding

14. A nurse caring for a pregnant client utilizes the RAFFT screening instrument to assess the possibility of substance abuse. What question does the "R" in RAFFT refer to?

a. "Do you use drugs as a form of recreation?"

b. "Do you drink or take drugs to relax?"

c. "Do you have any relatives that abuse drugs?"

d. "Do you ever rely on drugs to help you sleep? "

15. A nurse is caring for a pregnant client. The initial interview reveals that the client is accustomed to drinking coffee at regular intervals. What possible effect of maternal coffee consumption during pregnancy should the nurse make the client aware of?

a. Increased risk of heart disease

b. Increased risk of anemia

c. Increased risk of rickets

d. Increased risk of scurvy

16. The nurse is caring for a pregnant client who indicates that she is fond of meat, works with children, and has a pet cat. Which of the following instructions should the nurse give this client to prevent toxoplasmosis? Select all that apply.

a. Eat meat cooked to 160° F.

b. Avoid cleaning the cat's litter box.

c. Keep the cat outdoors at all times.

d. Avoid contact with children when they have a cold.

e. Avoid outdoor activities such as gardening.

17. A pregnant client has been diagnosed with gestational diabetes. Which of the following are risk factors for developing gestational diabetes? Select all that apply.

a. Maternal age less than 18 years

b. Genitourinary tract abnormalities

c. Obesity

d. Hypertension

e. Previous large for gestational age (LGA) infant

18. A nurse is caring for a pregnant client with sickle cell anemia. What should the nursing care for the client include? Select all that apply.

a. Teach the client meticulous hand-washing.

b. Assess serum electrolyte levels of the client at each visit.

c. Instruct client to consume protein-rich food.

d. Assess hydration status of the client at each visit.

e. Urge the client to drink 8 to 10 glasses of fluid daily.

19. A nurse is caring for a newborn with fetal alcohol spectrum disorder. What characteristic of the fetal alcohol spectrum disorder should the nurse assess for in the newborn?

a. Small head circumference

b. Decreased blood glucose level

c. Poor breathing pattern

d. Wide eyes

20. A nurse is documenting a dietary plan for a pregnant client with pregestational diabetes. What instructions should the nurse include in the dietary plan for this client?

a. Include more dairy products in the diet.

b. Include complex carbohydrates in the diet.

c. Eat only two meals per day.

d. Eat at least one egg per day.

CHAPTER 21

Nursing Management of Labor and Birth at Risk

Learning Objectives

Upon completion of the chapter, you will be able to:

- Propose at least five risk factors associated with dystocia.
- Differentiate the four major abnormalities or problems associated with dysfunctional labor patterns, giving examples of each problem.
- Examine the nursing management for the woman with dysfunctional labor experiencing a problem with the powers, passenger, passageway, and psyche.
- Devise a plan of care for the woman experiencing preterm labor.
- Relate the nursing assessment and management of the woman experiencing a postterm pregnancy.
- Assess four obstetric emergencies that can complicate labor and birth, including appropriate management for each.
- Compare and contrast the nursing management for the woman undergoing labor induction or augmentation, forceps, and vacuum-assisted birth.
- Summarize the plan of care for a woman who is to undergo a cesarean birth.
- Evaluate the key areas to be addressed when caring for a woman who is to undergo vaginal birth after cesarean.

SECTION I: ASSESSING YOUR UNDERSTANDING

Activity A FILL IN THE BLANKS

1. Abnormal or difficult labor is known as _____.

2. _____ presentation is frequently associated with multifetal pregnancies and grand multiparity.

3. _____ maneuver is used to identify deviations in fetal presentation or position.

4. _____ drugs promote uterine relaxation by interfering with uterine contraction.

5. _____ are given to enhance fetal lung maturity between 24 and 34 weeks of gestation.

6. Fetal _____, a glycoprotein produced by the chorion, is found at the junction of the chorion and decidua.

7. _____ score helps to identify women who would be most likely to achieve a successful induction.

8. _____ dilators absorb endocervical and local tissue fluids; as they enlarge, they expand the endocervix and provide controlled mechanical pressure.

9. An _____ involves inserting a cervical hook through the cervical os to artificially rupture the membranes.

10. _____ is produced naturally by the posterior pituitary gland and stimulates-contractions of the uterus.

Activity B **LABELING**

Consider the following figure. What is being depicted?

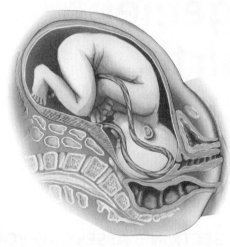

A

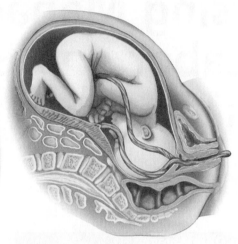

B

1. _____

_____

Activity C **MATCHING**

Match the tests in Column A with their purposes in Column B.

Column A

____ **1.** Ultrasound

____ **2.** Pelvimetry

____ **3.** Nonstress test

____ **4.** Phosphatidyl-glycerol level

____ **5.** Nitrazine paper and/or fern test

Column B

a. To rule out fetopelvic disproportion

b. To assess fetal lung maturity

c. To evaluate fetal size, position, and gestational age and to locate the placenta

d. To confirm ruptured membranes

e. To evaluate fetal well-being

Activity D **SEQUENCING**

Given below, in random order, are steps for administering oxytocin. Choose the correct sequence.

1. Use an infusion pump on a secondary line connected to the primary infusion.

2. Prepare the oxytocin infusion by diluting 10 units of oxytocin in 1,000 mL of lactated Ringer solution.

3. Perform or assist with periodic vaginal examinations to determine cervical dilation and fetal descent.

4. Start the oxytocin infusion in mU per minute or mL per hour as ordered.

5. Monitor the characteristics of the FHR, including baseline rate, baseline variability, and decelerations.

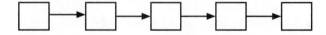

Activity E **SHORT ANSWERS**

Briefly answer the following.

1. What are symptoms of preterm labor?

   _____

   _____

   _____

2. What is cervical ripeness?

   _____

   _____

   _____

3. What is uterine rupture?

   _____

   _____

   _____

4. What are the indications and contraindications of amnioinfusion?

   _____

   _____

   _____

5. What care should the nurse take when assessing the client for risk of cord prolapse?

   _____

   _____

   _____

6. What are maternal and fetal complications in shoulder dystocia?

   _____

   _____

   _____

SECTION II: APPLYING YOUR KNOWLEDGE

Activity F **CASE STUDY**

Consider this scenario and answer the questions.

1. A nurse is caring for an antenatal mother who is advised to undergo amnioinfusion due to oligohydramnios. The nurse prepares the client for the procedure. What nursing interventions should the nurse follow when caring for the client to prevent maternal and fetal complications?

   _____

   _____

   _____

SECTION III: PRACTICING FOR NCLEX

Activity G **NCLEX-STYLE QUESTIONS**

Answer the following questions.

1. A nurse is assigned to care for a client who has to undergo a forceps and vacuum-assisted birth. The nurse understands that which of the following factors has contributed to a forceps and vacuum-assisted birth?
   a. A prolonged second stage of labor
   b. Oligohydramnios due to placental insufficiency
   c. Preterm labor with premature rupture of membranes
   d. Rupture of uterus

2. A nurse is assigned to care for a client who has been diagnosed with placental abruption. The nurse knows that which of the following could have led to placental abruption in the client?
   a. Obesity or excess weight gain
   b. CVD
   c. Gestational diabetes
   d. Gestational hypertension

3. A nurse is caring for a client who is experiencing acute onset of dyspnea and hypotension. The physician suspects the client has amniotic fluid embolism. What other sign or symptoms would alert the nurse to the presence of this condition in the client?
   a. Cyanosis
   b. Arrhythmia
   c. Hyperglycemia
   d. Hematuria
   e. Pulmonary edema

4. A nurse is caring for obstetric clients. The nurse should be aware of which of the following as an indication for labor induction?

   a. Chorioamnionitis

   b. Complete placenta previa

   c. Abruptio placenta

   d. Transverse fetal lie

5. A nurse is caring for a client who is scheduled to undergo amnioinfusion. The nurse knows that the client will not be able to have this procedure if which condition is present?

   a. The client has uterine hypertonicity

   b. The client has an active genital herpes infection

   c. The client has signs of abruptio placentae

   d. The client has invasive cervical cancer

6. A client is experiencing shoulder dystocia during delivery. Which of the following should the nurse identify as risks to the fetus in such a condition?

   a. Extensive lacerations

   b. Bladder injury

   c. Infection

   d. Nerve damage

7. A full-term pregnant client is being assessed for induction of labor. Her Bishop score is less than 6. Which of the following does it indicate?

   a. Cervical ripening method should be used.

   b. A cesarean may be required.

   c. Vaginal birth will be successful.

   d. Labor will occur spontaneously.

8. Which of the following postoperative interventions should a nurse perform when caring for a client who has undergone a cesarean section?

   a. Assess uterine tone to determine fundal firmness.

   b. Delay breastfeeding the newborn for a day.

   c. Ensure that the client does not cough or breathe deeply.

   d. Avoid early ambulation to prevent respiratory problems.

9. A client with full-term pregnancy who is not in active labor has been ordered oxytocin intravenously. Which of the following is a contraindication for oxytocin administration?

   a. Dysfunctional labor pattern

   b. Postterm status

   c. Prolonged ruptured membranes

   d. Overdistended uterus

10. A client who is in labor presents with shoulder dystocia of the fetus. Which of the following is an important nursing intervention?

    a. Assist with positioning the woman in squatting position.

    b. Assess for complaints of intense back pain in first stage of labor.

    c. Anticipate possible use of forceps to rotate to anterior position at birth.

    d. Assess for prolonged second stage of labor with arrest of descent.

11. A nurse is assessing the cause of multiple gestations in clients. Which of the following factors should the nurse assess as contributors to increased probability of multiple gestations?

    a. Infertility treatment

    b. Medications

    c. Advanced maternal age

    d. Adolescent pregnancies

12. A client is admitted to the health care facility with a gestational age of 42 weeks. The client is to undergo a cesarean section. Which of the following would be the fetal risk associated with postterm pregnancy?

    a. Underdeveloped suck reflex

    b. Congenital heart defects

    c. Intraventricular hemorrhage

    d. Cephalopelvic disproportion

13. A nurse is caring for a client who has been diagnosed with precipitous labor. For which of the following potential fetal complications should the nurse monitor as a result of precipitous labor?

    a. Facial nerve injury

    b. Cephalhematoma

    c. Intracranial hemorrhage

    d. Facial lacerations

14. A nurse is newly posted to the obstetric unit of the health care facility. Which of the following are the causes of intrauterine fetal demise in late pregnancy that the nurse should be aware of? Select all that apply.

a. Hydramnios

b. Multifetal gestation

c. Prolonged pregnancy

d. Malpresentation

e. Hypertension

15. A nurse is caring for an antenatal mother diagnosed with umbilical cord prolapse. Which of the following should the nurse monitor for in a fetus in cases of umbilical cord prolapse?

a. Fetal hypoxia

b. Preeclampsia

c. Coagulation defects

d. Placental pathology

Nursing Management of the Postpartum Woman at Risk

Learning Objectives

Upon completion of the chapter, you will be able to:

- Examine the major conditions that place the postpartum woman at risk.
- Analyze the risk factors, assessment, preventive measures, and nursing management of common postpartum complications.
- Differentiate the causes of postpartum hemorrhage based on the underlying pathophysiologic mechanisms.
- Outline the nurse's role in assessing and managing the care of a woman with a thromboembolic condition.
- Discuss the nursing management of a woman who develops a postpartum infection.
- Identify at least two affective disorders that can occur in women after birth, describing specific therapeutic management for each.

SECTION I: ASSESSING YOUR UNDERSTANDING

Activity A FILL IN THE BLANKS

1. Failure of the uterus to contract and retract immediately after birth is called uterine _____.

2. _____ refers to the incomplete involution of the uterus, or its failure to return to its normal size and condition after birth.

3. In von Willebrand disease, there is a _____ in von Willebrand factor, which is necessary for platelet adhesion and aggregation.

4. A blood clot within a blood vessel is called a _____.

5. Obstruction of a blood vessel by a blood clot carried by the circulation from the site of origin is called _____.

6. _____ is an infectious condition that involves the endometrium, decidua, and adjacent myometrium of the uterus.

7. Inflammation of the breast is called _____.

8. Excessive blood loss that occurs within 24 hours after birth is termed _____ postpartum hemorrhage.

9. Placenta _____ is a condition in which the chorionic villi adhere to the myometrium, causing the placenta to adhere abnormally to the uterus and not separate and deliver spontaneously.

10. A prolapse of the uterine fundus to or through the cervix, so that the uterus is turned inside out after birth, is called uterine _____.

Activity B MATCHING

Match the following causes of postpartum hemorrhage in Column A with their appropriate intervention in Column B.

Column A	Column B
___ 1. Uterine atony	a. Evacuation and oxytocics
___ 2. Retained placental tissue	b. Massage and oxytocics
___ 3. Lacerations or hematoma	c. Provide blood products
___ 4. Bleeding disorder	d. Surgical repair
___ 5. von Willebrand disease	e. Administration of desmopressin and plasma concentrates

Activity C SEQUENCING

Arrange the steps for the management of uterine inversion in the proper sequence.

1. Administration of oxytocin

2. Manually push back the uterus into proper position

3. Administration of general anesthetic

4. Administration of antibiotics

☐ → ☐ → ☐ → ☐ → ☐

Activity D SHORT ANSWERS

Briefly answer the following.

1. What are the causes of overdistention of the uterus?

   _____

   _____

   _____

2. What is idiopathic thrombocytopenia purpura?

   _____

   _____

   _____

3. Which microorganisms are responsible for postpartum infections?

   _____

   _____

   _____

4. What are baby blues?

   _____

   _____

   _____

5. What are the symptoms of postpartum psychosis?

   _____

   _____

   _____

6. What are the types of venous thrombosis?

   _____

   _____

   _____

SECTION II APPLYING YOUR KNOWLEDGE

Activity E CASE STUDY

Consider this scenario and answer the questions.

A 37-year-old client complains of calf pain following the vaginal delivery of her third child. On assessment, the nurse finds that the calf area is tender to the touch. The client is diagnosed with superficial venous thrombosis.

1. What are the risk factors for which a nurse should assess for the development of thromboembolic complications in a postpartum client?

   _____

   _____

   _____

2. What nursing interventions should the nurse perform to prevent thromboembolic complications in clients?

   _____

   _____

   _____

3. What interventions should the nurse perform to treat the client's condition of superficial venous thrombosis?

   _____

   _____

   _____

SECTION III: PRACTICING FOR NCLEX

Activity F **NCLEX-STYLE QUESTIONS**

Answer the following questions.

1. A nurse is caring for a postpartum client who has a history of thrombosis during pregnancy and is at high risk of developing a pulmonary embolism. For which sign or symptom should the nurse monitor the client to prevent the occurrence of pulmonary embolism?

   a. Sudden change in mental status

   b. Difficulty in breathing

   c. Calf swelling

   d. Sudden chest pain

2. A nurse is caring for a client who has been treated for a deep vein thrombosis. Which teaching point should the nurse stress when discharging the client?

   a. Avoid using compression stockings.

   b. Plan long rest periods throughout the day.

   c. Avoid using products containing aspirin.

   d. Avoid use of oral contraceptives.

3. A nurse is caring for a client with idiopathic thrombocytopenic purpura. The nurse is correct when performing which intervention?

   a. Administration of prescribed nonsteroidal anti-inflammatory drugs (NSAIDs)

   b. Administration of platelet transfusions as ordered

   c. Avoiding administration of oxytocics

   d. Continual firm massage of the uterus

4. Two weeks after a vaginal delivery, a client presents with low-grade fever. The client also complains of a loss of appetite and low energy levels. The physician suspects an infection of the episiotomy. What sign or symptom is most indicative of an episiotomy infection?

   a. Foul-smelling vaginal discharge

   b. Sudden onset of shortness of breath

   c. Pain in the lower leg

   d. Apprehension and diaphoresis

5. A nurse is caring for a postpartum client diagnosed with von Willebrand disease. What assessment finding will the nurse expect to find in the client?

   a. Prolonged bleeding time

   b. A fever of 100.4° F after the first 24 hours following childbirth

   c. Foul-smelling vaginal discharge

   d. Postpartum fundal height that is higher than expected

6. A nurse is assigned to care for a 38-year-old overweight client scheduled to undergo a cesarean section. The client is at an increased risk of thromboembolic complications. During assessment, what factor will help the nurse in the diagnosis of deep vein thrombosis of the leg?

   a. Sudden chest pain

   b. Dyspnea

   c. Tachypnea

   d. Calf tenderness

7. A nurse finds that a client is bleeding excessively after a vaginal delivery. Which assessment finding would indicate retained placental fragments as a cause of bleeding?

   a. Soft and boggy uterus that deviates from the midline

   b. Firm uterus with trickle of bright-red blood in perineum

   c. Firm uterus with a steady stream of bright-red blood

   d. Large uterus with painless dark-red blood mixed with clots

8. A client has had a forceps delivery which resulted in lacerations and bleeding. How can a nurse identify if the bleeding is due to laceration?

   a. Look for a contracted uterus with vaginal bleeding.

   b. Look for a subinvoluted uterus with vaginal bleeding.

   c. Look for a boggy uterus with vaginal bleeding.

   d. Look for an inverted uterus with vaginal bleeding.

9. A nurse is caring for a client who delivered vaginally 2 hours ago. What postpartum complication can the nurse assess within the first few hours following delivery?

   a. Postpartal infection

   b. Postpartal blues

   c. Postpartal hemorrhage

   d. Postpartum depression

10. A nurse is a caring for a postpartum client. What instruction should the nurse provide to the client as precautionary measures to prevent thromboembolic complications?

    a. Avoid performing any deep-breathing exercises.

    b. Try to relax with pillows under knees.

    c. Avoid sitting in one position for long periods of time.

    d. Refrain from elevating legs above heart level.

11. A postpartum client had a difficult labor. Which assessment finding will alert the nurse that the client is most likely hemorrhaging?

    a. Decreased heart rate

    b. Increased urinary output

    c. Decreased blood pressure

    d. Increased body temperature

12. A postpartum client who was discharged home returns to the primary health care facility after 2 weeks with complaints of fever and pain in the breast. The client is diagnosed with mastitis. What education should the nurse give to the client for managing and preventing mastitis?

    a. Discontinue breastfeeding to allow time for healing.

    b. Perform hand-washing before and after breastfeeding.

    c. Avoid hot or cold compresses on the breast.

    d. Discourage manual compression of breast for expressing milk.

13. A nurse is caring for a client who has had an intrauterine fetal death with prolonged retention of the fetus. Which of the following signs and symptoms should the nurse watch for in a client to assess for an increased risk of disseminated intravascular coagulation? Select all that apply.

    a. Hypertension

    b. Bleeding gums

    c. Tachycardia

    d. Acute renal failure

    e. Lochia less than usual

14. A client in her 7th week of the postpartum period is experiencing bouts of sadness and insomnia. The nurse suspects that the client may have developed postpartum depression. What signs or symptoms are indicative of postpartum depression? Select all that apply.

    a. Inability to concentrate

    b. Loss of confidence

    c. Manifestations of mania

    d. Decreased interest in life

    e. Bizarre behavior

15. A nurse is assessing a client with postpartal hemorrhage; the client is presently on IV oxytocin. Which of the following interventions should the nurse perform to evaluate the efficacy of the drug treatment? Select all that apply.

    a. Assess client's uterine tone

    b. Monitor client's vital signs

    c. Assess client's skin turgor

    d. Get a pad count

    e. Assess deep tendon reflexes

Nursing Care of the Newborn With Special Needs

Upon completion of the chapter, you will be able to:

- Examine factors that assist in identifying a newborn at risk due to variations in birth weight and gestational age.
- Detect contributing factors and common complications associated with dysmature infants and their management.
- Compare and contrast a small-for-gestational-age newborn and a large-for-gestational-age newborn; a post- and preterm newborn.
- Differentiate associated conditions that affect the newborn with variations in birth weight and gestational age, including appropriate management.
- Outline the nurse's role in helping parents experiencing perinatal grief or loss.
- Integrate knowledge of the risks associated with late preterm births into nursing interventions, discharge planning, and parent education.

SECTION I: ASSESSING YOUR UNDERSTANDING

Activity A FILL IN THE BLANKS

1. _____ is defined as a venous hematocrit of greater than 65%.

2. _____ feedings are used for compromised newborns to minimize energy expenditure from sucking during the feeding process.

3. A newborn who fails to establish adequate, sustained respiration after birth is said to have _____.

4. A _____ infant is born before the completion of 37 weeks.

5. One of the problems that affect the preterm infant's breathing ability and adjustment to extrauterine life includes an unstable chest wall, leading to _____.

6. A _____ newborn is an infant who is born from the first day of week 38 through 42 weeks.

7. _____ of prematurity is a potentially blinding eye disorder that occurs when abnormal blood vessels grow and spread through the retina, eventually leading to retinal detachment.

8. _____ assessment is considered the "fifth vital sign" and should be done as frequently as the other four vital signs.

9. Gestational age at birth is _____ correlated with the risk that the infant will experience physical, neurologic, or developmental sequelae.

10. Fetal growth is dependent on _____, placental, and maternal factors.

Activity B LABELING

Consider the following figure.

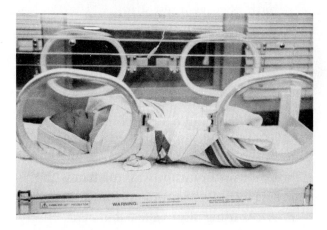

1. Identify the figure.

   _____

   _____

2. Why would a newborn be placed in an isolette?

   _____

   _____

Activity C MATCHING

Match the heat transfer mechanism in Column A with the ways to prevent heat loss in Column B.

Column A

____ **1.** Convection

____ **2.** Conduction

____ **3.** Radiation

____ **4.** Evaporation

Column B

a. Warm everything the newborn comes in contact with

b. Provide insulation to prevent heat transfer

c. Avoid drafts near the newborn

d. Delay the first bath until the baby's temperature is stable

Activity D SEQUENCING

Put the terms in correct sequence by writing the letters in the boxes provided below.

1. Given below, in random order, are a set of actions performed when resuscitating the newborn. Rearrange them in the correct sequence.

   a. Administer epinephrine and/or volume expansion.

   b. Position the head in a "sniffing" position.

   c. Clear the airway and stimulate breathing; use suction if necessary.

   d. Provide ventilation at a rate of 40 to 60 breaths per minute.

   e. Perform chest compressions if heart rate is below 60 beats per minute.

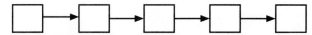

Activity E SHORT ANSWER

Briefly answer the following.

1. What are the physical characteristics of preterm newborns?

   _____

   _____

   _____

2. What are the signs of hypoglycemia in the newborn?

   _____

   _____

   _____

3. What is developmentally supportive care?

   _____

   _____

   _____

4. What are the risk factors to which a preterm infant is susceptible?

   _____

   _____

   _____

5. What are the characteristics of large-for-gestational-age newborns?

_____

_____

_____

6. What are the characteristics of postterm newborns?

_____

_____

_____

SECTION II: APPLYING YOUR KNOWLEDGE

Activity F CASE STUDY

Consider this scenario and answer the questions.

A nurse is caring for a preterm newborn who may not survive. The nurse is in the difficult situation of having to help the newborn's parents.

1. How can a nurse help the parents in the detachment process in the case of a dying newborn?

_____

_____

_____

2. What are the nursing interventions when caring for a family experiencing a perinatal loss?

_____

_____

_____

SECTION III: PRACTICING FOR NCLEX

Activity G NCLEX-STYLE QUESTIONS

Answer the following questions.

1. A nurse is caring for an infant born with polycythemia. Which intervention is most appropriate when caring for this infant?

a. Focus on decreasing blood viscosity by increasing fluid volume.

b. Check blood glucose within 2 hours of birth by reagent test strip.

c. Repeat screening every 2 to 3 hours or before feeds.

d. Focus on monitoring and maintaining blood glucose levels.

2. Which precautions should a nurse take to prevent infection in a newborn? Select all that apply.

a. Avoid coming to work when ill

b. Cover jewelry while washing hands

c. Use sterile gloves for an invasive procedure

d. Avoid using disposable equipment

e. Monitor laboratory test results for changes

3. When caring for a preterm infant, what intervention will most address the sensorimotor needs of the infant?

a. Rocking and massaging

b. Swaddling and positioning

c. Using minimal amount of tape

d. Using distraction through objects

4. Which of the following is a risk to newborns because of meconium in the amniotic fluid?

a. Bradycardia

b. Perinatal asphyxia

c. Acute respiratory complications

d. Polycythemia

5. A nurse has placed an infant with asphyxia on a radiant warmer. Which of the following signs indicate that the resuscitation methods have been successful?

a. Heart rate of 80 bpm

b. Tremors

c. Bluish tongue

d. Good cry

6. Which of the following interventions should a nurse perform to promote thermal regulation in a preterm newborn?

a. Assess the newborn's temperature every 5 hours until stable.

b. Set the temperature of the radiant warmer at a fixed level.

c. Observe for clinical signs of cold stress such as weak cry.

d. Check the blood pressure of the infant every 2 hours.

7. A nurse is caring for a preterm infant. Which intervention will prepare the preterm newborn's gut to overcome feeding difficulties?

   a. Administer Vitamin D supplements.

   b. Administer 0.5 mL of breast milk enterally.

   c. Administer iron supplements.

   d. Administer dextrose intravenously.

8. A nurse is caring for an infant born with hypoglycemia. What care should the nurse administer to a newborn with hypoglycemia?

   a. Maintain fluid and electrolyte balance.

   b. Give dextrose intravenously before oral feedings.

   c. Place infant on radiant warmer immediately.

   d. Focus on decreasing blood viscosity.

9. What assessment by the nurse will best monitor the nutrition and fluid balance in the postterm newborn?

   a. Measure weight once every 2 days.

   b. Assess for increased muscle tone.

   c. Assess for decrease in urinary output.

   d. Monitor for fall in temperature, indicative of dehydration.

10. Which maternal factors should the nurse consider that could lead to a newborn's being "large for gestational age"? Select all that apply.

    a. Diabetes mellitus

    b. Postdates gestation

    c. Alcohol use

    d. Glucose intolerance

    e. Renal infection

11. The nurse is performing a newborn assessment. What finding will alert the nurse to the development of polycythemia in the newborn?

    a. Jaundice

    b. Restlessness

c. Temperature instability

d. Wheezing

12. A nurse is assessing a term newborn and finds the blood glucose level is 23 mg per dL and the newborn has a weak cry, is irritable, and bradycardic. Which intervention is most appropriate?

    a. Administer dextrose intravenously.

    b. Monitor the infant's hematocrit levels closely.

    c. Administer IV glucose immediately.

    d. Place the infant on a radiant warmer.

13. A nurse is caring for an infant born with a high bilirubin level. When planning the infants care, what interventions will assist in reducing the bilirubin level? Select all that apply.

    a. Hydration

    b. Increase water intake

    c. Early feedings

    d. Administer vitamin supplements

    e. Phototherapy

14. Which of the following indicates meconium aspiration in a newborn?

    a. Bluish skin discoloration

    b. Listlessness or lethargy

    c. Stained umbilical cord

    d. Pink tongue

15. The nurse is caring for a client in the early stages of labor. What maternal factors will alert the nurse to plan for the possibility of a small-for-gestational-age newborn? Select all that apply.

    a. Smoking

    b. Hypotension

    c. Asthma

    d. Drug abuse

    e. Pregnancy weight gain of 20 lb

Nursing Management of the Newborn at Risk: Acquired and Congenital Newborn Conditions

Learning Objectives

Upon completion of the chapter, you will be able to:

- Assess the most common acquired conditions affecting the newborn.
- Construct the nursing management of a newborn experiencing respiratory distress syndrome.
- Outline the birthing room preparation and procedures necessary to prevent meconium aspiration syndrome in the newborn at birth.
- Discuss parent education for follow-up care needed by newborns with retinopathy of prematurity.
- Select risk factors for the development of necrotizing enterocolitis (NEC).
- Examine the impact of maternal diabetes on the newborn and care needed.
- Research the assessment and interventions for a newborn experiencing substance withdrawal after birth.
- Predict assessment and nursing management for newborns sustaining trauma and birth injuries.
- Plan the assessment, interventions, prevention, and management of hyperbilirubinemia in newborns.

- Summarize the interventions appropriate for a newborn with neonatal sepsis.
- Compare and contrast the four classifications of congenital heart disease.
- Evaluate the major acquired congenital anomalies affecting the central nervous system, respiratory system, gastrointestinal system, genitourinary system, and musculoskeletal system that can occur in a newborn.
- Distinguish between three inborn errors of metabolism.
- Formulate a plan of care for a newborn with an acquired or congenital condition.
- Characterize the importance of parental participation in care of the newborn with an acquired or congenital condition, including the nurse's role in facilitating parental involvement.

SECTION I: ASSESSING YOUR UNDERSTANDING

Activity A FILL IN THE BLANKS

1. An _____ is a defect of the umbilical ring that allows evisceration of abdominal contents into an external peritoneal sac.

2. _____ is a subperiosteal collection of blood secondary to the rupture of blood vessels between the skull and periosteum.

3. _____ is a condition in which total serum bilirubin level is above 5 mg per dL and exhibited as jaundice.

4. Presence of bacterial, fungal, or viral microorganisms or their toxins in blood or other tissues in newborns is known as neonatal _____.

5. _____ is a synthetic opiate narcotic that is used primarily as maintenance therapy for heroin addiction.

6. Immune hydrops is a severe form of _____ disease of the newborn that occurs when pathologic changes develop in the organs of the fetus secondary to severe anemia.

7. For the newborn with jaundice, regardless of its etiology, _____ is used to convert unconjugated bilirubin to the less toxic water-soluble form that can be excreted.

8. _____ is a herniation of abdominal contents through an abdominal wall defect.

9. Failure to establish adequate, sustained respiration after birth is known as neonatal _____.

10. _____ is a preventable neurologic disorder characterized by encephalopathy, motor abnormalities, hearing and vision loss, and death.

11. In bronchopulmonary dysplasia (BPD), high inspired oxygen concentrations cause an _____ process in the lungs that leads to parenchymal damage.

12. A _____ shunt is inserted from the ventricle in the brain and threaded down into the peritoneal cavity to allow drainage of excess cerebrospinal fluid (CSF).

Activity B MATCHING

Match the commonly abused substances in Column A with their effects on newborns in Column B.

Column A

____ 1. Marijuana

____ 2. Cocaine

____ 3. Methamphetamines

____ 4. Heroin

____ 5. Tobacco/nicotine

Column B

a. Altered responses to visual stimuli, sleep-pattern abnormalities, photophobia

b. Frantic fist sucking, high-pitched cry, and significant lassitude

c. Stiff and hyperextended positioning, limb defects, ambiguous genitalia

d. Smaller head circumference, piercing cry, genitourinary tract abnormalities

e. Low birthweight, small for gestational age, SIDS

Match the inborn errors of metabolism in Column A with their clinical picture in Column B.

Column A

____ 1. Phenylketonuria

____ 2. Maple syrup urine disease

____ 3. Galactosemia

____ 4. Congenital hypothyroidism

Column B

a. Large protruding tongue, slow reflexes, distended abdomen, large, open posterior fontanel, constipation, hypothermia, poor feeding, hoarse cry, dry skin, coarse hair, goiter, and jaundice

b. Lethargy, poor feeding, vomiting, weight loss, seizures, shrill cry, shallow respirations, loss of reflexes, and coma

c. Vomiting, hypoglycemia, liver damage, hyperbilirubinemia, poor weight gain, cataracts, and frequent infections

d. Newborns appear normal at birth but by 6 months of age signs of slow mental development evident

Activity C SHORT ANSWERS

Briefly answer the following.

1. What are the characteristics of an infant born to a diabetic mother?

_____

_____

_____

2. What are the most common types of malformations in infants of diabetic mothers?

_____

_____

_____

3. What does the treatment of infants born to diabetic mothers focus on?

_____

_____

_____

4. What are the causes of birth trauma?

_____

_____

_____

_____

5. What is meconium aspiration syndrome?

_____

_____

_____

6. What is periventricular/intraventricular hemorrhage (PVH/IVH)?

_____

_____

_____

7. What are the goals of therapy for a newborn with bladder exstrophy?

_____

_____

_____

8. As a nurse, how would you promote bonding between a newborn with a cleft lip and palate and its parents?

_____

_____

_____

SECTION II: APPLYING YOUR KNOWLEDGE

Activity D CASE STUDY

Consider the scenario and answer the questions.

A pregnant client visits a health care facility for regular checkups. During the examination, the client reveals that she is addicted to alcohol and tobacco. The client is concerned; she wants to provide a healthy environment for her unborn child and also know how to avoid harmful consequences.

1. What is the role of the nurse in handling substance-abusing mothers?

_____

_____

_____

2. How can the nurse use the "5 As" approach to help this client attempt to quit smoking?

_____

_____

_____

SECTION III: PRACTICING FOR NCLEX

Activity E NCLEX-STYLE QUESTIONS

Answer the following questions.

1. The nurse assessing a newborn suspects meconium aspiration syndrome. What sign or symptom would alert the nurse to this condition?

   a. High-pitched cry

   b. Bile-stained emesis

   c. Increased intracranial pressure

   d. End-expiratory grunting

2. A newborn in a family maternity center is suspected of having a cardiopulmonary disorder. Which of the following symptoms of persistent pulmonary hypertension should the nurse assess for in the newborn?

   a. Systolic ejection murmur

   b. Respiratory alkalosis

   c. Rhinorrhea

   d. Lacrimation

3. A nurse is caring for an infant born after a prolonged and difficult maternal labor. What are the nursing interventions involved when assessing for trauma and birth injuries in the newborn?

   a. Examine the newborn's skin for cyanosis.

   b. Be alert for signs of apathy and listlessness.

   c. Assess the baby for any temperature instability.

   d. Note any absence of or decrease in deep tendon reflexes.

4. A nurse is assigned to care for a newborn with hyperbilirubinemia. The newborn is relatively large in size and shows signs of listlessness. What would have most likely happened to have caused these conditions to occur in the infant?

   a. The infant's mother must have had a low birth weight.

   b. The infant's mother must have been a diabetic.

   c. The infant must have experienced birth trauma.

   d. The infant's mother must have abused alcohol.

5. A nurse is caring for a newborn with PVH/IVH in a local health care facility. Which of the following complications is/are likely to occur in a newborn with PVH/IVH that a nurse should assess for? Select all that apply.

   a. Hydrocephalus

   b. Acid–base imbalances

   c. Pneumonitis

   d. Vision or hearing deficits

   e. Cerebral palsy

6. A nurse is caring for a newborn whose chest x-ray reveals marked hyperaeration mixed with areas of atelectasis. The infant's arterial blood gas analysis indicates metabolic acidosis. The nurse should prepare for the assessment of which of the following dangerous conditions when providing care to this newborn?

   a. Choanal atresia

   b. NEC

   c. Meconium aspiration syndrome

   d. Hyperbilirubinemia

7. A nurse is caring for a newborn with transient tachypnea in a family maternity center. What is a priority nursing intervention for a newborn with transient tachypnea?

   a. Administer IV fluids; gavage feedings

   b. Maintain adequate hydration

   c. Monitor for signs of hypotonia

   d. Perform gentle suctioning

8. A nurse in a local family maternity center is caring for a newborn with asphyxia. What nursing management is involved when treating a newborn with asphyxia?

   a. Ensure adequate tissue perfusion.

   b. Ensure effective resuscitation measures.

   c. Administer IV fluids.

   d. Administer surfactant as ordered.

9. A nurse is caring for a newborn with esophageal atresia that had occurred during early fetal development. What should the preoperative nursing care for the newborn focus on?

   a. Document the amount and color of drainage.

   b. Administer antibiotics and total parenteral nutrition as ordered.

   c. Prevent aspiration by elevating the head of the bed.

   d. Provide colostomy care if required.

10. A client with a history of substance abuse during her pregnancy has delivered a newborn in a local health care facility. What is the most appropriate nursing intervention when caring for the newborn of this client?

   a. Encourage early initiation of feedings.

   b. Monitor newborn's cardiovascular status.

   c. Supplement breast milk with formula.

   d. Check newborn's skin turgor and fontanels.

11. A nurse is caring for a newborn with jaundice undergoing phototherapy. What intervention is appropriate when caring for the newborn?

   a. Expose the newborn's skin minimally.

   b. Shield the newborn's eyes.

   c. Discourage feeding the newborn.

   d. Discontinue therapy if stools are loose, green, and frequent.

12. A nurse is caring for a newborn with meconium aspiration syndrome. Which of the following interventions should the nurse perform when caring for this newborn? Select all that apply.

   a. Perform repeated suctioning and stimulation.

   b. Place the newborn under a radiant warmer or in a warmed Isolette.

   c. Handle and rub the newborn well with a dry towel.

   d. Administer oxygen therapy.

   e. Administer broad-spectrum antibiotics.

13. A newborn with feeding intolerance is suspected of having gastroschisis. Which of the following characteristics of gastroschisis should the nurse know when assessing the newborn?

   a. No peritoneal sac protecting herniated organs

   b. Normal herniated organs

   c. It is a defect of the umbilical ring

   d. Resolves with surgical correction

14. A nurse is caring for a newborn with NEC, scheduled to undergo surgery for bowel resection. The infant's parents wish to know the implications of the surgery. What information should the nurse provide to the parents regarding this surgery?

   a. Surgically treated NEC is a short process.

   b. Surgery will prevent long-term medical problems.

   c. Surgery requires placement of a proximal enterostomy.

   d. Surgery prevents the need for the use of long-term antibiotics.

15. BPD is the result of lung injury in the preterm newborn. What can be done to reduce the incidence of BPD in the preterm newborn?

   a. Antepartal administration of steroids to the mother

   b. Mechanical ventilation of the newborn with 100% oxygen content

   c. Steroid injection at birth to all infants at risk for BPD

   d. Exogenous surfactant given to the mother before the baby's birth

16. Congenital heart anomalies affect approximately 8 infants in every 1,000 live births. The nursing assessment should include what important information that might indicate heart failure in the infant?

   a. Capillary refill time

   b. Diminished peripheral pulses

   c. Color of hands and feet

   d. Blood glucose level

17. Providing nursing care to a newborn born with a congenital cardiac anomaly can be a challenging task. What is a priority component of providing nursing care to the newborn with a congenital cardiac anomaly?

   a. Oversee laboratory procedures.

   b. Accompany the newborn to all radiologic examinations.

   c. Prevent pain as much as possible.

   d. Teach the parents to take pulse and blood pressure measurements.

18. What is the most precise term used to describe a herniation through the skin of the back of a newborn when both the spinal cord and nerve roots are involved?

   a. Meningocele

   b. Spina bifida occulta

   c. Spina bifida cystica

   d. Myelomeningocele

19. Infants born with spina bifida are at increased risk for hydrocephalus. What is the priority nursing assessment for an infant at risk for hydrocephalus?

   a. Assess the level of irritability.

   b. Assess the weight.

   c. Assess head circumference.

   d. Assess movement of the lower extremities.

20. Infants born with a diaphragmatic hernia are given supportive treatment until they can have surgery to repair the defect. What are the medications usually given to these infants? Select all that apply.

    a. Steroids

    b. Inotropics

    c. Surfactant

    d. Plasma expanders

    e. Bronchodilators

21. The parents of a newborn with a cleft palate ask the nurse at what age the defect in the lip is usually repaired? Which response by the nurse is correct?

    a. 2 to 6 weeks

    b. 6 to 12 weeks

    c. 2 to 3 months

    d. 6 to 12 months

22. A relatively common birth defect, hypospadias, occurs when the urethral meatus is found on the underside of the penis instead of at the tip. What frequently accompanies this disorder that can lead to problems urinating?

    a. Chordee

    b. Prepuce

    c. Priapism

    d. Cholangi

23. The parents of an infant with congenital club foot ask the nurse what the treatment will consist of. What is the initial treatment for an infant born with a congenital club foot?

    a. Surgery

    b. Braces

    c. Physical therapy

    d. Serial casting

24. To properly assess for developmental dysplasia of the hip in the newborn, the nurse should perform what procedure to get the sensation of the dislocated hip going back into the acetabulum?

    a. Ortolani maneuver

    b. Barlow maneuver

    c. Pavlik maneuver

    d. Bill maneuver

25. What are the causes of retinopathy of the preterm newborn? Select all that apply.

    a. Insufficient oxygenation in an Isolette

    b. Assistive ventilation with high oxygen content

    c. Acidosis

    d. Alkalosis

    e. Shock

Growth and Development of the Newborn and Infant

Learning Objectives

- Identify normal developmental changes occurring in the newborn and infant.
- Identify the gross and fine motor milestones of the newborn and infant.
- Express an understanding of language development in the first year of life.
- Describe nutritional requirements of the newborn and infant.
- Develop a nutritional plan for the first year of life.
- Identify common issues related to growth and development in infancy.
- Demonstrate knowledge of appropriate anticipatory guidance for common developmental issues.

SECTION I: ASSESSING YOUR UNDERSTANDING

Activity A FILL IN THE BLANKS

1. Inconsolable crying, known as _____, lasts longer than 3 hours.

2. The education of parents about what to expect in the next phase of development is referred to as _____ guidance.

3. Milk production is stimulated by _____, a hormone secreted by the anterior pituitary.

4. The thin, yellowish fluid called _____ is produced by the breasts for the first 2 to 4 days after birth.

5. Stranger anxiety is an indicator that the infant is recognizing himself as _____ from others.

6. The sequential process by which infants and children gain various skills and function is referred to as _____.

7. The anterior fontanel normally remains open until _____ months of life.

Activity B LABELING

Label the tooth and age of eruption on the figure provided.

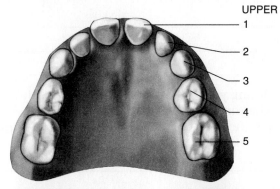

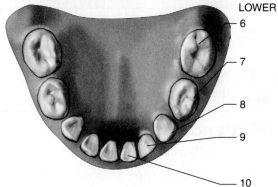

UPPER

1
2
3
4
5

LOWER

6
7
8
9
10

1. _____
2. _____
3. _____
4. _____
5. _____
6. _____
7. _____
8. _____
9. _____
10. _____

Activity C MATCHING

Match the infant age in Column A with the proper motor skill in Column B.

Column A

____ **1.** 1-month old

____ **2.** 2-month old

____ **3.** 3-month old

____ **4.** 4-month old

____ **5.** 5-month old

____ **6.** 6-month old

Column B

a. Raises head and chest

b. Hold open hand to face

c. Tripod sits

d. Grasps rattle or toy

e. Rolls from prone to supine

f. Lifts head while prone

Match the reflex in Column A with the description in Column B.

Column A

____ **1.** Asymmetric tonic neck

____ **2.** Babinski

____ **3.** Moro

____ **4.** Parachute

____ **5.** Root

Column B

a. Fanning and hyperextension

b. Fencing position

c. Prepare to "catch themselves"

d. Hands form "C"

e. Searches with the mouth

Activity D SEQUENCING

List the motor skills of the infant in order of occurrence.

1. Crawls on hands and knees

2. Pokes with index finger

3. Puts objects in container

4. Sits unsupported

5. Transfers object from one hand to the other

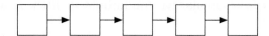

Activity E SHORT ANSWER

Briefly answer the following.

1. What are the nursing interventions that will help achieve the Healthy People 2020 objective of increasing the proportion of mothers who breastfeed?

_____

_____

_____

2. In what incidences is breastfeeding contraindicated?

_____

_____

_____

3. When providing education to a new parent about how to tell if her infant is hungry, what behavioral cues should be discussed as early cues of hunger?

_____

_____

_____

4. The nurse is reviewing the adjusted age of an infant. What is the adjusted age and how is it calculated?

_____

_____

_____

5. Identify four primitive reflexes present at birth.

_____

_____

_____

6. What changes normally take place in the cardiovascular system during the first year of life?

_____

_____

_____

SECTION II: APPLYING YOUR KNOWLEDGE

Activity F CASE STUDY

Consider the scenario and answer the questions.

Remember Allison Johnson, the 6-month old from Chapter 4, who was brought to the clinic by her mother and father for her 6-month check-up. As new parents, Allison's mother and father had many questions and concerns.

1. Allison's parents ask "What can we do to encourage Allison's development?".

_____

_____

2. Allison's dad states in college he took a psychology class and remembers there are different development theories. He asks how those relate to Allison right now.

_____

_____

_____

3. During your assessment, Allison's parents ask what findings would concern you. Discuss specific developmental warning signs you are assessing.

_____

_____

_____

SECTION III: PRACTICING FOR NCLEX

Activity G NCLEX-STYLE QUESTIONS

Answer the following questions.

1. The nurse is examining a 6-month-old girl who was born 8 weeks early. Which of the following findings is cause for concern?
   a. The child measures 21 inches in length
   b. The child exhibits palmar grasp reflex
   c. Head size increased 5 inches since birth
   d. The child weighs 10 pounds 2 ounces

2. The nurse is caring for the family of a 2-month-old boy with colic. The mother reports feeling very stressed by the baby's constant crying. Which of the following interventions would provide the most help in the short term?
   a. Urging the baby's mother to take time for herself away from the child
   b. Educating the parents about when colic stops
   c. Assessing the parents' care and feeding skills
   d. Watching how the parents respond to the child

3. The mother of 1-week-old baby boy voices concerns about her baby's weight loss since birth. At birth the baby weighed 7 pounds; the baby currently weighs 6 pounds 1 ounce. What response by the nurse is most appropriate?

   a. "All babies lose a substantial amount of weight after birth."

   b. "Your baby has lost too much weight and may need to be hospitalized."

   c. "Your baby's weight loss is well within the expected range."

   d. "Your baby has lost a bit more than the normal amount."

4. The nurse is teaching the parents of a 6-month-old boy about proper child dental care. Which of the following actions will the nurse indicate as the most likely to cause dental caries?

   a. Not cleaning a neonate's gums when he is done eating

   b. Putting the child to bed with a bottle of milk or juice

   c. Using a cloth instead of a brush for cleaning teeth

   d. Failure to clean the teeth with fluoridated toothpaste

5. The nurse is assessing the sleeping practices of the parents of a 4-month-old girl who wakes repeatedly during the night. Which of the following parent comments might reveal a cause for the night waking?

   a. They sing to her before she goes to sleep

   b. They put her to bed when she falls asleep

   c. If she is safe, they lie her down and leave

   d. The child has a regular, scheduled bedtime

6. The nurse is educating the mother of a 6-month-old boy about the symptoms for teething. Which of the following symptoms would the nurse identify?

   a. The child may run a mild fever or vomit

   b. The child avoids hard foods for soft ones

   c. The child increases biting and sucking

   d. The child has frequent loose stools

7. The nurse is teaching healthy eating habits to the parents of a 7-month-old girl. Which of the following recommendations is the most valuable advice?

   a. Let the child eat only the foods she prefers

   b. Actively urge the child to eat new foods

   c. Provide small portions that must be eaten

   d. Keep serving new foods several times

8. The nurse is providing helpful feeding tips to the mother of a 2-week-old boy. Which of the following recommendations will best help the child feed effectively?

   a. Maintaining a feed-on-demand approach

   b. Applying warm compresses to the breast

   c. Encouraging the infant to latch on properly

   d. Maintaining adequate diet and fluid intake

9. The nurse is providing anticipatory guidance to the mother of a 1-week-old girl. Which of the following is reason for the mother to contact her care provider?

   a. The dried umbilical cord stump falls off

   b. Rectal temperature is greater than 100.4°F

   c. The child is eating but still losing weight

   d. The child wets her diaper 8 times per day

10. The nurse is observing a 6-month-old boy for developmental progress. Which of the following milestones would be typical for him?

    a. Shifts a toy to his left hand and reaches for another

    b. Picks up an object using his thumb and finger tips

    c. Puts down a little ball to pick up a stuffed toy

    d. Enjoys hitting a plastic bowl with a large spoon

11. The nurse is assessing an infant at his 6 month well baby check-up. The nurse notes that at birth the baby weighed 8 pounds and was 20 inches in length. Which of the following findings is most consistent with the normal infant growth and development?

    a. The baby weighs 21 pounds and is 30 inches in length.

    b. The baby weighs 16 pounds and is 26 inches in length.

    c. The baby weighs 15 pounds and is 24 inches in length.

    d. The baby weighs 24 pounds and is 26 inches in length.

12. A 1-month-old infant's mother voices concern about her baby's respirations. She states they are rapid and irregular. What information should be provided by the nurse?

    a. The normal respiratory rate for an infant at this age is between 20 and 30 breaths per minute.

    b. The respirations of a 1-month-old infant are normally irregular and periodically pause.

    c. An infant at this age should have regular respirations.

    d. The physician should be notified about the irregularity of the infant's respirations.

13. The nurse is assessing the oral cavity of a 4-month-old infant. Which of the following findings are consistent with a child of this age?

    a. The infant has 1 to 3 natal teeth.

    b. The infant has no teeth.

    c. The infant has 1 to 2 lower teeth.

    d. The infant has 1 upper tooth.

14. The nurse is educating the mother of a newborn baby about feeding practices. The nurse correctly advises the mother:

    a. The best feeding schedule offers food every 4 to 6 hours.

    b. Most newborns need to eat about 4 times per day.

    c. The newborn's stomach can hold between one-half to 1 ounce.

    d. Demand scheduled feeding is associated with increased difficulty getting the baby to sleep through the night.

Growth and Development of the Toddler

- Explain normal physiologic, psychosocial, and cognitive changes occurring in the toddler.
- Identify the gross and fine motor milestones of the toddler.
- Demonstrate an understanding of language development in the toddler years.
- Discuss sensory development of the toddler.
- Demonstrate an understanding of emotional/ social development and moral/spiritual development during toddlerhood.
- Implement a nursing care plan to address common issues related to growth and development in toddlerhood.
- Encourage growth and learning through play.
- Develop a teaching plan for safety promotion in the toddler period.
- Demonstrate an understanding of toddler needs related to sleep and rest, as well as dental health.
- Develop a nutritional plan for the toddler based on average nutritional requirements.
- Provide appropriate anticipatory guidance for common developmental issues that arise in the toddler period.
- Demonstrate an understanding of appropriate methods of discipline for use during the toddler years.

- Identify the role of the parent in the toddler's life and determine ways to support, encourage, and educate the parents about toddler growth, development, and concerns during this period.

SECTION I: ASSESSING YOUR UNDERSTANDING

Activity A FILL IN THE BLANKS

1. When _____ of the spinal cord is achieved around age 2 years, the toddler is capable of exercising voluntary control over the sphincters.

2. The leading cause of unintentional injury and death in children in this country is due to _____.

3. The ability to understand what is being said or asked is called _____ language.

4. The _____ remains short in both the male and female toddler, making them more susceptible to urinary tract infections compared to adults.

5. During the _____ stage of development, according to Piaget, children begin to become more sophisticated with symbolic thought.

Activity B **MATCHING**

Match the word in Column A with the correct description in Column B.

Column A

___ **1.** Echolalia

___ **2.** Regression

___ **3.** Individuation

___ **4.** Ritualism

___ **5.** Egocentrism

___ **6.** Telegraphic speech

Column B

a. Self-interest due to an inability to focus on another's perspective

b. Familiar routine that provides structure and security for the toddler

c. Speech that uses essential words only

d. Repetition of words and phrases without understanding

e. Internalizing a sense of self and one's environment

f. Returning to a prior developmental stage

Match the nutrients in Column A with the appropriate food source in Column B.

Column A

___ **1.** Dietary fiber

___ **2.** Folate

___ **3.** Vitamin A

___ **4.** Vitamin C

___ **5.** Calcium

Column B

a. Avocados, broccoli, green peas, dark greens

b. Apricots, cantaloupe, carrots, sweet potatoes

c. Applesauce, carrots, corn, green beans

d. Dairy products, broccoli, tofu, legumes

e. Broccoli, oranges, strawberries, tomatoes

Activity C **SEQUENCING**

Place the following descriptions of expressive language in the order the toddler will display them:

1. Uses primarily descriptive words (hungry, hot)

2. Talks about something that happened in the past

3. Babbles in what sounds like sentences

4. Uses a finger to point to things

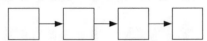

Activity D **SHORT ANSWERS**

Briefly answer the following.

1. Discuss ways to prevent temper tantrums in toddlers.

_____

_____

_____

2. Describe appropriate discipline for a toddler.

_____

_____

_____

3. Explain the care for the toddler's teeth and gums. How does the care change after the child reaches the age of 2?

_____

_____

_____

4. Discuss the changes in the genitourinary system in the toddler that allow for readiness for toilet training.

_____

_____

_____

5. Toddlers generally have a swayback appearance. What is the underlying cause of this manifestation?

_____

_____

_____

SECTION II: APPLYING YOUR KNOWLEDGE

Activity E CASE STUDY

Consider the scenario and answer the questions.

Jose Gonzales is a 2-year-old boy brought to the clinic by his mother and father for his 2-year-old check-up. The following questions refer to him.

1. Jose's parents state "We speak Spanish at home to Jose and are working to make him bilingual." What do you need to consider when assessing language development in Jose?

   _____

   _____

   _____

2. Jose's mother asks what they can do to encourage Jose's language development.

   _____

   _____

   _____

3. Jose's father states that Jose's favorite word is "No." He asks if this is normal at this age. How would you respond? (include a discussion on Erikson stage of development and suggestions for dealing with this)

   _____

   _____

   _____

SECTION III: PRACTICING FOR NCLEX

Activity F NCLEX-STYLE QUESTIONS

Answer the following questions.

1. The parents of an overweight 2-year-old boy admit that their child is a bit "chubby," but argue that he is a picky eater who will eat only junk food. Which is the best response by the nurse to facilitate a healthier diet?

   a. "You may have to serve a new food 10 or more times."

   b. "Serve only healthy foods. He'll eat when he's hungry."

   c. "Give him more healthy choices with less junk food available."

   d. "Calorie requirements for toddlers are less than infants."

2. The nurse is observing a 36-month-old boy during a well visit. Which motor skill has he most recently acquired?

   a. The child is able to undress himself

   b. He is able to push a toy lawnmower

   c. The child is able to kick a ball

   d. The child can pull a toy while walking

3. The nurse is providing anticipatory guidance to the parents of an 18-month-old girl. Which recommendation will be most helpful to the parents?

   a. Giving the child time out for 1 ½ minutes

   b. Ignoring bad behavior and praising good

   c. Slapping her hand using one or two fingers

   d. Describing proper behavior when she misbehaves

4. The nurse is teaching a first-time mother with a 14-month-old boy about child safety. Which is the most effective overall safety information to provide guidance for the mother?

   a. "Place a gate at the top of stairways."

   b. "Never let him out of your sight."

   c. "Put chemicals in a locked cabinet."

   d. "Don't smoke in the house or car."

5. The parents of a 2-year-old girl are concerned with her behavior. For which behavior would the nurse share their concern?

   a. The child refuses to share her toys with her sister

   b. She frequently babbles to herself when playing

   c. The child likes to change toys frequently

   d. She plays by herself even when other children are present

6. The nurse is discussing sensory development with the mother of a 2-year-old boy. Which parental comment suggests the child may have a sensory problem?

   a. "He wasn't bothered by the paint smell."

   b. "He was licking up the dishwashing soap."

   c. "He doesn't respond if I wave to him."

   d. "I dropped a pan behind him and he cried."

7. The nurse is assessing the language development of a 3-year-old girl. Which finding would suggest a problem?

   a. The child can make simple conversation

   b. She tells the nurse she saw Na-Na today

   c. The child speaks in 2- to 3-word sentences

   d. She can tell the nurse what her name is

8. The nurse is observing a 3-year-old boy in a daycare center. Which behavior might suggest an emotional problem?

   a. The child has persistent separation anxiety

   b. He goes from calm to tantrum suddenly

   c. The child sucks his thumb periodically

   d. He is unable to share toys with others

9. The nurse is teaching a mother of a 1-year-old girl about weaning her from the bottle and breast. Which recommendation would be part of the nurse's plan?

   a. Wean from breast by 18 months of age at the latest

   b. Give the child an iron-fortified cereal

   c. Switch the child to a no-spill sippy cup

   d. Wean from the bottle at 15 months of age

10. The parents of a 3-year-old boy have asked the nurse for advice about a preschool for their child. Which suggestion is most important for the nurse to make?

   a. "Look for a preschool that is clean and has a loving staff."

   b. "Check to make sure your child can attend with the sniffles."

   c. "Make sure that you can easily get an appointment to visit."

   d. "The staff should be trained in early childhood development."

11. The nurse is assessing a 2-year-old boy during a well-child visit. The nurse correctly identifies the child's current stage of Erickson's growth and development as:

   a. Trust versus mistrust

   b. Autonomy versus shame and doubt

   c. Initiative versus guilt

   d. Industry versus inferiority

12. The nurse is assessing a 3-year-old child. The nurse notes the child is able to understand that objects hidden from sight still exist. The nurse correctly documents the child is displaying:

   a. Tertiary circular reactions

   b. Mental combinations

   c. Preoperational thinking

   d. Concrete thinking

13. The nurse is discussing the activities of a 20-month-old child with his mother. The mother reports the children of her friends seem to have more advanced speech abilities than her child. After assessing the child, which of the following findings is cause for follow up?

   a. Inability to point to named body parts

   b. Inability to talk with the nurse about something that happened a few days ago

   c. Points to pictures in books when asked

   d. Understands approximately 75 to 100 words

14. The mother of an 18-month-old girl voices concerns about her child's social skills. She reports that the child does not play well with others and seems to ignore other children who are playing at the same time. What response by the nurse is indicated?

   a. "It is normal for children to engage in play alongside other children at this age."

   b. "Has your child displayed any aggressive tendencies toward other children?"

   c. "Perhaps you should consider a preschool to promote more socialization opportunities."

   d. "Does your child have opportunities to socialize much with other children?"

CHAPTER 27

Growth and Development of the Preschooler

Learning Objectives

- Identify normal physiologic, cognitive, and psychosocial changes occurring in the preschool-aged child.
- Express an understanding of language development in the preschool years.
- Implement a nursing care plan that addresses common concerns or delays in the preschooler's development.
- Integrate knowledge of preschool growth and development with nursing care and health promotion of the preschool-aged child.
- Develop a nutrition plan for the preschool-aged child.
- Identify common issues related to growth and development during the preschool years.
- Demonstrate knowledge of appropriate anticipatory guidance for common developmental issues that arise in the preschool period.

SECTION I: ASSESSING YOUR UNDERSTANDING

Activity A FILL IN THE BLANKS

1. The over-consumption of cow's milk may result in a deficiency of _____ due to the calcium blocking its absorption.

2. Communication in preschool children is _____ in nature, as they are not yet capable of abstract thought.

3. Preschool age children are more susceptible to bladder infections than are adults due to the length of the _____.

4. During a night _____ a child will scream and thrash but not awaken.

5. A nutrient _____ diet along with physical activity is the foundation for obesity prevention in the preschool child.

Activity B MATCHING

Match the theorist and stage in Column A with the proper activities/behaviors in Column B

Column A

_____ **1.** Erikson – Initiative versus guilt

_____ **2.** Piaget – Preconceptual

_____ **3.** Piaget – Intuitive

_____ **4.** Kohlberg – Punishment–obedience orientation

_____ **5.** Kohlberg – Preconventional morality

_____ **6.** Freud – Phallic stage

Column B

a. Displays animism

b. Able to classify and relate objects

c. Children may learn inappropriate behavior if the parent does not intervene to teach the behavior is wrong

d. Likes to please parents

e. Super-ego is developing and the conscience is emerging

f. Determines good and bad dependent upon associated punishment

Activity C SEQUENCING

Place the following motor skills in the order of acquisition.

1. Swings and climbs well

2. Copies circles and traces squares

3. Throws ball overhand

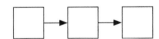

Activity D SHORT ANSWERS

Briefly answer the following.

1. Describe the cognitive abilities of a child in the intuitive phase.

_____

_____

_____

2. Explain the difference between nightmares and night terrors.

_____

_____

_____

3. Name three ways to promote healthy teeth and gums in preschoolers.

_____

_____

_____

4. What strategies should be used by the parents of a preschool-aged child who has lied?

_____

_____

_____

5. What is the primary social task of the preschool-aged child?

_____

_____

_____

SECTION II: APPLYING YOUR KNOWLEDGE

Activity E CASE STUDY

Consider the scenario and answer the questions.

Remember Nila Patel, the 4-year-old from Chapter 5, who was brought to the clinic by her parents for her school check-up.

1. Nila's mother states that "Nila loves to play make believe. She is constantly playing in a fantasy world. I am not sure if this is healthy behavior." How would you address Mrs. Patel's concerns?

   _____

   _____

   _____

2. Nila's parents express concerns about the transition to Kindergarten. What guidance can you give them regarding this?

   _____

   _____

   _____

3. During your assessment, Nila's mother asks what findings would concern you. Discuss specific developmental warning signs you are assessing for.

   _____

   _____

   _____

SECTION III: PRACTICING FOR NCLEX

Activity F NCLEX-STYLE QUESTIONS

Answer the following questions.

1. The nurse is conducting a well-child assessment of a 4-year-old. Which of the following assessment findings would warrant further investigation?

   a. Presence of 20 deciduous teeth

   b. Presence of 10 deciduous teeth

   c. Absence of dental caries

   d. Presence of 19 deciduous teeth

2. The nurse is conducting a health screening of a 5-year-old boy as required for kindergarten. The boy is fearful about going to a new school. The mother asks for the nurse's advice. Which is the best response by the nurse?

   a. "Kindergarten is a big step for a child. Be patient with him."

   b. "Talk to your son's new teacher and schedule a tour with him."

   c. "Be aware that he may have difficulty adjusting being away from home 5 days a week."

   d. "Remind him that kindergarten will be a lot of fun and he'll make new friends."

3. The nurse is conducting a well-child examination of a 4-year-old and is assessing the child's height. The nurse would expect that the child's height would have increased by which of the following since last year's examination?

   a. ½ to 1 inch

   b. 1 to 2 inches

   c. 2 ½ to 3 inches

   d. 3 ½ to 4 inches

4. A nurse is providing a routine wellness examination for a 5-year-old boy. Which of the following responses by the parents indicates a need for an additional referral or follow-up?

    a. "He can count to 30 but gets confused after that."

    b. "We often have to translate his speech to others."

    c. "He is always talking and telling detailed stories."

    d. "He knows his name and address."

5. The parents of a 4-year-old girl tell the nurse that their daughter is having frequent nightmares. Which of the following statements would indicate that the girl is having night terrors instead of nightmares?

    a. "She screams and thrashes when we try to touch her."

    b. "She is scared after she wakes up."

    c. "She comes and wakes us up after she awakens."

    d. "She has a hard time going back to sleep."

6. The nurse is providing teaching to the mother of a 4-year-old girl about bike safety. Which of the following statements indicates a need for further teaching?

    a. "The balls of her feet should reach both pedals while sitting."

    b. "Pedal back brakes are better for her age group."

    c. "She should always ride on the sidewalk."

    d. "She can ride on the street if I am riding with her."

7. The nurse is conducting a health screening for a 3-year-old boy as required by his new preschool. Which of the following statements by the parents would warrant further discussion and intervention?

    a. "The school has a looser environment which is a good match for his temperament."

    b. "The school requires processed foods and high sugar foods be avoided."

    c. "The school is quite structured and advocates corporal punishment."

    d. "There is a very low student teacher ratio and they do a lot of hands on projects."

8. A nurse is caring for a 4-year-old girl. The parents indicate that their daughter often reports that objects in the house are her friends. They are concerned because the girl says that the grandfather clock in the hallway smiles and sings to her. How should the nurse respond?

    a. "Your daughter is demonstrating animism which is common."

    b. "Attributing life-like qualities to inanimate objects is quite normal at this age."

    c. "Do you think your daughter is hallucinating?

    d. "Is there a family history of mental illness?"

9. The nurse is providing teaching about child safety to the parents of a 4-year-old girl. Which of the following statements by the parents would indicate a need for further teaching?

    a. "She should use a helmet when riding her bike."

    b. "She still needs a booster seat in the car."

    c. "We need to know the basics of CPR and first aid."

    d. "We need to continually remind her about safety rules."

10. The nurse is providing teaching about proper dental care for the parents of a 5-year-old girl. Which of the following responses indicates a need for further teaching?

    a. "Too much fluoride can contribute to fluorosis."

    b. "We should use only a pea-sized amount of toothpaste."

    c. "She needs to floss her teeth before brushing."

    d. "She should see a dentist every 6 months."

11. The father of a preschool boy reports concerns about the short stature of his son. The nurse reviews the child's history and notes the child is 4 years old and is presently 41 inches tall and has grown 2.5 inches in the past year. What response by the nurse is most appropriate?

    a. "Is there a reason you are concerned about your child's height?"

    b. "Your son is slightly below the normal height for his age group but may still grow to be a normal height in the coming year."

c. "Your son is slightly below the normal height for his age but he had demonstrated a normal growth rate this year."

d. "Both your son's height and rate of growth are within normal limits for his age."

12. The mother of a 4-year-old girl reports her daughter has episodes of wetting her pants. The nurse questions the mother about the frequency. The nurse determines these episodes occur about once every 1 to 2 weeks. What response by the nurse is indicated?

a. "You should consider restricting your daughter's fluid intake."

b. "Discipline should be applied after these times."

c. "At this age it is helpful to remind children to go to the bathroom."

d. "The frequency of these wetting episodes may be consistent with a low-grade urinary tract infection."

13. The nurse is caring for a 4-year-old child hospitalized in traction. The child talks about an invisible friend to the nurse. What action by the nurse is indicated?

a. The nurse should document the reports of hallucinations by the child.

b. The nurse should explain to the child that there are no friends present.

c. The nurse should discourage the child from talking about the imaginary friend.

d. The nurse should recognize this behavior as normal for the child's developmental age and do nothing.

14. The mother of a 4-year-old boy reports her son has voiced curiosity about her breasts. She asks the nurse what she should do. What is the best information that the nurse can give to the parent?

a. Advise the parent that sexual curiosity is unusual at this age.

b. Encourage the parent to provide a detailed discussion about human sexuality with the child.

c. Encourage the parent to determine what the child's specific questions are and answer them briefly.

d. Advise the parent to explain to the child that he is too young to discuss such things.

15. The mother of a 3-year-old child reports her son is afraid of dark. She asks the nurse for help. Which of the following is the best advice the nurse can offer?

a. Encourage the parent to allow a small night light.

b. Encourage the parent to consider allowing the child to sleep with her until he feels more able to sleep alone.

c. Encourage the mother to allow a night light until the child falls asleep and then recommend she turn it off.

d. Encourage the parent to avoid the use of night lights as they interfere with restful sleep in children.

28

Growth and Development of the School-Age Child

Learning Objectives

- Identify normal physiologic, cognitive, and moral changes occurring in the school-age child.
- Describe the role of peers and schools in the development and socialization of the school-age child.
- Identify the developmental milestones of the school-age child.
- Identify the role of the nurse in promoting safety for the school-age child.
- Demonstrate knowledge of the nutritional requirements of the school-age child.
- Identify common developmental concerns in the school-age child.
- Demonstrate knowledge of the appropriate nursing guidance for common developmental concerns.

SECTION I: ASSESSING YOUR UNDERSTANDING

Activity A FILL IN THE BLANKS

1. An 8-year-old who is the size of an 11-year-old will think and act like a(n) _____ year-old.

2. The Academy of Pediatrics recommends _____ hours or less of television viewing per day.

3. Brain growth is complete by the time the _____ birthday is celebrated.

4. Between the ages of 10 and 12 (the pubescent years for girls), _____ levels remain high, but are more controlled and focused than previously.

5. Motor vehicle accidents are a common cause of _____ in the school-aged child.

6. Most young children are not capable of handling _____ or making decisions on their own before 11 or 12 years of age.

7. Ways to develop self-worth is termed _____.

8. During school children are influenced by _____ and teachers.

9. Compared with the earlier years, caloric needs of the school-age child are _____.

10. The bladder capacity for a 10-year-old would be _____ ounces.

Activity B MATCHING

Match the terms with the descriptions.

Column A

____ **1.** Inferiority

____ **2.** Bruxism

____ **3.** Malocclusion

____ **4.** Caries

____ **5.** Secondary sexual characteristics

____ **6.** Principle of conservation

Column B

a. Gritting or grinding of teeth

b. Tooth decay

c. Feelings of inability or not measuring up to the abilities of others

d. Matter does not change when forms change

e. Improper teeth alignment

f. Changes in breast development and genitalia during late school age or early adolescent

Match the systems with the capacities.

Column A

____ **1.** Lymph system

____ **2.** Heart

____ **3.** Bones

Column B

a. Mineralization not complete until maturity

b. Smaller in size, in relation to the rest of the body, than any other developmental stage

c. Continues to grow until the child is 9 years old

Match the theorists with characteristics of their theories for the school-age child.

Column A

____ **1.** Kohlberg

____ **2.** Feud

____ **3.** Piaget

____ **4.** Erikson

Column B

a. Industry versus inferiority

b. Conventional: "good child, bad child"

c. Latency

d. Concrete operational

Activity C SEQUENCING

Place the following developmental milestones in the proper sequence.

1. Brain growth is complete

2. Fine motor skills develop

3. Frontal sinuses development is complete

4. Gross motor skills develop

5. Lymphatic tissue growth is complete

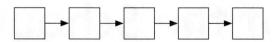

Activity D SHORT ANSWERS

Briefly answer the following.

1. Describe the development of children's gross motor skills as they correspond to age groups.

_____

_____

_____

2. Describe the child who is labeled "slow to warm."

_____

_____

_____

3. Define the nurse's role in school-age children's growth and development.

_____

_____

_____

4. Detail the sleep requirements for school-age children.

_____

_____

_____

5. Discuss the importance of body image on the school-aged child.

_____

_____

_____

SECTION II: APPLYING YOUR KNOWLEDGE

Activity E CASE STUDY

Olivia Anderson, 9 years old, is brought to the clinic by her mother for her annual check-up.

1. During your assessment you note the interaction between the mother and the daughter. While asking Olivia about her friends at school, the mother responds "Olivia does not have many friends. I have told her if she would just care more about her appearance, other children will want to spend time with her."

   How would you respond to the mother?

   _____

   _____

   _____

2. Olivia's mother expresses concerns regarding discipline and how best to approach this.

   How would you respond?

   _____

   _____

   _____

3. During your assessment, you discover that Olivia spends most of her time watching television and playing video games. What guidance can you give to Olivia and her mother regarding this?

   _____

   _____

   _____

SECTION III: PRACTICING FOR NCLEX

Activity F NCLEX-STYLE QUESTIONS

Answer the following questions.

1. The nurse is about to see a 9-year-old girl for a well-child check-up. Knowing that the child is in Piaget's period of concrete operational thought, which of the following characteristics will the child display?

   a. The child can consider an action and its consequences

   b. The child views the world in terms of her own experience

   c. The child makes generalized assumptions about groups of things

   d. The child knows lying is bad because she gets sent to her room for it.

2. The nurse is educating the parents of a 6-year-old boy how to manage the child's introduction into elementary school. The child has an easy temperament. Which of the following would the nurse most likely suggest?

   a. Comforting the child when he is frustrated

   b. Helping the child deal with minor stresses

   c. Schedule several visits to the school before classes start

   d. Being firm with the anticipated episodes of moodiness and irritability

3. The mother of a 7-year-old girl is asking the nurse's advice about getting her daughter a 2-wheel bike. Which of the following responses by the nurse is most important?

   a. "Teach her where she'll land on the grass if she falls."

   b. "Be sure to get the proper size bike."

   c. "She won't need a helmet if she has training wheels."

   d. "Learning to ride the bike will improve her coordination."

4. The school nurse is assessing the nutritional status of an overweight 12-year-old girl. Which of the following questions would be appropriate for the nurse to ask?

   a. Does your family have rules about foods and how they are prepared?

   b. What does your family do for exercise?

   c. How often does everyone in your family eat together?

   d. Have you gained weight recently?

5. The nurse has taken a health history and performed a physical exam for a 12-year-old boy. Which of the following findings will most likely be made?

   a. The child's body fat has decreased since last year

   b. The child has different diet preferences than his parents

   c. The child has a leaner body mass than a girl at this age

   d. The child described a somewhat reduced appetite

6. The nurse is teaching parents of an 11-year-old girl how to deal with the issues relating to peer pressure to use tobacco and alcohol. Which of the following suggestions provides the best course of action for the parents?

   a. Avoiding smoking in the house or in front of the child

   b. Hiding alcohol out of the child's reach

   c. Forbidding the child to have friends that smoke or drink

   d. Discuss tobacco and alcohol use with the child

7. The nurse is assessing the nutritional needs of an 8-year-old girl who weighs 65 pounds. Which of the following amounts would provide the proper daily caloric intake for this child?

   a. 1,895 calories per day

   b. 2,065 calories per day

   c. 2,245 calories per day

   d. 2,385 calories per day

8. The nurse is talking with the parents of an 8-year-old boy who has been cheating at school. Which of the following comments should be the primary message for the nurse to present?

   a. "The punishment should be severe and long lasting."

   b. "Make sure that your behavior around your son is exemplary."

   c. "Resolve this by providing an opportunity for him to cheat and then dealing with it."

   d. "You may be putting too much pressure on him to succeed."

9. A 9-year-old boy has arrived for a health maintenance visit. Which of the following milestones of physical growth would the nurse expect to observe?

   a. Brain growth is complete and the shape of the head is longer

   b. Lymphatic tissue growth is complete providing greater resistance to infections

   c. Frontal sinuses are developed while tonsils have decreased in size

   d. All deciduous teeth are replaced by 32 permanent teeth

10. The nurse is educating the parents of a 10-year-old girl in ways to help their child avoid tobacco. Which of the following suggestions would be part of the nurse's advice?

    a. "Keep your cigarettes where she can't get to them."

    b. "Always go outside when you have a cigarette."

    c. "Tell her only losers smoke and chew tobacco."

    d. "As parents, you need to be good role models."

11. The parents of a 7-year-old girl report concerns about her seemingly low self-esteem. The parents question how self-esteem is developed in a young girl. What response by the nurse is most appropriate?

    a. "The peers of a child at this age are the greatest influence on self-esteem."

    b. "Several interrelated factors are to blame for low self-esteem."

    c. "Your daughter's self-esteem is influenced by feedback from people they view as authorities at this age."

    d. "A child's self-esteem is greatly inborn and environmental influences guide it."

12. The parents of an 8-year-old boy report their son is being bullied and teased by a group of boys in the neighborhood. What information can be accurately provided by the nurse?

    a. "Perhaps teaching your son self-defense courses will help him to have a greater sense of control and safety."

    b. "Bullying can have lifelong effects on the self-esteem of a child."

    c. "Fortunately the scars of being picked on will fade as your son grows up."

    d. "Your son is at high risk for bullying other children as a result of this situation."

13. During a well-child check at the ambulatory clinic, the mother of a 10-year-old boy reports concerns about her son's frequent discussions about death and dying. Based upon knowledge of this age grout the nurse understands which of the following?

    a. Discussions about death and dying are not normal for this age group.

    b. Preoccupations about death and dying may hint at a psychological disorder.

    c. Preoccupation with thoughts related to death and dying in this age group are consistent with the later development of depression.

    d. Preoccupation with death and dying is common in the school-aged child.

14. The parents of a 9-year-old boy report they have been homeschooling their son and now plan to enroll him in the local public school. They voice concerns about the influence of the other children on their son's values. What information can be provided to the parents by the nurse?

    a. "At your son's age, values are most influenced by peers."

    b. "The values of the family will likely prevail for your son."

    c. "Values are largely inborn and will be impacted only in a limited way by environmental influences."

    d. "Teacher will begin to have the largest influence on a child's values at this age."

15. The nurse is caring for a hospitalized 5-year-old child. The child's mother has reported her child is becoming very "clingy." What advice can be provided to the parent by the nurse? Select all that apply.

    a. "Regression is normal during hospitalization."

    b. "Be careful not to coddle the child or it will result in regressive behaviors."

    c. "These behaviors are the result of a loss of self-control and are likely temporary."

    d. "Allowing the child to have some input in the care may be helpful in managing these behaviors."

CHAPTER 29

Growth and Development of the Adolescent

Learning Objectives

- Identify normal physiologic changes, including puberty, occurring in the adolescent.
- Discuss psychosocial, cognitive, and moral changes occurring in the adolescent.
- Identify changes in relationships with peers, family, teachers, and community during adolescence.
- Describe interventions to promote safety during adolescence.
- Demonstrate knowledge of the nutritional requirements of the adolescent.
- Demonstrate knowledge of the development of sexuality and its influence on dating during adolescence.
- Identify common developmental concerns of the adolescent.
- Demonstrate knowledge of the appropriate nursing guidance for common developmental concerns.

SECTION I: ASSESSING YOUR UNDERSTANDING

Activity A FILL IN THE BLANKS

1. Risk-taking behaviors of adolescents are those that could lead to physical or _____ injury.

2. Second only to growth during _____, adolescence provides the most rapid and dramatic changes in size and proportions.

3. Adolescents proceed from thinking in concrete terms to thinking in _____ terms.

4. Families who listen and continue to demonstrate affection for and acceptance of their adolescent have a more _____ outcome.

5. The prevalence of obesity is highest in _____ and African American teens between the ages of 12 and 19.

6. The family can experience a _____ if an adolescent's striving for independence is met with stricter parental limits.

7. According to Erikson, it is during adolescence that teenagers achieve a sense of _____.

8. The _____ of the skeletal system is completed earlier in girls than in boys.

9. During middle adolescence gross motor skills such as speed, accuracy, and _____ improve.

10. It is important for the nurse to take into consideration the effects culture, ethnicity, and _____ have on adolescents.

Activity B MATCHING

Match the illicit drug in Column A with the proper descriptive word or phrase in Column B.

Column A

_____ **1.** Amphetamines

_____ **2.** Barbiturates

_____ **3.** Cocaine

_____ **4.** Hallucinogens

_____ **5.** Opiates

_____ **6.** Phencyclidine hydrochloride (PCP)

Column B

a. Pressured speech and anorexia

b. Drowsiness, constricted pupils

c. Depression in children

d. Violence, irrational behavior

e. Hypertension, distorted perceptions

f. Hyperactivity in children

Match the type of contraceptive with the correct description.

Column A

_____ **1.** Condom

_____ **2.** Depo-Provera

_____ **3.** Diaphragm

_____ **4.** Emergency contraceptive pills

_____ **5.** Oral contraception

_____ **6.** Spermicides

Column B

a. Requires fitting and education

b. Effective if used with a barrier method

c. Injectable, administered every 3 months

d. Not appropriate for routine use

e. Inexpensive, protects against disease

f. Highly effective, expensive

Match the nutrient in Column A with the daily requirement in Column B.

Column A

_____ **1.** Calcium (boys and girls)

_____ **2.** Iron (boys)

_____ **3.** Iron (girls)

_____ **4.** Protein (boys)

_____ **5.** Protein (girls)

Column B

a. 12 mg/day

b. 45 to 59 g/day

c. 1,200 to 1,500 mg /day

d. 15 mg/day

e. 46 g/day

Activity C SEQUENCING

Beginning with early adolescence and ending with late adolescence, place the following physiological changes in sequential order.

1. Voice changes

2. Eruption of last four molars

3. Head, neck, hands, and feet reach adult proportions

4. Increase in shoulder, chest, and hip breadth

5. First menstrual period (average = 12.8 years)

6. Increase in percentage of body fat

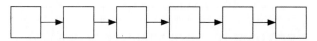

Activity D SHORT ANSWERS

Briefly answer the following.

1. List eight reasons why adolescents become pregnant.

_____

_____

_____

2. Describe the adolescent's achievement of his or her identity, including how previous developmental stages and culture play a role.

_____

_____

_____

3. Explain how the school experience comprises an integral component of the adolescent's preparation for the future.

_____

_____

_____

4. Explain the importance of sexuality discussions between parents and teens.

_____

_____

_____

5. Discuss the physical growth and development of the teenager. What factors influence the growth of teens? How has growth of teens changed over the past few decades?

_____

_____

_____

6. Discuss the cognitive development/capabilities of the teenaged child.

_____

_____

_____

SECTION II: APPLYING YOUR KNOWLEDGE

Activity E CASE STUDY

Cho Chung, a 15-year-old, is brought to the clinic by her mother for her annual school check-up.

1. During your assessment, Cho states she wants to get her belly button pierced but her parents refuse. She states, "They just don't understand that there is really no risk. I have at least 10 friends who have one, and none of them have had any problems." How would you address this?

_____

_____

_____

2. During your assessment, you find out Cho has recently become sexually active. How would you address sexually transmitted infections and teen pregnancy during Cho's visit?

_____

_____

_____

3. After the exam, Cho's mother expresses concerns about communicating with her daughter. How would you respond?

_____

_____

_____

SECTION III: PRACTICING FOR NCLEX

Activity F NCLEX-STYLE QUESTIONS

Answer the following questions.

1. The nurse knows that the 13-year-old girl in the exam room is in the process of developing her own set of values. Which of the following activities will this child be experiencing according to Kohlberg's theory?
   a. Wishing her parents were more understanding
   b. Assuming everyone is interested in her favorite pop star
   c. Wondering what is the meaning of life
   d. Comparing morals with those of peers

2. The nurse is promoting safe sex to a 14-year-old boy who is frequently dating. Which of the following points is most likely to be made during the talk?
   a. "Adolescents account for 25% of sexually transmitted infection (STI) cases."
   b. "Contraception is a shared responsibility."
   c. "Be careful or you'll wind up being a teenage dad."
   d. "Girls are more susceptible to STIs than boys."

3. The school nurse is providing nutritional guidance during a 9th grade health class. Which of the following foods would be recommended as a good source for calcium?
   a. Strawberries, watermelon, and raisins
   b. Beans, poultry, and fish
   c. Peanut butter, tomato juice, and whole grain bread
   d. Cheese, yogurt, and white beans

4. The nurse is talking to a 13-year-old boy about choosing friends. Which of the following functions do peer groups provide that can have a negative result?
   a. Following role models
   b. Sharing problems
   c. Negotiating differences
   d. Developing loyalties

5. The school nurse is assessing a 16-year-old girl who was removed from class because of disruptive behavior. She arrived in the nurse's office with dilated pupils and talking rapidly. Which of the following drugs might she be using?

   a. Opiates

   b. Barbiturates

   c. Amphetamines

   d. Marijuana

6. The nurse is providing anticipatory guidance for violence prevention to a group of parents with adolescent children. Which of the following actions would be most effective in preventing suicide?

   a. Watching for aggressive behavior or racist remarks

   b. Checking for signs of depression or lack of friends

   c. Becoming acquainted with the teen's friends

   d. Monitoring video games, TV shows, and music

7. A 16-year-old girl has arrived for her sports physical with a new piercing in her navel. What is the best approach for the nurse to use?

   a. "Be sure to clean the navel several times a day."

   b. "I hope for your sake the needle was clean."

   c. "This is a risk for hepatitis, tetanus, and AIDS."

   d. "This is a wound and can become infected."

8. Throughout a health surveillance visit, a 12-year-old boy complains to the nurse about his parents intruding on his personal space, but then says he is looking forward to the family vacation. Which of the following characteristics also suggests the boy has entered adolescence?

   a. Growing interest in attracting girls' attention

   b. Feels secure with his body image

   c. Experiences frequent mood changes

   d. Understands that actions have consequences

9. The nurse is performing a physical assessment on an 11-year-old girl during a health surveillance visit. Which of the following findings would suggest the child has reached adolescence?

   a. A significant muscle mass increase

   b. Eruption of last four molars

   c. Increased shoulder, chest and hip widths

   d. The child has higher blood pressure

10. The nurse is promoting nutrition to a teen who is going through a growth spurt. Knowing that the teen has a need for increased amounts of zinc, calcium, and iron, which of the following foods would be recommended for its high iron content?

    a. Fat-free milk

    b. Whole grain bread

    c. Organic carrots

    d. Fresh orange juice

11. The nurse is collecting data from a 15-year-old boy who is being seen at the ambulatory care clinic for immunizations. During the initial assessment, he voices concerns about being a few inches shorter than his peers. What response by the nurse is indicated?

    a. "Being short is nothing to be ashamed of."

    b. "I am sure you are not the shortest guy in your class."

    c. "Boys your age will often continue growing a few more years."

    d. "Are the other men in your family short?"

12. The nurse is meeting with a 16-year-old female child who reports being physically active on the track and basketball teams at school. The child reports a weight loss of 7 pounds since she began training for the track season. When reviewing her caloric needs the nurse recognizes the diet should include how many calories?

    a. 1,800 calories per day

    b. 2,000 calories per day

    c. 2,200 calories per day

    d. 2,400 calories per day

13. Which of the following behaviors by an 18-year-old is consistent with successful progression through the stages of Piaget's theory of development?

    a. There is a strong sense of understanding of internal identity.

    b. The individual reflects a strong moral code.

    c. The individual is able to use critical thought processes to handle a problem.

    d. The individual is able to be a part of a large group of peers while maintaining a sense of self.

14. The nurse is counseling an overweight, sedentary 15-year-old female child. The nurse is assisting her to make appropriate menu choices. Which of the following indicates the child understands the appropriate dietary selections to make?

    a. "I avoid all fat intake."

    b. "Because of my age, my dairy intake is unlimited."

    c. "I need to have 2 servings of fruit each day."

    d. "To lose weight my protein intake should be limited to 2 to 4 servings per day."

15. The nurse is performing an assessment on a 12-year-old male child. Which of the following findings is consistent with the child's age?

    a. Absence of pubic hair

    b. Presence of curling pubic hair

    c. Coarse pubic hair

    d. Presence of sparse pubic hair

Atraumatic and Family-Centered Care of Children

- Describe the major principles and concepts of atraumatic care.
- Incorporate atraumatic care to prevent and minimize physical stress for children and families.
- Discuss the major components and concepts of family-centered care.
- Utilize excellent therapeutic communication skills when interacting with children and their families.
- Use culturally competent communication when working with children and their families.
- Describe the process of health teaching as it relates to children and their families.

SECTION I: ASSESSING YOUR UNDERSTANDING

Activity A FILL IN THE BLANKS

1. Therapeutic care that decreases or eliminates the psychological and physical distress experienced by children and their families when receiving health care is referred to as _____ care.

2. Communication that is goal-directed, focused, and purposeful is considered _____ communication.

3. Things such as eye contact and body position are part of _____ communication.

4. A _____ nurse practitioner helps ensure that children and families receive atraumatic care.

5. Clarifying the parent's feelings by paraphrasing parts of a conversation is utilization of _____ communication.

6. Paying attention to what the child and parents are saying by nodding one's head and making eye contact is considered _____ listening.

7. When communicating with a family that speaks a different language than the nurse or with a child that is deaf may require the use of a reliable _____.

Activity B MATCHING

Match the development level in Column A with the communication technique in Column B appropriate for the developmental age.

Column A

___ **1.** Adolescents

___ **2.** Infants

___ **3.** Preschoolers

___ **4.** School-age children

___ **5.** Toddlers

Column B

a. Use a soothing voice

b. Prepare child just before procedure

c. Use diagrams and illustrations

d. Use storytelling and play

e. Define medical words as necessary

Activity C SEQUENCING

Place the following methods of learning in order from lowest percent of information remembered to the highest percent remembered after 2 weeks:

1. Actively discussing

2. Hearing

3. Performing an activity

4. Reading

5. Watching a demonstration

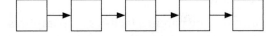

Activity D SHORT ANSWERS

Briefly answer the following.

1. Discuss how therapeutic hugging is beneficial during certain procedures?

_____

_____

_____

2. Describe four ways to evaluate the success of child and family education.

_____

_____

_____

3. What incidents would alert the nurse that a family may be suffering from health literacy difficulties?

_____

_____

_____

4. Name six suggestions to enhance learning if literacy problems exist.

_____

_____

_____

5. How can the nurse help prevent or minimize child and family separation during a child's hospitalization?

_____

_____

_____

SECTION II: APPLYING YOUR KNOWLEDGE

Activity E CASE STUDY

Consider the scenario and answer the questions.

Emma is a 4-year-old female admitted to your pediatric unit secondary to a suspected head injury from a fall. She was playing at a playground with her babysitter and fell from the top of the slide. Emma also has a laceration to her arm that will require stitches. She is scheduled for a CT scan. Her parents are with her and are very supportive and display no difficulties with health literacy.

1. How would you explain a head CT to Emma?

   _____

   _____

   _____

2. What technique should be used to restrain Emma while she receives her stitches?

   _____

   _____

   _____

SECTION III: PRACTICING FOR NCLEX

Activity F NCLEX-STYLE QUESTIONS

Answer the following questions.

1. The nurse is assessing the learning needs of the parents of 5-year-old girl who is scheduled for surgery. Which of the following nonverbal cues shows them that the nurse is interested in what the family members are saying?
   a. Sitting straight with feet flat on the floor
   b. Looking at child when the father is talking
   c. Nodding head while the mother speaks
   d. Standing several steps away from parents

2. The nurse is caring for a 3-year-old boy who must have a lumbar puncture. Which of the following actions would provide the greatest contribution toward atraumatic care?
   a. Having a child life nurse practitioner play with the child

   b. Explaining the lumbar puncture procedure
   c. Letting the child take his teddy bear with him
   d. Keeping the parents calm in front of the child

3. The nurse is caring for a 14-year-old boy, and his parents, who has just been diagnosed with a malignant tumor on his liver. Which of the following interventions is most important to this child and family?
   a. Arranging an additional meeting with the nurse practitioner
   b. Discussing treatment options with the child and parents
   c. Involving the child and family in decision making
   d. Describing postoperative home care for the child

4. The nurse is educating a 15-year-old girl with Grave's disease and her family about the disease and its treatment. Which of the following methods of evaluating learning is least effective?
   a. Having the child and family demonstrate skills
   b. Asking closed-ended questions for specific facts
   c. Requesting the parent to teach the child skills
   d. Setting up a scenario for them to talk through

5. The nurse is caring for a 14-year-old girl with terminal cancer and her family. Which of the following interventions would best provide therapeutic communication?
   a. Recognizing the parents' desire to use all options
   b. Supporting the child's desires for treatment
   c. Presenting options for treatment
   d. Informing the child in terms she can understand

6. The nurse is caring for a 6-year-old boy and his parents. The child will need chemotherapy for which informed consent is necessary. Which of the following is the most important nursing intervention?

   a. Teaching the parents about optional treatments

   b. Explaining the procedure and possible side effects

   c. Asking questions to determine the parents' understanding

   d. Witnessing the signing of the consent form

7. The nurse is caring for a 3-year-old girl with a ruptured appendix. Her parents have strong religious beliefs against certain types of medical treatment. Which of the following interventions best ensures that the child receives appropriate care?

   a. Recognizing the parents' religious beliefs

   b. Communicating using appropriate terms

   c. Educating the parents about the surgery and prognosis

   d. Assuring the parents that the surgeon is competent

8. The nurse is assessing the teaching needs of the parents of an 8-year-old boy with leukemia. Which of the following assessments would disclose a possible health literacy issue?

   a. The parents missed the last scheduled appointment

   b. The entire family is fluently bi-lingual

   c. The parents are taking notes on answers to their questions

   d. The mother seems to ask most of the questions regarding care

9. The nurse is teaching a 7-year-old girl about the tonsillectomy she will have. Which of the following techniques would be appropriate for this child? (Select all that apply)

   a. Allowing the child to do as much self-care as possible

   b. Explaining the procedure that will happen later in the day

   c. Offering choices of drinks and gelatin after the procedure

   d. Explaining that anesthesia is a lot like falling asleep

   e. Use plays or puppets to help explain the procedure

10. The nurse is educating the family of a 2-year-old Chinese boy with bronchiolitis about the disorder and its treatment. Which of the following actions, involving an interpreter, can jeopardize the family's trust?

    a. Allowing too little appointment time for the translation

    b. Using a person who is not a professional interpreter

    c. Asking the interpreter questions not meant for the family

    d. Using an older sibling to communicate with the parents

11. The child life nurse practitioner has been assigned to assist the hospitalized child and the child's parents. Which of the following are appropriate interventions for the child life nurse practitioner to perform? Select all that apply.

    a. The child life nurse practitioner talks to the family about a diagnostic test that the child is scheduled for later in the day

    b. The child life nurse practitioner gives the child an influenza vaccination

    c. The child life nurse practitioner starts the child's intravenous line

    d. The child life nurse practitioner shows the child where the pediatric play room is located

    e. The child life nurse practitioner speaks to the physician as the child's advocate

12. The child and her mother are receiving discharge instructions from the nurse. Which of the following statements by the child's mother are "red flags" that the mother may have poor literacy skills? Select all that apply.

    a. "I forgot my glasses today and can't seem to read this form."

    b. "I'm going to take a few notes while you're teaching us."

    c. "The receptionist told me that we missed another appointment."

    d. "I guess I just forgot to give her the medication the way you told me to."

    e. "I'm going to take these instructions home to read them."

13. The nurse is preparing to educate the child about a procedure that the child is scheduled for tomorrow morning. Which of the following techniques used by the nurse indicate the need for further education about communicating with a child? Select all that apply.

    a. The nurse stands at the foot of the child's bed while teaching the child.

    b. The nurse uses terms that the child will likely understand.

    c. The nurse speaks quickly.

    d. The nurse requests that the parents leave the room while the nurse educates the child.

    e. The nurse is patient with the child and looks for nonverbal cues.

14. The nurse is educating a young child about what to expect during an upcoming procedure. Which of the following statements by the nurse are appropriate to use? Select all that apply.

    a. "This little tube will go in your nose and down into your belly."

    b. "I'm going to give you this shot and it will put you to sleep."

    c. "You'll end up in 'ICU' where you'll wake up with some electrodes on your thorax."

    d. "When they come to get you, you'll get on a special rolling bed."

    e. "They're going to give you some special medicine to help the doctor see what's happening inside your belly."

15. The child has been admitted to a pediatric unit in a hospital. Which of the following nursing interventions indicate that atraumatic care principles are being used? Select all that apply.

    a. The nurse requests that parent assist the nurse by "holding the child down."

    b. The nurse applies a numbing cream prior to starting the child's intravenous line.

    c. The nurse asks the child if he would like to take a bath before or after he takes his medication.

    d. The nurse encourages the family to bring in the child's favorite stuffed animal from home.

    e. The nurse shows the parent how to unfold the chair in the child's room into a bed.

31

Health Supervision

Learning Objectives

- Describe the principles of health supervision.
- Identify challenges to health supervision for children with chronic illnesses.
- List the three components of a health supervision visit.
- Use instruments appropriately for developmental surveillance and screening of children.
- Demonstrate knowledge of the principles of immunization.
- Identify barriers to immunization.
- Identify the key components of health promotion.
- Describe the role of anticipatory guidance in health promotion.

SECTION I: ASSESSING YOUR UNDERSTANDING

Activity A FILL IN THE BLANKS

1. Because of the impact that hearing loss can have on _____, it is crucial that even slight hearing loss be identified by age 3 months.

2. Screening for iron deficiency at 6 months of age is important because the _____ iron stores of full-term infants are almost depleted.

3. If a client's family has difficulty accessing health care facilities, health promotion activities may be carried out in _____ settings such as schools and churches.

4. Health supervision has three components: screening, _____, and health promotion.

5. When obtaining an immunization history, asking _____ and where the last immunization was received provides more information than asking if immunizations are current.

6. The purpose of hyperlipidemia screening is to reduce the incidence of adult _____ disease.

7. The Weber test screens for hearing by assessing sound conducted via _____.

8. Vaccinations may be postponed if the child has a severe illness with high fever or _____, or has recently received blood products.

9. For children less than 3 years of age, vision screening based on the child's ability to _____ and follow objects.

10. _____ immunity is acquired when a person's own immune system generates the immune response.

Activity B MATCHING

Match the age and developmental warning sign in Column A with the possible developmental concern in Column B.

Column A

___ **1.** Rolls over before 3 months

___ **2.** Persistent head lag after 4 months

___ **3.** Not smiling at 6 months

___ **4.** Not babbling at 6 months

___ **5.** Not walking by 18 months

___ **6.** Hand dominance present before 18 months

Column B

a. Hemiplegia in opposite upper extremity

b. Hypertonia

c. Visual defect of attachment issue

d. Gross motor delay

e. Hypotonia

f. Hearing deficit

Match the developmental screening tool in Column A with the descriptive phrase in Column B.

Column A

___ **1.** Ages and Stages Questionnaire (ASQ)

___ **2.** Child Development Inventory (CDI)

___ **3.** Denver II

___ **4.** Goodenough Harris Drawing Test

___ **5.** Parent's Evaluation of Developmental Status (PEDS)

Column B

a. Simple questions about infant, toddler, or preschooler behaviors

b. Uses props provided in kit such as a baby doll, ball, and crayons to assess personal–social, fine motor–adaptive, language and gross motor skills

c. Assesses communication, gross and fine motor, personal–social, and problems-solving skills

d. Screens for developmental, behavioral, and family issues. Tool is available in Spanish.

e. Nonverbal screen for mental ability

Match the vision screening tool in Column A with the descriptive phrase in Column B.

Column A

___ **1.** Color Vision Testing Made Easy (CVTME)

___ **2.** Ishihara

___ **3.** LEA symbols or Allen figures

___ **4.** Snellen letters or numbers

___ **5.** Tumbling E

Column B

a. Uses pictures instead of the alphabet

b. Shapes embedded in dots

c. Used to assess the preschooler by asking him to point the direction the letter is pointing

d. Numbers hidden in dots

e. Used in children who know the alphabet

Activity C SEQUENCING

Beginning with an infant who is between birth and 3 months, and progressing in age, place the following developmental warning signs in sequential order.

1. Head lag disappears

2. Uses spoon or crayon

3. Uses imitative play

4. Rolls over

5. Says first word

6. Primitive reflex disappears

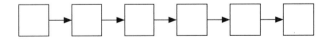

Activity D SHORT ANSWERS

Briefly answer the following.

1. Describe the proper technique for doing the Weber test, including what should be heard and where.

_____

_____

_____

2. What conditions seen in parents or grandparents who are less than 55 years of age would suggest screening for hyperlipidemia in the children?

_____

_____

_____

3. Describe the process of screening for hearing loss in older children, beginning with a history from the primary caregivers.

_____

_____

_____

4. Describe the potential impact of iron deficiency in children. During what periods of time is a child at the greatest risk for the development of the condition?

_____

_____

_____

5. Discuss the recommendations for screening children for hypertension. What factors increase the risk for the development of this condition?

_____

_____

_____

SECTION II: APPLYING YOUR KNOWLEDGE

Activity E CASE STUDY 1

Consider the scenario and answer the questions.

Jasmine Chase, a 15-year-old female, is seen in your clinic for her annual exam. During this health supervision visit, Jasmine expresses concerns about her weight. She states she has been attempting to diet and has reduced her number of meals a day by skipping breakfast. She also decided to give up meat, fish, and poultry, and eats mostly salads for lunch and dinner.

1. During the health interview and exam, what information do you want to elicit?

_____

_____

2. What screening test may be warranted for Jasmine and why?

_____

_____

_____

3. During today's exam, you determine Jasmine's height is 5 feet and her weight is 150 pounds. What can you do to help promote a healthy weight for Jasmine?

_____

_____

_____

CASE STUDY 2

Consider the scenario and answer the questions.

Claire Rosemount is a 5-year-old female who was recently diagnosed with Type I diabetes mellitus. Your clinic has been her medical home since birth. Health supervision of a child with a chronic illness can be challenging.

1. What can nurses do to meet these challenges and ensure proper care for Claire and other children with chronic illnesses?

_____

_____

_____

SECTION III: PRACTICING FOR NCLEX

Activity F NCLEX-STYLE QUESTIONS

Answer the following questions.

1. During the health history of a 2-month-old infant, the nurse identified a risk factor for developmental delay and is preparing to screen the child's development. Which of the following risks did the nurse find?

   a. The child had neonatal conjunctivitis

   b. The parents are both in college

   c. The child was born at 36 weeks

   d. The child has small eyes and chin

2. The nurse is promoting achieving the benefits of a healthy weight to an overweight 12-year-old child and her parents. Which of the following approaches is best?

   a. Showing the family the appropriate weight for the child

   b. Asking what activities she enjoys such as dance or sports

   c. Suggesting that the child join a little league softball team

   d. Pointing out fattening foods and excesses in their diet

3. The nurse is discussing Varicella immunization with a mother who is reluctant about vaccinating her 13-month-old because she feels it is "not necessary." Which of the following comments will be most persuasive for immunization?

   a. "Mild reactions occur in 5% to 10% of children."

   b. "Varicella is a highly contagious herpes virus."

   c. "Children not immunized are at risk if exposed to the disease."

   d. "Risk of Varicella is greater than the risk of vaccine."

4. The nurse is doing a health history for a 14-year-old boy during a health supervision visit. The boy says he has outgrown his clothes recently. Which of the following conditions needs to be checked for based on this information?

   a. Developmental problems

   b. Hyperlipidemia

   c. Iron deficiency anemia

   d. Systemic hypertension

5. A mother and her 2-week-old infant have arrived for a health supervision visit. Which of the following activities will the nurse perform?

   a. Assess the child for an upper respiratory infection

   b. Take a health history for a minor injury

   c. Administer a Varicella injection

   d. Warn against putting the baby to bed with a bottle

6. During a physical assessment of a 6-year-old child, the nurse observes the child has lost a tooth and uses the opportunity to promote oral health care. Which of the following comments would be included in this discussion?

   a. "Oral health can affect general health."

   b. "Fluoridated water has significantly reduced cavities."

   c. "Try to keep the child's hands out of the mouth."

   d. "Limit the amount of soft drinks in the child's diet."

7. The mother of a 5-year-old with eczema is getting a check-up for her child before school starts. Which of the following will the nurse do during the visit?

   a. Change the bandage on a cut on the child's hand

   b. Assess how the family is coping with the chronic illness

   c. Discuss systemic corticosteroid therapy

   d. Assess the child's fluid volume

8. The nurse is performing a vision screening for 6-year-old child. Which of the following screening charts would be best for determining the child's ability to discriminate color?

   a. Snellen

   b. Ishihara

   c. Allen figures

   d. CVTME

9. The nurse is anticipating that health supervision for a 5-year-old child will be challenging. Which of the following indicators supports this concern?

   a. Grandparents play a significant role in the family

   b. The child has a number of chores and responsibilities

   c. The mother dotes on the child

   d. The home is in a high-crime neighborhood

10. During the health history, the parent of a 10-year-old child mentions the child seems to have trouble hearing. Which of the following tests is the nurse likely to use?

    a. Rinne test

    b. Whisper test

    c. Evoked otoacoustic emissions test

    d. Auditory brain stem response test

11. The nurse is collecting data from the mother of a 3-year-old child. Which of the following reports will warrant further follow-up?

   a. The child cannot stack five blocks

   b. The child cannot grasp a crayon with the thumb and fingers

   c. The child cannot copy a circle

   d. The child is not able to throw a ball overhand

12. The student nurse is preparing to assist the registered nurse to perform the Denver II screening test. Which of the items will the student nurse correctly plan to use with the assessment? Select all that apply.

   a. Ball

   b. Four plastic rings

   c. Doll

   d. Crayon

   e. Crackers

13. The mother of a 2-year-old child questions when she will need to initially have her child's vision screened. What information should be provided by the nurse?

   a. Vision screening begins at 2 years of age

   b. Vision screening begins at 2 ½ years of age

   c. Vision screening begins at 3 years of age

   d. Vision screening begins just prior to kindergarten

14. The nurse is counseling a child about the health benefits associated with breastfeeding. Which of the following statements by the child indicates understanding?

   a. "Breastfeeding my baby passes on a type of active immunity."

   b. "Breastfeeding my baby passes on passive immunity."

   c. "Breastfeeding my baby provides lifelong immunity against certain diseases."

   d. "Breastfeeding my baby will help to stimulate my baby's immune system to activate."

15. Which of the following children poses the greatest risk for elevated lead levels?

   a. A Caucasian child who is 2 years of age

   b. An African American child who is 18 months of age

   c. A Caucasian child who is 10 years of age

   d. An Asian child who is 2 years of age

CHAPTER 32

Health Assessment of Children

Learning Objectives

- Demonstrate an understanding of the appropriate health history to obtain from the child and the parent or primary caregiver.
- Individualize elements of the health history depending upon the age of the child.
- Discuss important concepts related to health assessment in children.
- Perform a health assessment using approaches that relate to the age and developmental stage of the child.
- Describe the appropriate sequence of the physical examination in the context of the child's developmental stage.
- Distinguish normal variations in the physical examination from differences that may indicate serious alterations in health status.
- Determine the sexual maturity of females and males based upon evaluation of the secondary sex characteristics.

SECTION I: ASSESSING YOUR UNDERSTANDING

Activity A FILL IN THE BLANKS

1. _____ is an acronym that means pupils are equal, round, reactive to light and accommodation.

2. _____ is the measure of body weight relative to height.

3. The _____ is the area on an infant's head that is not protected by skull bone.

4. Auscultation is listening with a _____.

5. When assessing the thorax and lungs, an inspiratory high pitched sound is referred to as audible _____.

6. During assessment of the newborn the nurse notes small white papules on the infant's forehead, chin, nose, and cheeks. The nurse is correct in documenting this finding as _____.

7. Following inspection, _____ of the abdomen should be performed next during assessment of the abdomen.

Activity B LABELING

Consider the following figure.

Identify the point of maximal intensity (PMI) or apical impulse, for birth to 4 years, age 4 to 6 years, and 7 years and older.

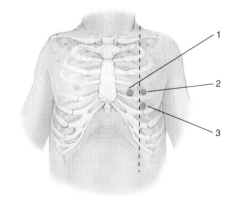

1. _____

2. _____

3. _____

Activity C **MATCHING**

Match the term in Column A with the proper definition in Column B.

Column A

____ **1.** Acrocyanosis

____ **2.** Cerumen

____ **3.** Lanugo

____ **4.** Stadiometer

____ **5.** Accommodation

Column B

a. Soft downy hair found on the newborn's body

b. Ability of the eyes to focus at different distances

c. Transient blueness in the hands and feet

d. Instrument to measure standing height

e. Waxy substance normally found lubricating and protecting the external ear canal

Activity D **SEQUENCING**

Place the following questions in the health interview of an adolescent in the proper sequence in the boxes provided below:

1. Are you sexually active?

2. What is your name?

3. What can I help you with today?

4. Do you have any allergies?

☐ → ☐ → ☐ → ☐

Activity E **SHORT ANSWERS**

Briefly answer the following.

1. Briefly describe the six grades of heart murmurs in children.

_____

_____

_____

2. Differentiate between ecchymosis, petechiae, and purpura.

_____

_____

3. Briefly describe the expected appearance of the healthy ear canal and tympanic membrane.

_____

_____

4. How does the heart rate vary according to a child's age?

_____

_____

5. What are some possible reasons for inaccurate pulse oximetry readings?

_____

_____

_____

6. Identify four risk factors that would indicate the need to assess the blood pressure of a child under the age of 3 years.

_____

_____

_____

SECTION II: APPLYING YOUR KNOWLEDGE

Activity F CASE STUDY

Consider the scenario and answer the questions.

As the nurse on a pediatric unit you are assigned to care for three children. You receive the following information on each child in report. Based on this information, rank in order of priority when to assess each child. Provide rationale for your answers.

1. A 5-year-old hospitalized with an acute asthma attack. Vital signs are: heart rate 124, respiratory rate 28 to 30, blood pressure 93/48, and axillary temperature of 98.6F.

   _____

   _____

   _____

2. A 3-month-old hospitalized for rule out sepsis secondary to fever. Vital signs are: heart rate 165, respiratory rate 34, blood pressure 108/64, and rectal temperature of 102.5F taken immediately before report. No intervention was initiated.

   _____

   _____

   _____

3. A 7-month-old hospitalized with pneumonia. Vital signs are: heart rate of 165 with brief episodes of dropping into the 60's during the previous shift, respiratory rate of 78, blood pressure 112/72, and axillary temperature of 99.5F.

   _____

   _____

   _____

SECTION III: PRACTICING FOR NCLEX

Activity G NCLEX-STYLE QUESTIONS

Answer the following questions.

1. The nurse is examining the genitals of a healthy newborn girl. The nurse would expect to observe which of the following normal findings?

   a. Swollen labia minora

   b. Lesions on the external genitalia

   c. Labial adhesions

   d. Swollen labia majora

2. The nurse is caring for a 13-year-old girl. As part of a routine health assessment the nurse needs to address areas relating to sexuality and substance abuse. Which of the following should the nurse say first to encourage communication?

   a. Do you smoke cigarettes or marijuana?

   b. I promise not to tell your mother any of your responses.

   c. Tell me about some of your current activities at school.

   d. Are you considering sexual activity?

3. The nurse is caring for a 10-year-old girl and is trying to obtain clues about the child's state of physical, emotional, and moral development. Which of the following questions would most likely elicit the desired information?

   a. "Do you like your school and your teacher?"

   b. "Would you say that you are a good student?"

   c. "Tell me about your favorite activity at school?"

   d. "Do you have a lot of friends at school?"

4. A nurse is caring for a very shy 4-year-old girl. During the course of a well-child assessment the nurse must take the girl's blood pressure. Which of the following is the best approach?

   a. "May I take your blood pressure?"

   b. "Your sister did a great job when I took hers"

   c. "Help me take your dolls blood pressure"

   d. "Will you let me put this cuff on your arm?"

5. The nurse is preparing to see a 14-month-old child and needs to establish the chief complaint or purpose of the visit. Which of the following would be the best approach with the parents?

   a. "What is your chief complaint?"

   b. "What can I help you with today?"

   c. "Is your child feeling sick?"

   d. "Has your child been exposed to infectious agents?"

6. A nurse is conducting a physical examination of an uncooperative preschooler. In order to encourage deep breathing during lung auscultation what could the nurse say?

   a. "You must breathe deeply so I can hear your lungs"

   b. "You may not leave until I listen to your breathing"

   c. "Do you think you can blow out my light bulb on this pen?"

   d. "Do you want your mother to listen to your lungs?"

7. The nurse is conducting a physical examination of a healthy 6-year-old. Which of the following would the nurse do first?

   a. Observe the skin for its overall color and characteristics.

   b. Tap with the knee with a reflex hammer to check for deep tendon reflexes.

   c. Palpate the skin for texture and hydration status.

   d. Auscultate the heart, lungs, and the abdomen.

8. A nurse is assessing an infant's reflexes. The nurse places his or her thumb to the ball of the infant's foot to elicit which reflex?

   a. Parachute

   b. Plantar grasp

   c. Babinski

   d. Palmar grasp

9. The emergency department nurse is caring for a child who is showing signs of anaphylaxis. The nurse evaluates how comprehensive the history of the child should be and determines that which action takes priority?

   a. Taking a problem-focused history

   b. Obtaining a complete and detailed history

   c. Stabilizing the child's physical status

   d. Getting the child's history from other providers

10. The nurse is conducting a physical examination of a 5-year-old girl. The nurse asks the girl to stand still with her eyes closed and arms down by her side. The girl immediately begins to lean. This tells the nurse which information?

    a. The child has poor coordination and poor balance

    b. The child warrants further testing for cerebellar dysfunction

    c. The child has a negative Romberg test; no further testing is necessary

    d. The child has a possible inner ear infection

11. The nurse needs to calculate the child's body mass index (BMI). The child's weight is 42 kg and is 142 cm tall. Calculate the child's BMI using the metric method, round answer to the nearest whole number.

12. The experienced nurse is assessing the child's lungs. Rank the following steps in the proper order of assessment:

    a. The nurse percusses over the child's lungs.

    b. The nurse visually inspects the child's thorax.

    c. The nurse palpates the child's thorax.

    d. The nurse auscultates the child's lungs.

CHAPTER 33

Caring for Children in Diverse Settings

Learning Objectives

- Identify the major stressors of illness and hospitalization for children.
- Identify the reactions and responses of children and their families during illness and hospitalization.
- Explain the factors that influence the reactions and responses of children and their families during illness and hospitalization.
- Describe the nursing care that minimizes stressors for children who are ill or hospitalized.
- Discuss the major components of admission for children to the hospital.
- Discuss appropriate safety measures to use when caring for children of all ages.
- Review nursing responsibilities related to child discharge from the hospital.
- Describe the various roles of community and home care nurses.
- Discuss the variety of settings in which community-based care occurs.
- Discuss the advantages and disadvantages of home health care.

SECTION I: ASSESSING YOUR UNDERSTANDING

Activity A FILL IN THE BLANKS

1. Therapeutic _____ is the use of a holding position that promotes close physical contact between the child and a parent or caregiver that is used when the child needs to remain still for procedures such as IV insertion.

2. Restraints should be checked every _____ minutes following initial placement, then every hour for proper placement.

3. A good time to assess the skin is during _____ time.

4. Forcing a child to _____ can exacerbate any nausea or vomiting.

5. _____ play allows a child to express his or her feelings and fears, as well as providing a means to promote energy expenditure.

6. Nurses in the school setting develop _____ to plan how the school staff will collaborate with the student and family in meeting the needs of students with complex health care issues.

7. _____ nurses focus on health supervision services and connecting children to needed community resources.

Activity B MATCHING

Match the term in Column A with the proper definition in Column B.

Column A	Column B
____ **1.** Denial	**a.** Increased stimulation for the child
____ **2.** Regression	**b.** Defense mechanism used by children to avoid unpleasant realities
____ **3.** Sensory overload	**c.** Distress related to being removed from primary caregivers and familiar surroundings
____ **4.** Separation anxiety	**d.** Lack of stimulation
____ **5.** Sensory deprivation	**e.** Defense mechanism used by children to avoid dealing with conflict by returning to a previous stage that may be more comfortable to the child

Activity C SEQUENCING

Place the three stages of separation anxiety in the proper sequence.

1. Despair

2. Denial

3. Protest

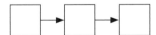

Activity D SHORT ANSWERS

Briefly answer the following.

1. How can the nurse address and minimize separation anxiety in the hospitalized child?

_____

_____

_____

2. When does discharge planning begin? Why?

_____

_____

_____

3. What are some common behaviors or methods children use for coping with hospitalization?

_____

_____

_____

4. What are the most common reasons for children to be hospitalized?

_____

_____

_____

5. What are some ways the home care nurse can establish a trusting relationship with the child and caregivers?

_____

_____

_____

SECTION II: APPLYING YOUR KNOWLEDGE

Activity E CASE STUDY

Consider the scenario and answer the questions.

A variety of reactions and responses are seen as a result of the stressors children experience in relation to hospitalization. Nurses often spend more time with children and their families compared to other physicians during hospitalization. Therefore, it is essential that nurses establish strategies to care and intervene in order to help children cope with their experience. Nurses must examine effects of hospitalization within the child's developmental stage and understand the reactions and responses of the child and family to hospitalization.

While working on the pediatric unit, your child care assignment involves children of differing developmental ages. Read the below reactions and identify interventions and rationales for each of the following children in your care.

1. Leslie Lucas, a 6-month-old female with a club foot repair, is hospitalized post-surgery. She has been irritable and difficult to console.

   _____

   _____

   _____

2. Eli Castle, an 18-month-old male admitted with pneumonia, has not slept more than 1 hour without waking.

   _____

   _____

   _____

3. Amelia Lionhart, a 4-year-old female admitted with dehydration, repeatedly wakes up crying after having nightmares.

   _____

   _____

   _____

4. Jamal Anderson, a 10-year-old male, hospitalized secondary to asthma, has eaten very little from his meal trays for the past few days.

   _____

   _____

   _____

5. Cheryl Erikson, a 16-year-old female with lymphoma, expresses a desire to be left alone in her darkened room.

   _____

   _____

   _____

SECTION III: PRACTICING FOR NCLEX

Activity F NCLEX-STYLE QUESTIONS

Answer the following questions.

1. The nurse is caring for an 18-month-old boy hospitalized with a gastrointestinal disorder. The nurse knows that the child is at risk for separation anxiety. The nurse understands to watch carefully for which of the following behaviors, indicating that the first phase of separation anxiety is occurring?

   a. Crying and acting out

   b. Embracing others who attempt to comfort him

   c. Disinterest in play and food

   d. Exhibiting apathy and withdrawing from others

2. The nurse is caring for a preschooler who is hospitalized with a suspected blood disorder and receives an order to draw a blood sample. Which of the following would be the best way to approach the child for this procedure?

   a. "I need to take some blood."

   b. "We need to put a little hole in your arm."

   c. "I need to remove a little blood."

   d. "Why don't you sit on your mom's lap?"

3. The nurse is caring for a child hospitalized with complications from asthma. Which of the following statements by the parents indicates a need for careful observation of the child's anxiety level?

   a. "My mother passed away here after surgery."

   b. "Our twins were born here 18 months ago."

   c. "My son was born at this hospital."

   d. "We attended a 'living with asthma' class here."

4. A nurse is caring for a 6-year-old boy hospitalized due to an infection requiring intravenous antibiotic therapy. The child's motor activity is restricted and he is acting out, yelling, kicking, and screaming. Which of the following responses by the nurse would help promote positive coping?

   a. "Your medicine is the only way you will get better."

   b. "Let me explain why you need to sit still."

   c. "Would you like to read or play video games?"

   d. "Do I need to call your parents?"

5. A nurse is telling the parents how to help their 10-year-old daughter deal with an extended hospital stay due to surgery, followed by traction. Which of the following responses indicates a need for further teaching?

   a. "I should not tell her how long she will be here."

   b. "She will watch our reactions carefully."

   c. "We must prepare her in advance."

   d. "She will be sensitive to our concerns."

6. A nurse is preparing to admit a child for a tonsillectomy. How should the nurse establish rapport?

   a. "Let's take a look at your tonsils."

   b. "Do you understand why you are here?"

   c. "Are you scared about having your tonsils out?"

   d. "Tell me about your cute stuffed dog you have."

7. The nurse is preparing to admit a 4-year-old who will be having tympanostomy tubes placed in both ears. Which of the following strategies would most likely reduce the child's fears of the procedure?

   a. "The doctor is going to insert tympanostomy tubes in your ears"

   b. "Don't worry, you will be asleep the whole time"

   c. "Let me show you how tiny these tubes are"

   d. "Let me show you the operating room"

8. A nurse is developing a preoperative plan of care for a 2-year-old. The nurse understands to pay particular attention to which of the child's age-related fears?

   a. Separation from friends

   b. Separation from parents

   c. Loss of control

   d. Loss of independence

9. The nurse is providing teaching for the parents of a 7-year-old boy, scheduled for surgery, to help prepare the child for hospitalization. Which of the following statements by the parents indicates a need for further teaching?

   a. "We should talk about going to the hospital and what it will be like coming home"

   b. "We should visit the hospital and go through the preadmission tour in advance"

   c. "It is best to wait and let her bring up the surgery or any questions she has"

   d. "It is a good idea to read stories about experiences with hospitals or surgery"

10. The nurse is caring for a 7-year-old boy in a body cast. He is shy and seems fearful of the numerous personnel in and out of his room. How can the nurse help reduce his fear?

    a. Remind the boy he will be out of the hospital and going home soon.

    b. Encourage the boy's parents to stay with him at all times to reduce his fears.

    c. Write the name of his nurse on a board and identify all staff on each shift, every day.

    d. Tell him not to worry; explain that everyone is here to care for him.

11. The nurse is providing care for a hospitalized child. Rank the following phases in the order of occurrence based on the nurse's statements.

    a. "Let's sit over here and play a game of 'Go Fish'."

    b. "You handled that procedure so well! Would you like me to get Mr. Snuggles for you?"

    c. "Would you like your medicine before or after your mom helps take a bath?"

    d. "Hi, my name is Cindy and I'm going to be your nurse for today."

12. The nurse has applied a restraint to the child's right wrist to prevent the child from pulling out an intravenous line. Which of the following assessment findings are important to note to ensure that there is proper circulation to the child's right arm?

    a. Capillary refill is less than 2 seconds in upper extremities bilaterally

    b. Fingers are pink and warm bilaterally

    c. Lungs are clear throughout

    d. Radial pulses are easily palpable bilaterally

    e. Bowel sounds present in all four quadrants

13. The student nurse is assisting the more experienced pediatric nurse. Which of the following statements by the student indicate further education is required?

    a. "Could you give the nauseated child some medicine before it is time for him to start thinking about ordering lunch?"

    b. "I'm going to redress the child's IV site while she is in the playroom."

    c. "I took our new teenaged child down to show him the playroom."

    d. "It would be easy to perform a straight catheterization while the baby is in his crib."

    e. "I told the child's mom to go ahead and bring in his blanket and stuffed animal."

14. The nurse is documenting the child's intake. The child ate four cups of ice during this shift. How many cups of fluid did the child ingest?

    a. 4 cups of fluid

    b. 1 cup of fluid

    c. ½ cup of fluid

    d. 2 cups of fluid

Caring for the Special Needs Child

Learning Objectives

- Analyze the impact that being a child with special needs has on the child and family.
- Identify anticipated times when the child and family will require additional support.
- Describe ways that nurses assist children with special needs and their families to obtain optimal functioning.
- Discuss early intervention and public school education for the special needs child.
- Plan for transition of the special needs child from the inpatient facility to the home, and from pediatric to adult medical care.
- Discuss key elements related to pediatric end-of-life care.
- Differentiate developmental responses to death and appropriate interventions.

SECTION I: ASSESSING YOUR UNDERSTANDING

Activity A FILL IN THE BLANKS

1. The Individuals with Disabilities Education Act (IDEA) of 2004 mandates government-funded care coordination and special education for children up to _____ years of age.

2. _____ care provides an opportunity for families to take a break from the daily intensive care giving responsibilities.

3. When working with a dying child, always focus on the _____ as the unit of care.

4. _____ remains the leading cause of death from disease in all children over the age of 1 year.

5. A _____ consent is necessary for organ donation, so the family must be appropriately informed and educated.

6. _____ care provides the best quality of life possible at the end of life while alleviating physical, psychological, emotional, and spiritual suffering.

7. During the last stages of a terminal illness, _____ care allows for family-centered care in the child's home or appropriate facility.

Activity B   MATCHING

Match the child's stage in Column A with their needs as they go through the dying process in Column B.

Column A

_____ **1.** Toddler (1 to 3 years)

_____ **2.** 3 to 5 years

_____ **3.** 5 to 10 years

_____ **4.** 10 to 14 years

_____ **5.** 14 to 18 years

Column B

a. Need to know death is not a punishment; need to know that although they will be missed, the family will function without them

b. Specific honest details; old enough to help in some decision making

c. Reinforcement of self-esteem; privacy and time alone, time with peers; participation in decision making

d. Support through honest, detailed explanations; wants to feel truly involved and listened to

e. Need familiarity, routine, favorite toys and physical comfort

Activity C   SEQUENCING

Place the Adolescent Health Transition Project (AHTP) recommendations schedule for transitioning child care to adult care for the child with special health care needs in the proper sequence.

1. Explore health care financing for young adults. If needed, notify the local division of vocational rehabilitation by the autumn before the teen is to graduate from high school of the impending transition. Initiate guardianship procedures if appropriate.

2. Ensure that a transition plan is initiated and that the individualized education plan (IEP) reflects post-high school plans.

3. Ensure that the young adult has registered with the Division of Developmental Disabilities for adult services if applicable.

4. Notify the teen that all rights transfer to him or her at the age of majority. Check the teen's eligibility for SSI the month the child turns 18. Determine if the child is eligible for SSI work incentives.

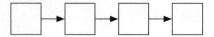

Activity D   SHORT ANSWERS

Briefly answer the following.

1. Name four different complementary therapies that might be adopted for treatment of children with chronic illness.

_____

_____

_____

2. Explain dietary requirements and how they are best met for formerly premature infants who need to "catch-up" on weight.

_____

_____

_____

3. How should the nurse explain DNR orders (do not resuscitate) to a family when they are trying to make this decision regarding a terminally ill child?

_____

_____

_____

4. List the principles that the Last Acts Palliative Care Task Force has established regarding the care of children with a terminal illness.

_____

_____

_____

5. Since the body requires less nutrition during the dying process, what are some important care measures to keep in mind for the dying child?

_____

_____

_____

SECTION II: APPLYING YOUR KNOWLEDGE

Activity E CASE STUDY

Consider the scenario and answer the questions.

1. Preet Singh is a 2-year-old boy born at 27 weeks gestation and has a history of hydrocephalus and developmental delay. What role can the nurse play in assisting the family to obtain optimal functioning?

   _____

   _____

   _____

2. Georgia Lansing, a 7-year-old girl, has been diagnosed with lymphoma. She recently had a relapse and has not responded to treatment. The family has decided on palliative care. Discuss ways the nurse can support the dying child and family.

   Include the type of support and education that the dying child needs according to the developmental stage.

   _____

   _____

   _____

SECTION III: PRACTICING FOR NCLEX

Activity F NCLEX-STYLE QUESTIONS

Answer the following questions.

1. The nurse is caring for the family of a medically fragile 2-year-old girl. Which activity is most effective in building a therapeutic relationship?
   a. Helping access an early intervention program.
   b. Teaching physiotherapy techniques.
   c. Listening to parents' triumphs and failures.
   d. Getting free samples of the child's medications.

2. A 14-year-old boy is aware that he is dying. Which action best meets the child's need for self-esteem and sense of worth?
   a. Providing full participation in decision making.
   b. Initiating conversations about his feelings.
   c. Giving direct, honest answers to his questions.
   d. Listening to his fears and concerns about dying.

3. A 10-year-old girl with bone cancer is near death. Which action would best minimize her 8-year-old sister's anxiety?
   a. Correcting her when she says her sister won't die.
   b. Telling her that her sister won't need food any more.
   c. Discouraging the child's questions about death.
   d. Explaining how the morphine drip works.

4. A 15-year-old boy with special needs is attending high school. Which nursing intervention will be most beneficial to his education?
   a. Collaborating with the school nurse about his care.
   b. Serving on his individualized education plan (IEP) committee.
   c. Advocating for financial aid for a motorized wheelchair.
   d. Assessing how attending school will affect his health.

5. A 6-month-old girl is significantly underweight. Which assessment finding will point to an inorganic cause of failure to thrive?
   a. Examining to see if the infant refuses the nipple.
   b. Observing to see if the child avoids eye contact.
   c. Asking the mother if the birth was premature.
   d. Checking the health history for risk factors.

6. The nurse is caring for the family of a 9-year-old boy with cerebral palsy. Which intervention will best improve communication between the nurse and the family?

a. Giving direct, understandable answers.

b. Sharing cell phone numbers with the parents.

c. Using reflective listening techniques.

d. Saying the same thing in different ways.

7. It is difficult for the father of a technologically dependent 7-year-old girl to leave his work. Which nursing intervention would best involve him in family-centered care?

a. Leave a voice mail for the father at work.

b. Email a status report to the father's office.

c. Urge the father to come to the hospital at lunch.

d. Schedule education sessions in the evening.

8. The nurse is caring for the family of a medically fragile child in the hospital. Which intervention is most important to the parents?

a. Educating the parents about the course of treatment.

b. Evaluating the emotional strength of the parents.

c. Preparing a list of supplies the family will need.

d. Assessing the adequacy of the home environment.

9. The nurse at a hospice care facility is caring for a 12-year-old girl. Which intervention best meets the needs of this child?

a. Assuring her the illness is not her fault.

b. Urging her to invite her friends to visit.

c. Acting as the child's personal confidant.

d. Explaining her condition to her in detail.

10. The nurse is caring for a 15-year-old boy with cystic fibrosis. Which intervention will help avert risky behavior?

a. Assessing for signs of depression.

b. Encouraging participation in activities.

c. Monitoring compliance with treatment.

d. Urging that he join a support group.

11. The infant was born prematurely. Which of the following assessment findings may indicate that the child is suffering from a medical condition associated with being born prematurely?

a. The child's parents stated that the child began losing baby teeth earlier than their other children.

b. The child's hearing is not within normal limits and the child requires a hearing aid.

c. The child eyes deviate inward.

d. The child is noted to be above the 95th percentile for height and at the 85th percentile for weight.

e. The child started speaking multi-word sentences at 18 months old.

12. The infant was born at 32 weeks gestation and is now 9 months old. What is the infant's corrected age?

13. The child has been hospitalized for failure to thrive. The child weighs 23.2 kg. The child is to receive 120 kilocalories per kg of weight per day. How many kilocalories should the child eat each day?

14. Rank the following psychosocial development stages in the proper order of occurrence.

a. Initiative

b. Autonomy

c. Industry

d. Trust

15. The child has been diagnosed with vulnerable child syndrome. Which of the following statements by the child's parent is associated with the presence of this syndrome?

   a. "I discipline all of three of my kids very fairly."

   b. "He was always a sweet and happy baby."

   c. "For the first few weeks of his life, he was so yellow I was afraid he would glow."

   d. "When she was a toddler she developed meningitis and the doctors told me they didn't think she'd make it."

   e. "She was born with a cleft lip and palate. I was so afraid she wasn't getting enough formula."

Key Pediatric Nursing Interventions

Learning Objectives

- Describe the "eight rights" of pediatric medication administration.
- Explain the physiologic differences in children affecting a medication's pharmacodynamic and pharmacokinetic properties.
- Accurately determine recommended pediatric medication doses.
- Demonstrate the proper technique for administering medication to children via the oral, rectal, ophthalmic, otic, intravenous, intramuscular, and subcutaneous routes.
- Integrate the concepts of atraumatic care in medication administration for children.
- Identify the preferred sites for peripheral and central intravenous medication administration.
- Describe nursing management related to maintenance of intravenous infusions in children, as well as prevention of complications.
- Explain nursing care related to enteral tube feedings.
- Describe nursing management of the child receiving total parenteral nutrition.

SECTION I: ASSESSING YOUR UNDERSTANDING

Activity A FILL IN THE BLANKS

1. A Port-A-Cath is a type of _____ central venous access device.

2. _____ is the behavior of a medication at the cellular level.

3. Encouraging the child to count aloud or asking a child to blow bubbles during a medical procedure is a method to create a _____.

4. When inserting a rectal suppository for any child under the age of 3, the nurse should use the _____ finger.

5. _____ typically occurs with too rapid cessation of TPN (total parenteral nutrition).

6. _____ tubes are inserted through the nose and terminate in the stomach and are used for short-term enteral feeding.

7. Administration of medication into the eyes is referred to as the _____ route.

Activity B LABELING

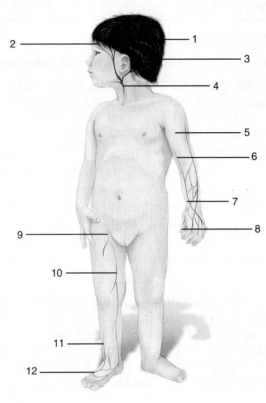

1. _____
2. _____
3. _____
4. _____
5. _____
6. _____
7. _____
8. _____
9. _____
10. _____
11. _____
12. _____

Provide labels for the preferred peripheral sites for IV insertion.

a. Dorsal arch
b. Great saphenous
c. Basilic
d. Superficial temporal
e. Femoral
f. Cephalic
g. Frontal
h. Dorsal arch
i. External jugular
j. Occipital
k. Digital
l. Small saphenous

Activity C MATCHING

Match the term in Column A with the proper definition in Column B.

Column A

____ **1.** Gavage feedings

____ **2.** Enteral nutrition

____ **3.** Bolus feeding

____ **4.** Parenteral nutrition

____ **5.** Residual

Column B

a. Nutrition delivered directly into the intestinal tract

b. Administration of a specified feeding solution at specific intervals, usually over a short period of time

c. Intravenous delivery of nutritional substances

d. The amounts of contents remaining in the stomach indicating gastric emptying time

e. Feeding administered via a tube into the stomach or intestines

Activity D SEQUENCING

Place the steps of administering a gavage enteral feeding in the proper sequence.

1. Measure the amount of gastric residual.

2. Flush the tube with water and administer the feeding.

3. Check tube for placement.

4. Flush the tube with water.

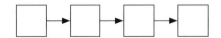

Activity E SHORT ANSWERS

Briefly answer the following.

1. What is the rationale for performing all invasive procedures outside of the child's hospital room?

_____

_____

_____

2. There are eight rights of pediatric medication administration. How can the nurse ensure that the medication is being administered to the right child?

_____

_____

_____

3. What are the key measures to reduce the risk of complications related to the use of central venous access devices and total parenteral nutrition?

_____

_____

_____

4. What are the eight rights of medication administration for children?

_____

_____

_____

5. Briefly explain the methods for verifying proper feeding tube placement.

_____

_____

_____

SECTION II: APPLYING YOUR KNOWLEDGE

Activity F CASE STUDY

Consider the scenario and answer the questions.

Jennifer Michels, a 7-month-old, has a rectal temperature of 102.5 F. As the nurse caring for her, you are preparing to administer oral acetaminophen per the physicians order. Jennifer's weight is 15 lbs.

1. Discuss the steps you will take for administering a PRN dose of oral acetaminophen for Jennifer. Include rationale for your actions.

_____

_____

_____

2. The physician ordered 70 mg po every 4 hours for fever or discomfort. Calculate the correct dose for Jennifer's weight based on recommended dosing for acetaminophen of 10 to 15 mg/kg every 4 to 6 hours. Is the physician's order a safe and therapeutic dose?

_____

_____

_____

3. Obtain the amount to be drawn up using a concentration of acetaminophen infant drops 80 mg/0.8 ml.

_____

_____

_____

SECTION III: PRACTICING FOR NCLEX

Activity G NCLEX-STYLE QUESTIONS

Answer the following questions.

1. The nurse is caring for a 4-year-old who requires a venipuncture. Which of the following explanations to prepare the child for the procedure is most appropriate?

   a. "The doctor will look at your blood to see why you are sick."

   b. "The doctor wants to see if you have strep throat."

   c. "The doctor needs to take your blood to see why you are sick."

   d. "The doctor needs to culture your blood to see if you have strep."

2. The nurse is caring for a child with an intravenous device in his hand. Which of the following signs would alert the nurse that infiltration is occurring?

   a. Warmth, redness

   b. Cool, puffy skin

   c. Induration

   d. Tender skin

3. The nurse is preparing to administer a medication via a syringe pump as ordered for a 2-month-old girl. What is the priority nursing action?

   a. Gather the medication

   b. Verify the medication order

   c. Gather the necessary equipment and supplies

   d. Wash hands and put on gloves

4. A nurse is teaching the parents of a 5-year-old boy who requires daily oral medication how to administer it. Which of the following responses indicates a need for further teaching?

   a. "I should never refer to the medicine as candy."

   b. "We should never bribe our child to take the medicine."

   c. "He needs to take his medicine or he will lose a privilege."

   d. "We checked that the medicine can be mixed with yogurt or applesauce."

5. A nurse is preparing to administer an ordered IM injection to an infant. The nurse knows that the most appropriate injection site for this child is the:

   a. Deltoid

   b. Ventrogluteal

   c. Dorsogluteal

   d. Vastus lateralis

6. The nurse is preparing to remove an IV device from the arm of a 6-year-old girl. Which of the following is the best approach to minimize fear and anxiety?

   a. "This won't be painful; you'll just feel a tug and a pinch."

   b. "The first step is for you to help me remove this dressing from your IV."

   c. "Be sure to keep your hands clear of the scissors so I don't cut you."

   d. "Please be a big girl and don't cry when I remove this."

7. The nurse is teaching the parents of a 5-month-old how to administer an oral antibiotic. Which of the following responses indicates a need for further teaching?

   a. "We can mix the antibiotics into his formula or food."

   b. "We can follow his medicine with some applesauce or yogurt."

   c. "We can place the medicine along the inside of his cheek."

   d. "We should not forcibly squirt the medication in the back of his throat."

8. A nurse is caring for a child who requires intravenous maintenance fluid. The child weighs 30 kg. The nurse calculates the child's daily maintenance fluid requirement to be:

   a. 1,500 mL

   b. 1,600 mL

   c. 1,700 mL

   d. 1,800 mL

9. The nurse is assessing the aspirate of a gavage feeding tube to confirm placement. Which of the following assessment findings indicates intestinal placement?

   a. Clear aspirate

   b. Yellow aspirate

   c. Tan aspirate

   d. Green aspirate

10. The nurse is preparing to administer medication to a 10-year-old who weighs 70 pounds. The prescribed single dose is 3 to 4 mg/kg per day. Which of the following is the appropriate dose range for this child?

    a. 96 to 128 mg

    b. 105 to 140 mg

    c. 210 to 280 mg

    d. 420 to 560 mg

11. The child weighs 47 pounds. How many kilograms does the child weigh? Round the answer to the nearest tenth.

12. The child weighs 27 kg. Using the following formula, calculate how many milliliters of intravenous fluids should be administered to the child in a 24 hour period.

Formula:

   100 milliliters per kilogram of body weight for the first 10 kilograms
   50 milliliters per kilogram of body weight for the next 10 kilograms
   20 milliliters per kilogram of body weight for the remainder of body weight in kilograms

13. The adolescent weighs 113 pounds. The nurse closely monitors the child's urine output. How many milliliters of urine is the least amount that the adolescent should make during an 8-hour shift? Round to the nearest whole number.

14. The nurse is calculating the urinary output for the infant. The infant's diaper weighed 40 grams prior to placing the diaper on the infant. After removal of the wet diaper, the diaper weighed 75 grams. How many milliliters of urine can the nurse document as urinary output?

15. Age affects how the medication is distributed throughout the body. Which of the following are factors that affect how medication distribution is altered in infants and young children? Select all that apply.

    a. Infants and young children have an increased percentage of water in their bodies

    b. Infants and young children have an increased percentage of body fat

    c. Infants and young children have an increased number of plasma proteins available for binding to drugs

    d. The blood–brain barrier in infants and young children does not easily allow permeation by many medications

    e. The livers in infants and young children are immature

CHAPTER 36

Pain Management in Children

Learning Objectives

- Identify the major physiologic events associated with the perception of pain.
- Discuss the factors that influence the pain response.
- Identify the developmental considerations of the effects and management of pain in the infant, toddler, preschooler, school-age child, and adolescent.
- Explain the principles of pain assessment as they relate to children.
- Understand the use of the various pain rating scales and physiologic monitoring for children.
- Establish a nursing care plan for children related to management of pain, including pharmacologic and nonpharmacologic techniques and strategies.

SECTION I: ASSESSING YOUR UNDERSTANDING

Activity A FILL IN THE BLANKS

1. Two of the most commonly used agents for conscious sedation are _____ and fentanyl.

2. EMLA should be applied _____ minutes before a superficial procedure such as a heel stick or venipuncture.

3. Conscious sedation is a medically controlled state of _____ consciousness.

4. _____ is considered the "gold standard" for all opioid agonists and is the drug to which all other opioids are compared.

5. Patient controlled analgesia is usually reserved for use by children _____ years of age and older.

6. The point at which an individual feels the lowest intensity of the painful stimulus is referred to as the _____.

7. _____ is the pain rating scale that is used for children that uses photographs of facial expressions.

Activity B MATCHING

Match the term in Column A with the proper definition in Column B.

Column A

___ 1. Somatic pain

___ 2. Transduction

___ 3. Nociceptive pain

___ 4. Neuromodulators

___ 5. Epidural

Column B

a. Process of nociceptor activation

b. Pain due to the activation of the A delta fibers and C fibers by noxious stimulant

c. Situated within the spinal canal, on or outside the dura mater

d. Pain that develops in the tissues

e. Substances that modify the perception of pain

Match the medication in Column A with its action in Column B.

Column A

_____ **1.** Morphine

_____ **2.** Pentazocine

_____ **3.** Ibuprofen

_____ **4.** Acetaminophen

Column B

a. Inhibition of prostaglandin synthesis

b. Opioid agonist acting primarily at μ receptor sites

c. Direct action of hypothalamic heat regulating center

d. Antagonist at μ receptor sites agonist at κ receptor sites

Activity C SEQUENCING

Place the physiologic events that lead to the sensation of pain in the proper sequence.

1. Modulation

2. Transmission

3. Transduction

4. Perception

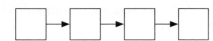

Activity D SHORT ANSWERS

Briefly answer the following.

1. What is the difference between superficial somatic pain and deep somatic pain?

_____

_____

_____

2. What are the three general principles that guide pain management in children?

_____

_____

_____

3. Which of the factors that influence a child's perception of pain can be changed?

_____

_____

_____

4. What is conscious sedation? What are the advantages of conscious sedation? What agents may be used to achieve conscious sedation?

_____

_____

_____

5. Discuss the administration of epidural anesthesia.

_____

_____

_____

SECTION II: APPLYING YOUR KNOWLEDGE

Activity E CASE STUDY

Owen Nelson, 6 months old, is admitted to your unit post club foot repair. His parents' are at the bedside and concerned about Owen's comfort. They state "We have heard that infants do not feel pain like adults do but we want to make sure Owen is not in pain. How do we do this?"

1. How would you address Owen's parents concerns?

_____

_____

_____

2. During your assessment you find that Owen is lying in his crib with his legs elevated, his face is relaxed, he appears restless but moves easily, cries occasionally but is consoled by his mother's or father's touch and voice. Using the appropriate pain assessment tool for Owen's age and development, assess Owen's pain level based on the above information. What further assessment information may be helpful in determining if Owen is in pain?

_____

_____

_____

3. Based on your above assessment, you intervene by providing pain medication to Owen per the physician's order to. What nonpharmacological interventions can you discuss with the parents to help decrease Owen's discomfort?

_____

_____

_____

SECTION III: PRACTICING FOR NCLEX

Activity F NCLEX-STYLE QUESTIONS

Answer the following questions.

1. The nurse is providing postsurgical care for a 5-year-old. The nurse knows to avoid which of the following questions when assessing the child's pain level?
   a. Would you say that the pain you are feeling is sharp or dull?
   b. Would you point to the cartoon face that best describes your pain?
   c. Would you point to the spot where your pain is?
   d. Would you please show me with photograph and number best describes your hurt?

2. The nurse is assisting with the administration of parenteral opioids for a child for an initial dose. What action should the nurse take first?
   a. Ensure naloxone is readily available
   b. Assess for any adverse reaction
   c. Assess the status of bowel sounds
   d. Premedicate with acetaminophen

3. The nurse is caring for a child who has received postoperative epidural analgesia. What is the priority nursing assessment?
   a. Urinary retention
   b. Pruritus
   c. Nausea and vomiting
   d. Respiratory depression

4. A nurse is applying EMLA as ordered. The nurse understands that EMLA is contraindicated in which of the following situations?
   a. Infants less than 6 weeks of age
   b. Children with darker skin
   c. Infants less than 12 months receiving methemoglobin-inducing agents
   d. Children undergoing venous cannulation or intramuscular injections

5. A nurse is caring for a 4-year-old child who is exhibiting extreme anxiety and behavior upset prior to receiving stitches for a deep chin laceration. Which of the following is the priority nursing intervention?
   a. Ensuring that emergency equipment is readily available
   b. Serving as an advocate for the family to ensure appropriate pharmacologic agents are chosen
   c. Conducting an initial assessment of pain to serve as a baseline from which options for relief can be chosen
   d. Ensuring the lighting is adequate for the procedure but not so bright to cause discomfort

6. A nurse is interviewing the mother of a sleeping 10-year-old girl in order to assess the level of the child's postoperative pain. Which of the following comments would trigger additional questions and necessitate further teaching?
   a. "She is asleep, so she must not be in pain."
   b. "She has never had surgery before."
   c. "She is very articulate and will tell you how she feels."
   d. "She has a very easy going temperament."

7. The nurse is providing teaching the parents of a 9-year-old boy with episodes of chronic pain how to help him manage his pain nonpharmacologically. Which of the following statements indicates a need for further teaching?
   a. "We should perform the techniques along with him."
   b. "We should start the method as soon as he feels pain."
   c. "We need to identify the ways in which he shows pain."
   d. "We should select a method that he likes the best."

8. A nurse is assessing the pain level of an infant. Which of the following findings is not a typical physiologic indicator of pain?

   a. Decreased oxygen saturation

   b. Decreased heart rate

   c. Palmar sweating

   d. Plantar sweating

9. The nurse is preparing to assess the postsurgical pain level of a 6-year-old. The child has appeared unwilling or unable to accurately report his pain level. Which of the following assessment tools would be most appropriate for this child?

   a. FACES Pain Rating Scale

   b. FLACC Behavioral scale

   c. Oucher Pain rating

   d. Visual Analog and Numerical scales

10. The nurse is preparing to assess the pain of a developmentally and cognitively delayed 8-year-old. Which of the pain rating scales should the nurse choose?

    a. FACES pain rating scale

    b. Word Graphic Rating Scale

    c. Adolescent Pediatric Pain Tool

    d. Visual Analog and Numerical Scales

11. The nurse is caring for a patient who is 30 weeks gestation. The patient is preparing to undergo an invasive procedure on her unborn baby. The patient discusses the likelihood that her fetus will experience pain. Which of the following statements indicates an understanding of the influences of stimuli on the unborn fetus?

    a. "Unborn babies do not feel painful sensations."

    b. "Since my child is a boy the amount of pain that he can experience is lessened."

    c. "Painful stimuli can be felt by the fetus only in the hours prior to delivery."

    d. "The physiological maturity needed for the fetus to sense pain is present by about 23 weeks gestation."

12. A pregnant teen voices concerns related to potential paralysis about the plans for an epidural anesthetic to be administered. What information can be provided to the teen?

    a. "Paralysis is not a serious concern for the procedure."

    b. "The spinal cord will not be damaged by the insertion of the epidural catheter."

    c. "The spinal cord ends above the area where the epidural is inserted."

    d. "The risk of paralysis is limited because your physician is skilled in the administration of epidurals."

13. The nurse is assigned to care for a 14-year-old child who is hospitalized in traction for serious leg fractures after an automobile accident. The parents ask the nurse to avoid administering analgesics to their child to help prevent him from becoming addicted. What response by the nurse is indicated?

    a. "We can talk with the physician to see about reducing the amount of medications given to reduce the potential for addiction."

    b. "If there is no history of drug abuse in the family there should be no increased risk for the development of addiction."

    c. "Administering medications to manage complaints of pain is not going to cause addition."

    d. "Your child is too young to experience drug addiction."

14. The nurse is caring for a 5-year-old child who underwent a painful surgical procedure earlier in the day. The nurse notes the child has not reported pain to any of the nursing staff. What action by the nurse is indicated?

    a. Contact the physician to report the child's condition.

    b. Administer prophylactic analgesics.

    c. Observe for behavioral cues consistent with pain.

    d. Encourage the child to report pain.

15. The nurse is preparing to administer a dose of Toradol (ketorolac) to a 15-year-old child. The nurse should do which of the following to reduce the potential for gastrointestinal upset?

    a. Administer the medication before meals.

    b. Administer the medication with milk

    c. Administer the medication with meals

    d. Administer the medication with a citrus beverage

Nursing Care of the Child with an Infectious or Communicable Disorder

Learning Objectives

- Discuss anatomic and physiologic differences in children versus adults in relation to the infectious process.
- Identify nursing interventions related to common laboratory and diagnostic tests used in the diagnosis and management of infectious conditions.
- Identify appropriate nursing assessments and interventions related to medications and treatments for childhood infectious and communicable disorders.
- Distinguish various infectious illnesses occurring in childhood.
- Devise an individualized nursing care plan for the child with an infectious or communicable disorder.
- Develop child/family teaching plans for the child with an infectious or communicable disorder.

SECTION I: ASSESSING YOUR UNDERSTANDING

Activity A FILL IN THE BLANKS

1. The trigger of prostaglandins to increase the body's temperature set point is caused by
_____.

2. Monocytes use _____ as a means to eliminate pathogens.

3. B cells use _____ to attack specific foreign substances.

4. Fever can increase the production of _____ and slow the growth of bacteria and viruses.

5. Acetaminophen and _____, administered at the appropriate dose and interval, are safe and effective for reducing fever in children.

Activity B **MATCHING**

Match the infection chain link in Column A
with the proper word or phrase in Column B.

Column A

___ **1.** Infectious agent

___ **2.** Mode of
     transmission

___ **3.** Portal of entry

___ **4.** Portal of exit

___ **5.** Reservoir

___ **6.** Susceptible host

Column B

a. Child

b. Rickettsiae

c. Gastrointestinal
     tract

d. Animal

e. Fomite

f. Respiratory tract

Match the vector-borne illness in Column A
with Column B.

Column A

___ **1.** Endemic typhus

___ **2.** Pediculosis pubis

___ **3.** Rickettsialpox

___ **4.** Roundworm

___ **5.** Scabies

Column B

a. Mouse mite bite

b. Rat flea feces

c. Sexual contact

d. Close, prolonged
     contact

e. Ingested fecal
     matter

Activity C **SEQUENCING**

Place the following stages of an infectious
disease in the proper order:

1. Convalescence

2. Illness

3. Incubation

4. Prodromal

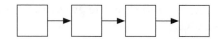

Activity D **SHORT ANSWERS**

Briefly answer the following.

1. Name five risk factors for sepsis that are
     related to pregnancy and labor.

_____

_____

_____

2. Describe the nursing management of
     mumps.

_____

_____

_____

3. Explain postexposure prophylaxis after an
     animal bite.

_____

_____

_____

4. Explain the role of fever in the child with an
     infection.

_____

_____

_____

5. Explain sepsis. What is septic shock?

_____

_____

_____

SECTION II: APPLYING YOUR KNOWLEDGE

Activity E CASE STUDY

Jennifer Mikelson, a 16-year-old female, is seen in your clinic. She presents with complaints of abnormal vaginal discharge and pain with urination. Jennifer is visibly upset and not very willing to answer questions at this time. She states "can't you just give me some medicine to take."

1. How would you proceed with your assessment?

_____

_____

_____

2. Jennifer is diagnosed with Chlamydia. What home care instructions and education should you provide?

_____

_____

_____

3. By the end of the assessment Jennifer is opening up. She states she recently began having sexual relations with her boyfriend. He does not like condoms so the majority of the sexual interactions have been unprotected. How would you respond?

_____

_____

_____

SECTION III: PRACTICING FOR NCLEX

Activity F NCLEX-STYLE QUESTIONS

Answer the following questions.

1. A 10-year-old girl with long hair is brought to the emergency room because she began acting irritable, complained of headache, and is very sleepy. What question would be most appropriate to ask the parents?

   a. "Has she done this before?"

   b. "How long has she been acting like this?"

   c. "What were you doing prior to her beginning to feel sick?"

   d. "What medications is she currently taking?"

2. A 6-year-old boy is suspected of having late-stage Lyme disease. Which of the following assessments would produce findings supporting this concern?

   a. Inspection for erythema migrans

   b. Asking the child if his knees hurt

   c. Observation of facial palsy

   d. Examination for conjunctivitis

3. The nurse is preparing to administer acetaminophen to a 4-year-old girl to provide comfort to the child. Which of the following precautions is very specific with antipyretics?

   a. Check for medicine allergies

   b. Take entire course of medication

   c. Ensure proper dose and interval

   d. Warn of possible drowsiness

4. A 10-year-old boy has an unknown infection and will need a urine for culture and sensitivity. To assure that the sensitivity results is accurate, which of the of the following steps is most important?

   a. Ensure that the specimen is obtained from proper area

   b. May need to collect three specimens on three different days

   c. Use aseptic technique when getting the specimen

   d. Obtain specimen before antibiotics are given

5. The nurse at an outpatient facility is obtaining a blood specimen from a 9-year-old girl. Which of the following techniques would most likely be used?

   a. Puncturing a vein on the dorsal side of the hand

   b. Administration of sucrose prior to beginning

   c. Accessing an indwelling venous access device

   d. Using an automatic lancet device on the heel

6. Which child needs to be seen immediately in the physician's office?
   a. A 10-month-old with a fever and petechiae who is grunting
   b. A 2-month-old with a slight fever and irritability after getting immunizations the previous day
   c. A 4-month-old with a cough, elevated temperature and wetting eight diapers every 24 hours
   d. An 8-month-old who is restless, irritable, and afebrile

7. The nurse is administering a chicken pox vaccination to a 12-month-old girl. Which of the following is a unique concern with Varicella?
   a. This disease can reactivate years later causing shingles
   b. Vitamin A is indicated for children younger than 2 years
   c. Dehydration is caused by mouth lesions
   d. Avoid exposure to pregnant women

8. The pediatric nurse knows that there are a number of anatomic and physiologic differences between children and adults. Which of the following statements about the immune systems of infants and young children is true?
   a. Children have an immature immune response
   b. Cellular immunity is not functional in children
   c. Children have an increased inflammatory response
   d. Passive immunity overlaps immunizations

9. The nurse is taking a health history for an 8-year-old boy who is hospitalized. Which of the following is a risk factor for sepsis in a hospitalized child?
   a. A maternal infection or fever
   b. Use of immunosuppression drugs
   c. Lack of juvenile immunizations
   d. Resuscitation or invasive procedures

10. The nurse is caring for a 5-year-old girl with scarlet fever. Which of the following interventions will most likely be part of her care?
    a. Exercising both standard and droplet precautions
    b. Palpating for and noting enlarged lymph nodes

    c. Monitoring for changes in respiratory status
    d. Teaching proper administration of Penicillin V

11. The nurse is caring for a 10-year-old child with a skin rash. The nurse should include which of the following interventions to manage the associated pruritus?
    a. Encourage warm baths
    b. Apply hot compresses
    c. Press the pruritic area
    d. Rub powder on the pruritic area

12. The student nurse is discussing the plan of care for a child admitted to the hospital for treatment of an infection. Which of the following actions should be taken first?
    a. Obtain blood cultures
    b. Initiate antibiotic therapy
    c. Obtain urine specimen for analysis
    d. Initiate intravenous therapy

13. The nurse is reviewing the assessment data from a 4-year-old admitted to the hospital for management of early onset sepsis. Which of the following findings are supportive of the diagnosis?
    a. The child complains about having to stay in bed
    b. The child's tympanic temperature is 98.8 F
    c. The child is hypotensive
    d. The child is irritable

14. The nurse is preparing to perform a finger stick on a child. Which of the following actions indicates the need for further instruction?
    a. The nurse cleans the finger with an alcohol-based solution prior to the finger stick.
    b. The nurse presses the collection tube against the skin of the finger during specimen collection.
    c. The nurse uses the outer side of the finger for performing the stick.
    d. The nurse wears gloves during the collection of the specimen.

Activity B LABELING

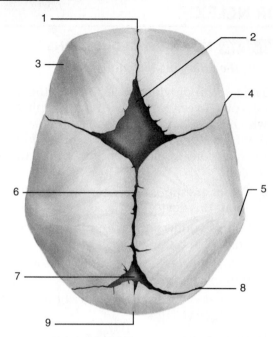

Label the skull structures in the infant.

1. _____
2. _____
3. _____
4. _____
5. _____
6. _____
7. _____
8. _____
9. _____

Activity C MATCHING

Match the term in Column A with the proper definition in Column B.

Column A

_____ 1. Febrile seizures

_____ 2. Reye's syndrome

_____ 3. Craniosynostosis

_____ 4. Aseptic meningitis

_____ 5. Positional plagiocephaly

Column B

a. Treat aggressively with intravenous antibiotics initially

b. Position the infant so that the flatten area is up

c. Surgical correction to allow brain growth

d. Rectal diazepam

e. Maintain cerebral perfusion, manage ICP, manage hydration, and safety measures

Activity D SEQUENCING

Place the following levels of consciousness in the proper order from lowest to highest using the boxes provided below:

1. Coma

2. Confusion

3. Full consciousness

4. Obtunded

5. Stupor

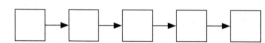

Activity E SHORT ANSWERS

Briefly answer the following.

1. Describe how to test for Kernig sign, what indicates a positive sign, and what disorder is indicated.

   _____

   _____

   _____

2. Describe the opisthotonic position, what age a child would assume this position, and what neurologic disorder is implicated.

   _____

   _____

   _____

3. What are the proper positions for a lumbar puncture for an infant and child?

   _____

   _____

   _____

4. What is the purpose of a ventriculoperitoneal (VP) shunt, what causes it to malfunction, and what are the symptoms the malfunction produces?

   _____

   _____

   _____

5. In regards to the Glasgow Coma Scale, what are the three major areas of assessment, and what does a low score indicate?

_____

_____

_____

SECTION II: APPLYING YOUR KNOWLEDGE

Activity F CASE STUDY

Jessica Clark, 5 years old, is admitted to the neurologic unit at a pediatric hospital after having a seizure at school. Her mother reports that Jessica has a history of seizures and is taking phenobarbital to control them. The mother states, "Ever since Jessica started school this year, it has been more difficult to get her to take her medicine."

1. What diagnostic and laboratory tests can you anticipate?

_____

_____

_____

2. Minutes after leaving the room, the mother calls you back because Jessica is having another seizure. Identify nursing interventions related to the care of this child during and immediately following a seizure. List in order of priority.

_____

_____

_____

3. What teaching will the nurse do with this child's family? Include a discussion on ways to increase compliance with the seizure medication.

_____

_____

_____

SECTION III: PRACTICING FOR NCLEX

Activity G NCLEX-STYLE QUESTIONS

Answer the following questions.

1. The nurse is providing education to the parents of a 3-year-old girl with hydrocephalus who has just had an external ventricular drainage system placed. Which of the following questions would best begin the teaching session?
   a. "What questions or concerns do you have about this device?"
   b. "Do you understand why you clamp the drain before she sits up?"
   c. "What do you know about her autoregulation mechanism failing?"
   d. "Why do you always keep her head raised 30 degrees?"

2. During physical assessment of a 2-month-old infant, the nurse suspects the child may have a lesion on the brain stem. Which of the following signs or symptoms was observed?
   a. Only one eye is dilated and reactive
   b. A sudden increase in head circumference
   c. Horizontal nystagmus
   d. The posterior fontanel is closed

3. After a difficult birth, the nurse observes that a newborn has swelling on part of his head. Which of the following signs suggests cephalohematoma?
   a. Swelling does not cross the midline or suture lines
   b. The swelling crosses the midline of the infant's scalp
   c. The infant had a low birth weight when born at 37 weeks
   d. The infant has facial abnormalities

4. The nurse is caring for an 8-year-old girl who was in a car accident. Which of the following symptoms would suggest the child has a cerebral contusion?
   a. She has trouble focusing when reading
   b. She has difficulty concentrating
   c. She has had some vomiting
   d. She is bleeding from the ear

5. The nurse caring for an infant with craniosynostosis, specifically positional plagiocephaly, would prioritize which of the following activities?
   a. Moving the infant's head every 2 hours
   b. Measuring the intake and output every shift
   c. Massaging the scalp gently very 4 hours
   d. Giving the infant small feedings whenever he is fussy

6. Premature infants have more fragile capillaries in the periventricular area than term infants. Which of the following problems does this put them at risk for?
   a. Moderate closed-head injury
   b. Early closure of the fontanels
   c. Congenital hydrocephalus
   d. Intracranial hemorrhaging

7. The nurse is caring for a near-term pregnant woman who has not taken prenatal vitamins or folic acid supplements. Which of the following congenital defects is most likely to occur based on the mother's prenatal history?
   a. Neonatal conjunctivitis
   b. Facial deformities
   c. A neural tube defect
   d. Incomplete myelinization

8. The nurse is caring for a 3-year-old boy who is experiencing seizure activity. Which of the following diagnostic tests will determine the seizure area in the brain?
   a. Cerebral angiography
   b. Lumbar puncture
   c. Video electroencephalogram
   d. Computed tomography

9. A pregnant patient asks if there is any danger to the development of her fetus in the first few weeks of her pregnancy. The nurse would be correct in responding:
   a. "As long as you were taking good care of your health before becoming pregnant, your fetus should be fine during the first few weeks of pregnancy."
   b. "Bones begin to harden in the first 5 to 6 weeks of pregnancy so vitamin D consumption is particularly important."
   c. "During the first 3 to 4 weeks of pregnancy brain and spinal cord development occur and are affected by nutrition, drugs, infection, or trauma."
   d. "The respiratory system matures during this time so good prenatal care during the first weeks of pregnancy is very important."

10. The nurse has developed a nursing plan for the care of a 6-year-old girl with congenital hydrocephalus whose shunt has become infected. The most important discharge teaching point for this family is:
    a. Maintaining effective cerebral perfusion
    b. Educating the parents how to properly give antibiotics
    c. Establishing seizure precautions for the child
    d. Encouraging development of motor skills

11. The young child has been diagnosed with bacterial meningitis. Which of the following nursing interventions are appropriate?
    a. Initiate droplet isolation
    b. Identify close contacts of the child who will require postexposure prophylactic medication
    c. Administer antibiotics as ordered
    d. Monitor the child for signs and symptoms associated with decreased intracranial pressure
    e. Initiate seizure precautions

12. The meningococcal vaccine should be offered to high-risk populations. Which of the following people who have never been vaccinated have an increased risk of becoming infected with meningococcal meningitis?

    a. An 18-year-old student who is preparing for college in the fall and has signed up to live in a dormitory with two other suite mates

    b. A child who is 12 years old

    c. A 5-year-old child who routinely travels in the summer with her parents on mission trips to Haiti

    d. A child who was diagnosed with diabetes mellitus when he was 7 years old

    e. A child who is 8 years old

13. An 11-year-old child was recently diagnosed with chickenpox. His parents gave him aspirin for a fever and the child is now hospitalized. Which of the following nursing interventions are commonly associated with the management of Reye's syndrome?

    a. Request order for an antiemetic

    b. Assess intake and output every shift

    c. Assess child's skin for the development of distinctive rash every 4 hours

    d. Request order for anticonvulsant

    e. Monitor the child's laboratory values related to pancreatic function

14. The young child was involved in a motor vehicle accident and was admitted to the pediatric intensive care unit with changes in level of consciousness and a high-pitched cry. Which of the following are late signs of increased intracranial pressure?

    a. The child states that he feels a little "dizzy."

    b. The child's toes are pointed downward, his head and neck are arched backwards, and his arms and legs are extended.

    c. The sclera of the eyes is visible above the iris.

    d. The child's heart rate is 56 beats per minute.

    e. The child's pupils are fixed and dilated.

Nursing Care of the Child with a Disorder of the Eyes or Ears

Learning Objectives

- Differentiate between the anatomic and physiologic differences of the eyes and ears in children as compared with adults.
- Identify various factors associated with disorders of the eyes and ears in infants and children.
- Discuss common laboratory and other diagnostic tests useful in the diagnosis of disorders of the eyes and ears.
- Discuss common medications and other treatments used for treatment and palliation of conditions affecting the eyes and ears.
- Recognize risk factors associated with various disorders of the eyes and ears.
- Distinguish between different disorders of the eyes and ears based on the signs and symptoms associated with them.
- Discuss nursing interventions commonly used in regard to disorders of the eyes and ears.
- Devise an individualized nursing care plan for the child with a sensory impairment or other disorder of the eyes or ears.
- Develop patient/family teaching plans for the child with a disorder of the eyes or ears.
- Describe the psychosocial impact of sensory impairments on children.

SECTION I: ASSESSING YOUR UNDERSTANDING

Activity A FILL IN THE BLANKS

1. According to *Healthy People 2020* recommendations, visual acuity testing should begin at _____ years of age.

2. Short length and _____ position of eustachian tubes leads to greater susceptibility of acute otitis media in children less than 2 years of age.

3. Systemic _____ are used to treat periorbital cellulitis.

4. Permanent visual _____ can be averted with early identification and treatment of amblyopia.

5. Vision or hearing impairment impedes _____ progress.

6. The spherical shape of the newborn's lens does not allow for _____ accommodation.

Activity B MATCHING

Match the term in Column A with the proper definition in Column B.

Column A

_____ **1.** Contusion

_____ **2.** Corneal abrasion

_____ **3.** Eyelid injury

_____ **4.** Foreign body

_____ **5.** Scleral hemorrhage

Column B

a. Vision is usually unaffected

b. Discoloration and edema of eyelid

c. Erythema that resolves gradually without intervention

d. May require ointment to sooth injury or antibiotic ointment

e. Requires careful removal only by a health care professional

Activity C SEQUENCING

Place the following vision and hearing milestones in the proper order:

1. Binocular vision

2. Eye color

3. Functional hearing

4. Visual acuity of 20/20

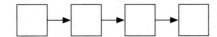

Activity D SHORT ANSWERS

Briefly answer the following.

1. List at least five signs and symptoms of children with hearing loss at (a) infant, (b) young child, and (c) older child stages.

_____

_____

_____

2. Describe how to interact with a visually impaired child, especially the use of one's voice and ways to act as the child's eyes.

_____

_____

_____

3. List at least three signs and symptoms that would lead the nurse to suspect a child is visually impaired at (a) infant, (b) young child, or (c) older child stages.

_____

_____

_____

4. List at least five factors that increase the risk of a child developing acute otitis media.

_____

_____

_____

5. Discuss the characteristics that increase the risk of a child having difficulty with the development of speech or language, or having learning difficulties.

_____

_____

_____

SECTION II: APPLYING YOUR KNOWLEDGE

Activity E CASE STUDY

Brandon, age 6 months, has been brought to the pediatrician's office for a well-baby checkup. Brandon's mother tells the nurse that she is concerned about Brandon's left eye. She tells the nurse that Brandon's eyes do not seem to be looking in the same place. Upon assessment the nurse finds asymmetry of the corneal light reflex. Brandon is referred for further assessment to an ophthalmologist.

1. Brandon is diagnosed with amblyopia. What information would the nurse know to include in a teaching plan for Brandon's family at this first visit?

2. Why is it important to treat amblyopia as soon as it is found and what treatments might be used in the treatment of Brandon's condition?

SECTION III: PRACTICING FOR NCLEX

Activity F NCLEX-STYLE QUESTIONS

Answer the following questions.

1. The nurse is caring for a 2-year-old girl with persistent otitis media with effusion. Which of the following interventions is most important to the developmental health of the child?
   a. Informing the parents to avoid nonprescription drugs
   b. Telling parents not to smoke in the house
   c. Educating the parents about proper antibiotic use
   d. Reassessing for language acquisition

2. The nurse is explaining information to the parents of a 3-year-old boy who may have strabismus. Which of the following examinations would the nurse expect to assist with first in order to find out if he has strabismus?
   a. Refractive examination
   b. Visual acuity test
   c. Corneal light reflex test
   d. Ophthalmologic examination

3. The nurse is caring for a 10-year-old girl with acute periorbital cellulitis. Which of the following will be the primary nursing intervention (therapy) for this disorder?
   a. Application of heated aqua pad to site
   b. Administering Rocephin IV as ordered
   c. Administering Morphine Sulfate as ordered
   d. Monitoring for increased intracranial pressure

4. The nurse is caring for a 24-month-old boy with regressed retinopathy of prematurity. Which of the following interventions would be priority for this child?
   a. Assessing the child for asymmetric corneal light reflex
   b. Observing for rubbing or shutting the eyes or squinting
   c. Referring the child to the local district of Early Intervention
   d. Teaching the parents to check how the child's glasses fit

5. The nurse is caring for an 8-year-old boy with otitis media with effusion. Which of the following situations may have caused this disorder?
   a. He frequently goes swimming
   b. He has good attendance at school
   c. He is experiencing recurrent nasal congestion
   d. He had recent bacterial conjunctivitis

6. The nurse is caring for a 7-year-old girl in an outpatient clinic diagnosed with amblyopia that is unrelated to any other disorder. Which of the following interventions would be most helpful at this time?

   a. Discouraging the child from roughhousing

   b. Explaining postsurgical treatment of the eye

   c. Ensuring follow-up visits with the ophthalmologist

   d. Educating parents on how to use prescribed atropine drops

7. The nurse is teaching the parents of a 4-year-old boy with strabismus. Teaching for the parents would include:

   a. The need for ultraviolet-protective glasses postoperatively

   b. The importance of completing the full course of oral antibiotics

   c. The possibility that multiple operations may be necessary

   d. That it is critical to comply with patching as prescribed

8. The nurse is educating the parents of a 5-year-old girl with infectious conjunctivitis about the disorder. Which of the following is most important to prevent the spread of the disorder?

   a. Properly applying the prescribed antibiotic

   b. Staying home from school

   c. Washing hands frequently

   d. Keeping hands away from eyes

9. A 10-year-old boy has just been treated for otitis externa and now the nurse is teaching the boy and his parents about prevention. Which of the following recommendations would be included as part of the education?

   a. Using alcohol and vinegar for soreness

   b. Using cotton swabs to keep the inner ear dry

   c. Using a hair dryer on cool to dry the ears

   d. Washing his hair only when necessary

10. The nurse is teaching parents of a 9-year-old girl about the importance of her wearing her prescribed glasses. Which of the following subjects is least important to promoting compliance?

    a. Getting scheduled eye examinations on time

    b. Checking condition and fit of glasses monthly

    c. Watching for signs that prescription needs changing

    d. Encouraging the use of eye protection for sports

11. The pediatric office nurse notes that several of the young children that are waiting to see the physician may have conjunctivitis. Which of the following findings are consistent with bacterial conjunctivitis?

    a. Only the right eye is involved.

    b. The drainage is yellow and thick.

    c. The drainage is white.

    d. There is clear, watery drainage from both eyes.

    e. The child suffers from seasonal allergies.

12. A child has been diagnosed with bacterial conjunctivitis. Which of the following statements by the child's parent indicate the need for further education?

    a. "I'll continue to use Visine to help with the redness."

    b. "All of us at home need to wash our hands really well."

    c. "We should not use a towel that he has used."

    d. "He can go back to school in 4 hours after that thick yellow drainage is gone."

    e. "This is really contagious."

13. The young child has been diagnosed with a corneal abrasion. Which of the following findings are most consistent with this diagnosis?

    a. The child's pupils are equal, round, reactive to light and accommodation.

    b. The child denies any eye pain.

    c. The child complains that it hurts to look towards bright light.

    d. The child has a large purple bruise over the eye and edema on the eyelid.

    e. The child's eye is draining clear fluid and the child says it feels like it is full of tears.

14. The nurse works in a pediatrician office. Which of the following children who have been diagnosed with acute otitis media does the nurse expect the physician to treat with antibiotics?

    a. The 12-year-old child is complaining that he has some mild ear pain with a temperature of 101.4 F.

    b. The 8-year-old child who is crying due to ear pain and has a temperature of 103 F.

    c. The 2-month-old child who is having difficulty sleeping and has a fever of 102.6 F.

    d. The 5-month-old child who is fussy and pulling at her ears.

    e. The 22-month-old who is irritable with the presence of purulent drainage from her right ear.

CHAPTER 40

Nursing Care of the Child with a Respiratory Disorder

Learning Objectives

- Distinguish between the anatomy and physiology of the respiratory system in children versus adults.
- Identify various factors associated with respiratory illness in infants and children.
- Discuss common laboratory and other diagnostic tests useful in the diagnosis of respiratory conditions.
- Describe nursing care related to common medications and other treatments used for management and palliation of respiratory conditions.
- Recognize risk factors associated with various respiratory disorders.
- Distinguish different respiratory disorders based on their signs and symptoms.
- Discuss nursing interventions commonly used for respiratory illnesses.
- Devise an individualized nursing care plan for the child with a respiratory disorder.
- Develop child/family teaching plans for the child with a respiratory disorder.
- Describe the psychosocial impact of chronic respiratory disorders on children.

SECTION I: ASSESSING YOUR UNDERSTANDING

Activity A FILL IN THE BLANKS

1. A _____ is a surgical construction of a respiratory opening in the trachea.

2. Allergic rhinitis is associated with _____ dermatitis and asthma.

3. Cough and _____ are symptoms of influenza for both children and adults.

4. Pulse oximetry is an _____ measurement of oxygen saturation in arterial blood.

5. Auscultation of the lungs might reveal _____ or rales in the younger child with pneumonia.

6. Tuberculin skin testing is also known as a _____ test.

7. Pseudoephedrine is an example of a _____ used for the treatment of runny or stuffy nose associated with the common cold.

Activity B LABELING

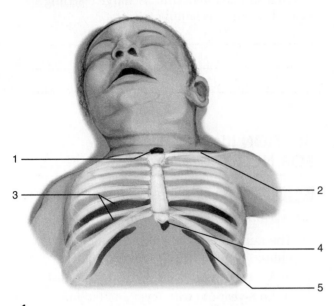

1. _____
2. _____
3. _____
4. _____
5. _____

Label the image using the following terms:

Intercostal
Substernal
Supraclavicular
Subcostal
Suprasternal

Activity C MATCHING

Match the term in Column A with the proper definition in Column B.

Column A

_____ **1.** Nasal cannula

_____ **2.** Non-rebreather mask

_____ **3.** Partial rebreather mask

_____ **4.** Simple face mask

_____ **5.** Venturi mask

Column B

a. Minimum flow rate of 6 L/min

b. Oxygen reservoir bag

c. Mixes room air and oxygen

d. Must have patent nasal passages

e. One-way valve

Activity D SEQUENCING

Place the following steps for using a bulb syringe in the proper order:

1. Clean the bulb syringe

2. Compress the bulb

3. Empty the bulb

4. Instill saline nose drops

5. Place the bulb in the nose

6. Release pressure on bulb

7. Remove the bulb from nose

8. Tilt the infant's head back

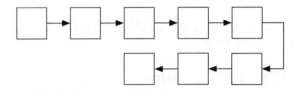

Activity E SHORT ANSWERS

Briefly answer the following.

1. Discuss common signs and symptoms that are seen with sinusitis.

   _____

   _____

   _____

2. Discuss common laboratory and diagnostic tests that the nurse anticipates to be ordered for a child suspected of having cystic fibrosis and identify findings that indicate cystic fibrosis.

   _____

   _____

   _____

3. Compare the similarities and differences of croup and epiglottitis.

   _____

   _____

   _____

4. Discuss the therapeutic management of the common cold.

_____

_____

_____

5. What is the most common cause of bronchiolitis and discuss the peak incidence of the disorder.

_____

_____

_____

SECTION II: APPLYING YOUR KNOWLEDGE

Activity F   **CASE STUDY**

James Jackson, an 8-year-old boy, is admitted to the pediatric hospital because of dyspnea, coughing, and wheezing. James states "my chest feels really tight." Physical findings include pallor, tachypnea, tachycardia, and bilateral wheezing on auscultation. This is the first time James has experienced these symptoms.

1. What health history information is important for the nurse to collect?

_____

_____

_____

2. List four nursing diagnoses that would pertain to James. Prioritize and provide rationale.

James has been diagnosed with asthma and is prescribed a bronchodilator and a metered dose inhaler while in the health care facility and for home. His breathing becomes easier and he states the tightness has gone away.

_____

_____

_____

3. Since this is James' first episode of asthma, what will be important discharge teaching for him and his family?

_____

_____

_____

SECTION III: PRACTICING FOR NCLEX

Activity G   **NCLEX-STYLE QUESTIONS**

Answer the following questions.

1. The nurse is assessing several children. Which child is most at risk for dysphagia?

  a. A 7-month-old with erythematous rash

  b. An 8-year-old with fever and fatigue

  c. A 4-year-old with pharyngitis

  d. A 2-month-old with toxic appearance

2. The nurse is caring for a 14-month-old boy with cystic fibrosis. Which of these signs of ineffective family coping requires the most urgent intervention?

  a. Compliance with therapy is diminished

  b. The family becomes over vigilant

  c. The child feels fearful and isolated

  d. Siblings are jealous and worried

3. The nurse is taking a health history for a 3-year-old girl suspected of having pneumonia who presents with a fever, chest pain, and cough. Which of the following is a risk factor for pneumonia?

  a. The child is a triplet

  b. The child was a postmaturity date infant

  c. The child has diabetes

  d. The child attends day care

4. The nurse is auscultating the lungs of a lethargic, irritable 6-year-old boy and hears wheezing. The nurse will most likely be including which teaching point if the child is suspected of having asthma.

   a. "I'm going to have the respiratory therapist get some of the mucus from your lungs."

   b. "I'm going to have this hospital worker take a picture of your lungs."

   c. "We're going to go take a look at your lungs to see if there are any sores on them."

   d. "I'm going to hold your hand while the phlebotomist gets blood from your arm."

5. The nurse is caring for a 3-year-old girl who is cyanotic and breathing rapidly. Which of the following would best relieve these symptoms?

   a. Suctioning

   b. Oxygen

   c. Saline lavage

   d. Saline gargles

6. The nurse knows that respiratory disorders in children are sometimes attributed to differences in anatomy and physiology. Which of the following is an accurate statement?

   a. Adults have twice as many alveoli as newborns

   b. The tongue is proportionately smaller in infants than in adults

   c. Infants consume twice as much oxygen as adults

   d. Hypoxemia occurs later in children than adults

7. The nurse is caring for a 5-year-old girl who shows signs and symptoms of epiglottis. The nurse recognizes a common complication of the disorder is for the child to:

   a. Complain of ear pain

   b. Experience nuchal rigidity

   c. Have unilateral breath sounds upon auscultation

   d. Be at risk for respiratory distress

8. The nurse is developing a teaching plan for the parents of a 10-year-old boy with cystic fibrosis. The plan should include teaching of:

   a. Use of a flutter valve device

   b. Use of a metered dose inhaler

   c. Proper use of a nebulizer

   d. How to work a peak flow meter

9. The nurse is caring for a neonate being treated for respiratory distress syndrome who is on a ventilator. Early assessment of the complication of mucus plugging can be determined by:

   a. Promoting adequate gas exchange

   b. Monitoring for adequate lung expansion

   c. Maintaining adequate fluid volume

   d. Preventing infection

10. The nurse is caring for a 10-year-old girl with allergic rhinitis. Which intervention helps prevent secondary bacterial infection?

    a. Using normal saline nasal washes

    b. Teaching parents how to avoid allergens

    c. Discussing anti-inflammatory nasal sprays

    d. Teaching parents about oral antihistamines

11. The young child is wearing a nasal cannula. The oxygen is set at 3 L/minute. Calculate how much oxygen the child is receiving?

12. The child has been diagnosed with asthma and the child's physician is using a stepwise approach. Rank the following in order of occurrence as the child's condition worsens.

    a. The nurse administers a medium-dose inhaled corticosteroid and salmeterol

    b. The nurse administers albuterol as needed

    c. The nurse administers a medium-dose inhaled corticosteroid

    d. The nurse administers a low-dose inhaled corticosteroid

13. The student nurse is discussing the differences between children's respiratory systems and adults'. Which of the following statements by the student nurse are accurate? Select all that apply.

    a. "Children are less likely to develop problems associated with swelling of the airways."

    b. "When compared to adults, children's tongues are proportionally smaller."

    c. "The only time that newborns can breathe through their mouths is when they cry."

    d. "A newborn's respiratory tract is drier because the newborn doesn't make very much mucus."

    e. "Children under the age of 6 years are more prone to developing sinus infections."

14. The young child has been diagnosed with group A streptococcal pharyngitis. The physician orders amoxicillin 45 mg/kg in three equally divided doses. The child weighs 23 pounds. Calculate how many milligrams the child will receive with each dose of amoxicillin (round to the nearest whole milligram).

15. The child has been admitted to the hospital with a possible diagnosis of pneumonia. Which of the following findings are consistent with this diagnosis?

    a. The child's temperature is 98.4 F

    b. The child's chest X-ray indicates the presence of perihilar infiltrates

    c. The child's white blood cell count is elevated

    d. The child's respiratory rate is rapid

    e. The child is producing yellow purulent sputum

CHAPTER 41

Nursing Care of the Child with a Cardiovascular Disorder

Learning Objectives

- Compare anatomic and physiologic differences of the cardiovascular system in infants and children versus adults.
- Describe nursing care related to common laboratory and diagnostic tests used in the medical diagnosis of pediatric cardiovascular conditions.
- Distinguish cardiovascular disorders common in infants, children, and adolescents.
- Identify appropriate nursing assessments and interventions related to medications and treatments for pediatric cardiovascular disorders.
- Develop an individualized nursing care plan for the child with a cardiovascular disorder.
- Describe the psychosocial impact of chronic cardiovascular disorders on children.
- Devise a nutrition plan for the child with cardiovascular disease.
- Develop patient/family teaching plans for the child with a cardiovascular disorder.

SECTION I: ASSESSING YOUR UNDERSTANDING

Activity A FILL IN THE BLANKS

1. Cardiac _____ is the radiographic study of the heart and coronary vessels after injection of contrast medium.

2. Cardiac catheterization may be categorized as diagnostic, interventional, or _____.

3. Coarctation of the aorta is defined as _____ of the aorta.

4. Examples of defects with increased _____ blood flow are patent ductus arteriosus (PDA), atrial septal defect (ASD), and ventricular septal defect (VSD).

5. Eighty percent of all cases of heart failure in children with congenital heart defects occur by the age of _____.

6. Cardiac disorders that are not congenital are considered _____ disorders.

7. _____ is a delayed disorder resulting from group A streptococcal pharyngeal infection.

Activity B MATCHING

Match the term in Column A with the proper definition in Column B.

Column A

____ **1.** Alprostadil

____ **2.** Furosemide

____ **3.** Heparin

____ **4.** Ace inhibitors

____ **5.** Niacin

Column B

a. Management of edema associated with heart failure

b. Temporary maintenance of ductus arterious patency in infants with ductal-dependent congenital heart defects

c. Management of hypertension

d. Prophylaxis and treatment of thromboembolic disorders especially after cardiac surgery

e. Medication to lower blood cholesterol levels

Activity C SEQUENCING

Place the following changes that occur in the cardiopulmonary system immediately following birth in proper order:

1. Drop in pulmonary artery pressure

2. Reduction of pulmonary vascular resistance to blood flow

3. Decreased pressure in the right atrium

4. Lungs inflate

5. Closure of the ductus arteriosus

6. Closure of the foramen ovale

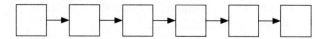

Activity D SHORT ANSWERS

Briefly answer the following.

1. Describe the action and indications for digoxin (Lanoxin). What are the key considerations when administering digoxin?

_____

_____

_____

2. Heart murmurs must be evaluated on the basis of what characteristics?

_____

_____

_____

3. What are the three types of atrial septal defects?

_____

_____

_____

4. Discuss the incidence of ventricular septal defect (VSD) and common assessment findings.

_____

_____

_____

5. What are the risk factors for the development of infective endocarditis?

_____

_____

_____

SECTION II: APPLYING YOUR KNOWLEDGE

Activity E CASE STUDY

The nurse is caring for a 2-year-old girl who was admitted to the hospital to undergo a cardiac catheterization for a suspected cardiac defect.

1. Discuss preprocedure nursing care for the child and family.

_____

_____

_____

2. Discuss postprocedure nursing care following a cardiac catheterization.

_____

_____

_____

SECTION III: PRACTICING FOR NCLEX

Activity F NCLEX-STYLE QUESTIONS

Answer the following questions.

1. The nurse is caring for an 8-month-old infant with a suspected congenital heart defect. The nurse examines the child and documents the following expected finding:

  a. Steady weight gain since birth

  b. Softening of the nail beds

  c. Appropriate mastery of developmental milestones

  d. Intact rooting reflex

2. The nurse is assessing the heart rate of a healthy 6-month-old. The nurse would expect which heart rate range?

  a. 60 to 68 bpm

  b. 70 to 80 bpm

  c. 80 to 105 bpm

  d. 120 to 130 bpm

3. The nurse is conducting a physical examination of a 7-year-old girl prior to a cardiac catheterization. The nurse knows to pay particular attention to assessing the child's pedal pulses. How can the nurse best facilitate their assessment after the procedure?

  a. Mark the location of the child's peripheral pulses with an indelible marker

  b. Mark the child's pedal pulses with an indelible marker, then document

  c. Document the location and quality of the child's pedal pulses

  d. Assess the location and quality of the child's peripheral pulses

4. The nurse is assessing the past medical history of an infant with a suspected cardiovascular disorder. Which of the following responses by the mother warrants further investigation?

  a. "His Apgar score was an eight"

  b. "I was really nauseous throughout my whole pregnancy"

  c. "I am on a low dose of lithium"

  d. "I had the flu during my last trimester"

5. A nurse is assessing the skin of a 12-year-old with suspected right ventricular heart failure. Which of the following findings would the nurse expect to note?

  a. Edema of the lower extremities

  b. Edema of the face

  c. Edema in the presacral region

  d. Edema of the hands

6. A nurse is palpating the pulse of a child with suspected aortic regurgitation. Which of the following assessment findings would the nurse expect to note?

  a. Appropriate mastery of developmental milestones

  b. Bounding pulse

  c. Preference to resting on the right side

  d. Pitting periorbital edema

7. The nurse is conducting a physical examination of a baby with a suspected cardiovascular disorder. Which of the following assessment findings is suggestive of sudden ventricular distention?

   a. Decreased blood pressure
   b. A heart murmur
   c. Cool, clammy, pale extremities
   d. Accentuated third heart sound

8. The nurse performs a cardiac assessment and notes a loud heart murmur with a precordial thrill. This murmur would be classified as a:

   a. Grade I
   b. Grade II
   c. Grade III
   d. Grade IV

9. The nurse is assessing the blood pressure of an adolescent. Which blood pressure measurement would be expected for a healthy 13-year-old boy?

   a. 80/40 mm Hg
   b. 80 to 100/64 mm Hg
   c. 94 to 112/56 to 60 mm Hg
   d. 100 to 120/50 to 70 mm Hg

10. The nurse is auscultating heart sounds of a child with a mitral valve prolapse. The nurse would expect which assessment finding?

    a. A mild to late ejection click at the apex
    b. Abnormal splitting of S2 sounds
    c. Clicks on the upper left sternal border
    d. Intensifying of S2 sounds

11. The infant has been hospitalized and develops hypercyanosis. The physician has ordered the nurse to administer 0.1 mg of morphine sulfate per every kilogram of the infant's body weight. The infant weighs 15.2 pounds. Calculate the infant's morphine sulfate dose. Round your answer to the nearest tenth.

12. The young child had a chest tube placed during cardiac surgery. Which of the following findings may indicate the development of cardiac tamponade? Select all that apply.

    a. The chest tube drainage had been averaging 15 to 25 mL out per hour and now there is no drainage from the chest tube
    b. The child's heart rate has increased from 88 beats per minute to 126 beats per minute
    c. The child's right atrial filling pressure has decreased
    d. The child is resting quietly
    e. The child's apical heart rate is strong and easily auscultated

13. The pediatric nurse has digoxin ordered for each of the five children. The nurse will withhold digoxin for which of the following children? Select all that apply.

    a. The 4-month-old child's apical heart rate is 102 beats per minute
    b. The 12-year-old's digoxin level was 0.9 ng/mL from a blood draw this morning
    c. The 16-year-old child has a heart rate of 54 beats per minute
    d. The 2-year-old child has a digoxin level of 2.4 ng/mL from a blood draw this morning
    e. The 5-year-old child has developed vomiting, diarrhea and is difficult to arouse

14. Identify which of the following findings are major criteria used to help the physician diagnose acute rheumatic fever? Select all that apply.

    a. The young child has an elevated erythrocyte sedimentation rate
    b. The young child has a temperature of 101.2 F
    c. The child has painless nodules located on his wrists
    d. The child has developed pericarditis with the presence of a new heart murmur
    e. The child has developed heart block with a prolonged PR interval

15. The child has returned to the nurse's unit following a cardiac catheterization. The insertion site is located at the right groin. Peripheral pulses were easily palpated in bilateral lower extremities prior to the procedure. Which of the following findings should be reported to the child's physician?

a. The right groin is soft without edema

b. The child's right foot is cool with a pulse assessed only with the use of a Doppler

c. The child has a temperature of 102.4 °F

d. The child is complaining of nausea

e. The child has a runny nose

CHAPTER 42

Nursing Care of the Child with a Gastrointestinal Disorder

Learning Objectives

■ Compare the differences in the anatomy and physiology of the gastrointestinal system between children and adults.

■ Discuss common medical treatments for infants and children with gastrointestinal disorders.

■ Discuss common laboratory and diagnostic tests used to identify disorders of the gastrointestinal tract.

■ Discuss medication therapy used in infants and children with gastrointestinal disorders.

■ Recognize risk factors associated with various gastrointestinal illnesses.

■ Differentiate between acute and chronic gastrointestinal disorders.

■ Distinguish common gastrointestinal illnesses of childhood.

■ Discuss nursing interventions commonly used for gastrointestinal illnesses.

■ Devise an individualized nursing care plan for infants/children with a gastrointestinal disorder.

■ Develop teaching plans for family/patient education for children with gastrointestinal illnesses.

■ Describe the psychosocial impact that chronic gastrointestinal illnesses have on children.

SECTION I: ASSESSING YOUR UNDERSTANDING

Activity A   FILL IN THE BLANKS

1. Vomiting is a reflex with three different phases. The first phase is the prodromal period, the second phase is _____, and the third phase is vomiting.

2. Biliary _____ is an absence of some or all of the major biliary ducts, resulting in obstruction of bile flow.

3. Chronic diarrhea is diarrhea that lasts for more than _____ weeks.

4. Oral candidiasis is a _____ infection of the oral mucosa.

5. Cholelithiasis is the presence of _____ in the gallbladder.

6. _____ supplementation while a child is taking antibiotics for other disorders may reduce the incidence of antibiotic-related diarrhea.

7. The proximal segment of the bowel telescoping into a more distal segment of the bowel is known as _____.

Activity B LABELING

Identify which is the colostomy and which is the ileostomy.

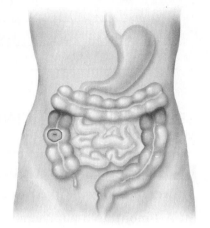 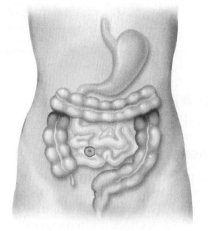

1. _____   2. _____

Activity C MATCHING

Match the term in Column A with the proper definition in Column B.

Column A

____ **1.** Bowel prep

____ **2.** Cleansing enema

____ **3.** Icteric

____ **4.** Total parenteral nutrition (TPN)

____ **5.** Ostomy

Column B

a. Long-term NPO status, swallowing or absorption difficulties

b. Colonoscopy or bowel surgery

c. Severe constipation or impaction

d. Jaundiced or yellow in color

e. Imperforate anus, gastroschisis, Hirschsprung's disease

Activity D SEQUENCING

Place the steps of abdominal assessment in the proper sequence.

1. Palpation

2. Inspection

3. Percussion

4. Auscultation

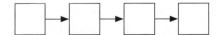

Activity E SHORT ANSWERS

Briefly answer the following.

1. What does the acronym S.T.O.M.A. stand for?

_____

_____

_____

2. Infants and children repeatedly put objects to their mouth for exploration. Why is this considered a risk factor for gastrointestinal illnesses?

_____

_____

_____

3. How is acute hepatitis typically treated?

_____

_____

_____

4. What complications are of most concern during infancy for the child with a cleft palate?

_____

_____

_____

5. Discuss the signs and symptoms that would indicate that an infant had pyloric stenosis.

_____

_____

_____

SECTION II: APPLYING YOUR KNOWLEDGE

Activity F CASE STUDY

Nico Taylor, a 1-month-old boy who was born at 33 weeks gestation is seen in your clinic. His birth weight was 4 pounds 12 ounces and length was 18 inches. At his 2 week check-up he weighed 5 pounds 4 ounces and was 18.5 inches in length. His mother reports that he has always spit up quite a bit, but eats well. A few days ago she noted increased irritability with a hoarse cry and arching of his back with feedings. On physical exam he weighs 4 pounds 14 ounces with a length of 19 inches. His head is round with a sunken anterior fontanel, and his mucous membranes are sticky. Heart rate is 152 without a murmur, and breath sounds are clear with a respiratory rate of 42. His abdomen is soft and nondistended with positive bowel sounds in all four quadrants. Nico's skin turgor is poor.

1. Which part of your physical assessment findings is concerning to you?

_____

_____

_____

2. What interventions are anticipated for Nico?

_____

_____

_____

3. How would you evaluate Nico's progress?

_____

_____

_____

4. Nico is diagnosed with gastroesophageal reflux. What education will you provide for the family regarding Nico's care?

_____

_____

_____

SECTION III: PRACTICING FOR NCLEX

Activity G NCLEX-STYLE QUESTIONS

Answer the following questions.

1. A 4-month-old has had a fever, vomiting, and loose watery stools every few hours for 2 days. The mother calls the physician's office and asks the nurse what she should do. What is the most appropriate response from the nurse?

   a. "Do not give the child anything to drink for 4r hours. If the fever goes down and the loose stools stop, you can resume breastfeeding."

   b. "Continue breastfeeding as you have been doing. The fluid from the breast milk is important to maintain fluid balance."

   c. "Give a clear pediatric electrolyte replacement for the next few hours, then call back to report on how your daughter is doing."

   d. "Bring her to the office today so we can evaluate her fluid balance and determine how we can treat her."

2. The nurse is caring for a 13-year-old girl with suspected autoimmune hepatitis. The girl inquires about the testing required to evaluate the condition. How should the nurse respond?

   a. "You will most likely have a blood test to check for certain antibodies."

   b. "You will most likely have an ultrasound evaluation."

   c. "You will most likely have viral studies."

   d. "You will most likely be tested for ammonia levels."

3. The nurse is obtaining the history of an infant with a suspected intestinal obstruction. Which of the following responses regarding newborn stool patterns would indicate a need for further evaluation for Hirschsprung's disease?

a. The infant passed a meconium stool in the first 24 to 48 hours of life

b. The infant has had diarrhea for 3 days

c. The infant has been constipated and passing gas for 2 days

d. The infant passed a meconium plug

4. A nurse is caring for a 6-year-old girl recently diagnosed with celiac disease and is discussing dietary restrictions with the girl's mother. Which of the following responses indicates a need for further teaching?

a. "My daughter is eating more vegetables."

b. "There is gluten hidden in unexpected foods."

c. "There are many types of flour besides wheat."

d. "My daughter can eat any kind of fruit."

5. The nurse is providing instructions to the parents of a 10-year-old boy who has undergone a barium swallow/upper and lower GI for suspected inflammatory bowel disease. Which of the following instructions is most important?

a. "Please be aware of any signs of infection."

b. "It is very important to drink lots of water and fluids after the test is finished."

c. "Your child could have diarrhea for several days afterward."

d. "Your child might have lighter stools for the next few days."

6. A nurse is caring for a 13-year-old boy recently diagnosed with Crohn's disease. He says he feels isolated and that there is no one who understands the challenges of his disease. How should the nurse respond?

a. "You need to remember that Crohn's disease goes into periods of remission."

b. "This is something that you will eventually accept with time."

c. "There are a lot of kids experiencing similar feelings at the Crohn's support group."

d. "You have to go to a support group; it will be very helpful."

7. The nurse is assessing a 10-day-old infant for dehydration. Which of the following findings indicates severe dehydration?

a. Pale and slightly dry mucosa

b. Blood pressure of 80/42

c. Tenting of skin

d. Soft and flat fontanels

8. A nurse is caring for a 6-year-old boy with a history of encopresis. What is the best way to approach the parents to assess for proper laxative use?

a. "Tell me about his daily stool patterns."

b. "Are you giving him the laxatives properly?"

c. "Are the laxatives working?"

d. "Describe his bowel movements for the past week."

9. Which of the following exhibits features most suggestive of ulcerative colitis rather than Crohn's disease?

a. A 16-year-old female with continuous distribution of disease in the colon, distal to proximal

b. A 14-year-old female with full-thickness chronic inflammation of the intestinal mucosa

c. An 18-year-old male with abdominal pain

d. A 12-year-old with oral temperature of 101.6 F

10. The nurse is conducting a physical examination of an infant with suspected pyloric stenosis. Which of the following findings indicates pyloric stenosis?

a. Olive-shaped mass in upper right abdomen

b. Perianal fissures and skin tags

c. Abdominal pain and irritability

d. Hard, moveable "olive-like mass" in the upper right quadrant

11. The infant is listless with sunken fontanels and has been diagnosed with dehydration. The infant is still producing at least 1 mL/kg each hour of urine. The infant weighs 13.2 pounds. At the minimum, how many milliliters of urine will the infant produce during the next 8-hour shift?

12. The young child has been diagnosed with hepatitis B. Which of the following statements by the child's mother indicates that further education is required?

    a. "We went swimming in a local lake 2 months ago and I just knew she drank some of the lake water."

    b. "Could I have this virus in my body, too?"

    c. "The virus is the reason her skin looks a little yellowish."

    d. "The only way you can get this virus is from intravenous drug use."

    e. "Her fever and rash are probably related to this virus."

13. The adolescent child has been diagnosed with gastroesophageal reflux disease. Which of the following statements by the child indicates that adequate learning has occurred?

    a. "This famotidine may make me tired."

    b. "The omeprazole could give me a headache."

    c. "It sounds like the physician is reluctant to give me a prokinetic because of the side effects."

    d. "I will probably need a laxative because of the omeprazole."

    e. "I should try to lie down right after I eat."

14. The child has been diagnosed with severe dehydration. The physician has ordered the nurse to administer a bolus of 20 mL/kg of normal saline over a 2-hour period. The child weighs 63.5 pounds. How should the nurse set the child's intravenous administration pump? (mL/hour) Round to the nearest whole number.

15. The newborn was diagnosed with esophageal atresia. Which of the following findings is most consistent with this condition?

    a. The newborn's mouth was very dry.

    b. The newborn coughed excessively during attempts to feed.

    c. The newborn's skin was very jaundiced.

    d. Coarse crackles were auscultated throughout all lung fields.

    e. With X-ray, the nasogastric tube that the nurse attempted to insert previously was found coiled in the upper esophagus.

Nursing Care of the Child with a Genitourinary Disorder

Learning Objectives

■ Compare anatomic and physiologic differences of the genitourinary system in infants and children versus adults.

■ Describe nursing care related to common laboratory and diagnostic testing used in the medical diagnosis of pediatric genitourinary conditions.

■ Distinguish genitourinary disorders common in infants, children, and adolescents.

■ Identify appropriate nursing assessments and interventions related to medications and treatments for pediatric genitourinary disorders.

■ Develop an individualized nursing care plan for the child with a genitourinary disorder.

■ Describe the psychosocial impact of chronic genitourinary disorders on children.

■ Devise a nutrition plan for the child with renal insufficiency.

■ Develop child/family teaching plans for the child with a genitourinary disorder.

SECTION I: ASSESSING YOUR UNDERSTANDING

Activity A FILL IN THE BLANKS

1. Cytotoxic drugs cause bone marrow _____.

2. Human chorionic gonadotropin is used to precipitate _____ descent.

3. A creatinine (serum) clearance test is used to diagnose impaired _____ function.

4. Urodynamic studies measures the urine _____ during micturition.

5. Desmopressin is a medication commonly used to treat nocturnal _____.

6. Bladder capacity of the newborn is _____.

Activity B LABELING

Indicate which image represents:

1. Hypospadias
2. Epispadias

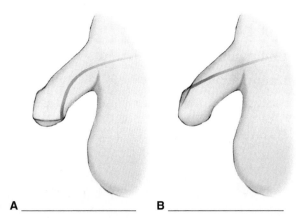

A _____   B _____

Activity C MATCHING

Match the term in Column A with the proper definition in Column B.

Column A

_____ **1.** Anuria

_____ **2.** Anasarca

_____ **3.** Menorrhagia

_____ **4.** Oliguria

_____ **5.** Hyperlipidemia

Column B

a. Profuse menstrual bleeding

b. Significant decrease in urinary output

c. Elevated lipid levels in the blood stream

d. Severe generalized edema

e. Absence of urine formation

Match the treatment in Column A with the appropriate indication in Column B.

Column A

_____ **1.** Peritoneal dialysis

_____ **2.** Foley catheter

_____ **3.** Nephrostomy tube

_____ **4.** Bladder augmentation

Column B

a. Decreased bladder capacity

b. Used to drain an obstructed kidney

c. Acute or chronic renal failure

d. Unable to void postoperatively

Activity D SEQUENCING

Review the steps of care needed for the child scheduled to undergo a voiding cystourethrogram (VCUG).

1. Bladder filled with contrast material

2. Insertion of urinary catheter

3. Bladder emptied

4. Child scanned with fluoroscope

5. Fluoroscope completed

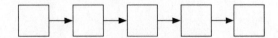

Activity E SHORT ANSWERS

Briefly answer the following.

1. How will the urine appear after a bladder augmentation is done?

_____

_____

_____

2. What are the key nursing implications following cystoscopy?

_____

_____

_____

3. What medications/ supplements are commonly used to treat the complications of end-stage renal disease?

_____

_____

_____

4. Discuss testicular torsion.

_____

_____

_____

5. The nurse has completed the newborn assessment for a baby boy. The assessment reveals the right testicle is undescended. How will this condition be managed?

_____

_____

_____

SECTION II: APPLYING YOUR KNOWLEDGE

Activity F CASE STUDY

Corey Bond is a 5-year-old introduced female. She was brought to the clinic by her mother. She presented with fever and lethargy for the past 24 hours. A urinalysis and culture confirmed that Corey has a urinary tract infection. This is Corey's first urinary tract infection and her mother is concerned and states "I do not understand how a 5-year-old can get a urinary tract infection?"

1. How will you address the mother's concerns?

   _____

   _____

   _____

2. Corey is started on oral antibiotics at home. What education can you provide the family regarding treatment and providing comfort?

   _____

   _____

   _____

3. What can Corey and her family do to try to prevent the recurrence of a urinary tract infection?

   _____

   _____

   _____

SECTION III: PRACTICING FOR NCLEX

Activity G NCLEX-STYLE QUESTIONS

Answer the following questions.

1. The nurse is caring for a 10-year-old girl presenting with fever, dysuria, flank pain, urgency, and hematuria. The nurse would expect to help obtain which of the following tests first to reveal preliminary information about the urinary tract?

   a. Total protein, globulin, and albumin

   b. Creatinine clearance

   c. Urinalysis

   d. Urine culture and sensitivity

2. The nurse is caring for a 12-year-old boy diagnosed with acute glomerulonephritis. When reviewing the boy's health history which of the following will likely be noted?

   a. The boy has a history of recurrent urinary tract infections

   b. The boy has a family history of renal disorders

   c. The boy has a recent history of an upper respiratory infection.

   d. The boy has a history of hypotension.

3. The nurse is caring for a child who is undergoing peritoneal dialysis. Immediately after draining the dialysate, what is the immediate action the nurse should take?

   a. Empty the old dialysate

   b. Weigh the old dialysate

   c. Weigh the new dialysate

   d. Start the process over again with a fresh bag

4. A nurse is caring for a 12-year-old girl recently diagnosed with end-stage renal disease. The nurse is discussing dietary restrictions with the girl's mother. Which of the following responses indicates a need for further teaching?

   a. "My daughter can eat what she wants when she is hooked to the machine."

   b. "My daughter must avoid a high sodium diet."

   c. "She needs to restrict her potassium intake."

   d. "She can eat whatever she wants on dialysis days."

5. The nurse is administering cyclophosphamide as ordered for a 12-year-old boy with nephrotic syndrome. Which of the following instructions is most accurate regarding administration of this cytotoxic drug?

   a. Administer in the evening on an empty stomach

   b. Provide adequate hydration and encourage voiding

   c. Administer in the morning, encourage fluids and voiding during and after administration

   d. Encourage fluids, adequate food intake, and voiding before and after administration

6. A nurse is caring for a 10-year-old boy with nocturnal enuresis with no physiologic cause. He says he is embarrassed and wishes he could stop the bedwetting immediately. How should the nurse respond?

   a. "You will grow out of this eventually; you just need to be patient."

   b. "There are several things we can do to help you achieve this goal."

   c. "There are almost 5 million people that have enuresis."

   d. "The pull-ups look just like underwear; no one has to know."

7. The nurse is assessing an infant with suspected hemolytic uremic syndrome. Which of the following characteristics of this condition would the nurse expect to assess, including information from the chart review?

   a. Hemolytic anemia, acute renal failure, and hypotension

   b. Dirty green colored urine, elevated erythrocyte sedimentation, and depressed serum complement level

   c. Hemolytic anemia, thrombocytopenia, and acute renal failure

   d. Thrombocytopenia, hemolytic anemia, and nocturia several times each night

8. A nurse is caring for a 13-year-old boy with end-stage renal disease who is preparing to have his hemodialysis treatment in the dialysis unit. Which of the following is the appropriate nursing action?

   a. Administer his routine medications as scheduled

   b. Take his blood pressure measurement in extremity with AV fistula

   c. Withhold his routine medication until after dialysis is completed

   d. Assess the Tenckhoff catheter site

9. The nurse is conducting a follow-up visit for a 13-year-old girl who has been treated for pelvic inflammatory disease. Which of the following remarks indicates a need for further teaching?

   a. "I should be tested for other sexually transmitted diseases."

   b. "Douching is not necessary and can cause bacteria to flourish."

   c. "I cannot have sex again until my partner is treated."

   d. "My partner needs to be treated with antibiotics."

10. The nurse is caring for a child who receives dialysis via an AV fistula. Which of the following findings indicates an immediate need to notify the physician?

    a. Presence of a bruit

    b. Presence of a thrill

    c. Dialysate without fibrin or cloudiness

    d. Absence of a thrill

11. The nurse is caring for a child diagnosed with hydronephrosis. Which of the following manifestations is consistent with complications of the disorder?

    a. Hypertension

    b. Hypotension

    c. Hypothermia

    d. Tachycardia

12. The nurse is caring for a child who has been admitted to the acute care facility with manifestations consistent with hydronephrosis. Which of the following diagnostic tests can the nurse anticipate will be performed to confirm diagnosis? Select all that apply.

    a. Intravenous pyelogram (IVP)

    b. Urinalysis

    c. Voiding cystourethrogram (VCUG)

    d. Complete blood cell count

    e. Renal ultrasound

13. The nurse is caring for the parents of a newborn who has an undescended testicle. Which of the following comments by the parents indicates understanding of the condition?

    a. "Our son may need surgery on his testes before we are discharged to go home."

    b. "Our son may have to go through life without two testes."

    c. "Our son's condition may resolve on its own."

    d. "Our son will likely have a high risk of cancer in his teen years as a result of this condition."

14. The nurse is caring for a child with epididymitis. When planning care which of the following interventions may be included?

   a. Scrotal elevation

   b. Warm compresses

   c. Corticosteroid therapy

   d. Catheterization

15. The nurse is planning the discharge instructions for the parents of a 1-month-old child who has had a circumcision completed.

Which of the following should be included in the education provided?

   a. Use Vaseline on the head of the penis for the first 2 weeks after the procedure.

   b. Report any bleeding to the physician.

   c. Reduce the child's fluid intake to reduce voiding during the first 24 hours.

   d. Report redness or swelling on the penile shaft.

CHAPTER 44

Nursing Care of the Child with a Neuromuscular Disorder

Learning Objectives

■ Compare differences between the anatomy and physiology of the neuromuscular system in children versus adults.

■ Identify nursing interventions related to common laboratory and diagnostic tests used in the diagnosis and management of neuromuscular conditions.

■ Identify appropriate nursing assessments and interventions related to medications and treatments used for childhood neuromuscular conditions.

■ Distinguish various neuromuscular illnesses occurring in childhood.

■ Devise an individualized nursing care plan for the child with a neuromuscular disorder.

■ Develop patient/family teaching plans for the child with a neuromuscular disorder.

■ Describe the psychosocial impact of chronic neuromuscular disorders on the growth and development of children.

SECTION I: ASSESSING YOUR UNDERSTANDING

Activity A FILL IN THE BLANKS

1. Dermatomyositis is a(n) _____ disease that results in inflammation of the muscles or associated tissues.

2. Due to hypertonicity, sustained _____ may be present after forced dorsiflexion.

3. Atrophy is a _____ or wasting in size of a muscle.

4. Spasticity is _____ muscle contractions that are not coordinated with other muscles.

5. Decreased muscle tone is called _____.

6. The structural disorders of spina bifida occulta, meningocele, and myelomeningocele are all considered _____.

7. _____ syndrome is also called acute inflammatory demyelinating polyradiculoneuropathy.

Activity B LABELING

Provide the appropriate labels for the following images.

1. Normal spine
2. Spine showing spina bifida occulta
3. Spine showing meningocele
4. Spine showing myelomeningocele

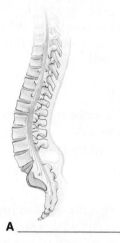 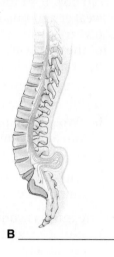 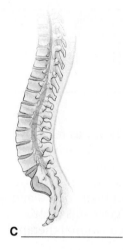 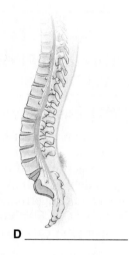

A _____ B _____ C _____ D _____

Activity C MATCHING

Match the medication in Column A with the appropriate action in Column B.

Column A

____ **1.** Baclofen

____ **2.** Corticosteroids

____ **3.** Botulin toxin

____ **4.** Benzodiazepines

____ **5.** Oxybutynin

Column B

a. Central acting skeletal muscle relaxant

b. Anticonvulsant

c. Anti-inflammatory

d. Neurotoxin

e. Antispasmodic

Activity D SHORT ANSWERS

Briefly answer the following.

1. What are the four classifications of cerebral palsy? Which is the most common form? Which is the rarest form?

_____

_____

_____

2. According to the text, what is the appropriate nursing management focus for a child with myelomeningocele?

_____

_____

_____

3. What are the common symptoms of Guillain–Barré syndrome in children?

_____

_____

_____

4. What factors increase the risk of a fetus developing a neural tube defect?

_____

_____

_____

5. Discuss the commonalities of the various forms of muscular dystrophy. What is the most common childhood type of muscular dystrophy?

_____

_____

_____

SECTION II: APPLYING YOUR KNOWLEDGE

Activity E CASE STUDY

Elijah Jefferson, a 2-year-old boy, was recently diagnosed with cerebral palsy (CP). He was born at 28 weeks gestation after a complicated and prolonged delivery. Elijah's parents have many questions and concerns about their son's diagnosis. They ask "Can Elijah outgrow this disorder with proper physical and occupational therapy?"

1. How can you help Elijah's parents to have an accurate perception of CP?

_____

_____

_____

2. What are some assessment findings on exam that are characteristic of CP?

_____

_____

_____

3. Discuss the focus of nursing management when caring for a child with CP.

_____

_____

_____

SECTION III: PRACTICING FOR NCLEX

Activity F NCLEX-STYLE QUESTIONS

Answer the following questions.

1. The nurse is taking the history of a 4-year-old boy. His mother mentions that he seems weaker and unable to keep up with his 6-year-old sister on the playground. Which of the following questions will elicit the most helpful information?

   a. "Has he achieved his developmental milestones on time?"

   b. "Would you please describe the weakness you are seeing in your son?"

   c. "Do you think he is simply fatigued?"

   d. "Has his pace of achieving milestones diminished?"

2. The nurse is conducting a physical examination of a 9-month-old baby with a suspected neuromuscular disorder. Which of the following findings would warrant further evaluation?

   a. Presence of symmetrical spontaneous movement

   b. Absence of Moro reflex

   c. Absence of tonic neck reflex

   d. Presence of Moro reflex

3. The nurse is conducting a wellness examination of a 6-month-old child. The mother points out some dimpling and skin discoloration in the child's lumbosacral area. How should the nurse respond?

   a. "This could be an indicator of spina bifida; we need to evaluate this further."

   b. "This can be considered a normal variant with no indication of a problem; however, the doctor will want to take a closer look."

   c. "Dimpling, skin discoloration, and abnormal patches of hair are often indicators of spina bifida occulta."

   d. "This is often an indicator of spina bifida occulta as opposed to spina bifida cystica."

4. A nurse is caring for an infant with a meningocele. Which of the following would alert the nurse that the lesion is increasing in size?

   a. Leaking cerebrospinal fluid

   b. Increasing ICP

   c. Constipation and bladder dysfunction

   d. Increasing head circumference

5. A nurse is teaching the parents of a boy with a neurogenic bladder about clean intermittent catheterization. Which of the following responses indicates a need for further teaching?

   a. "We must be careful to use latex-free catheters."

   b. "The very first step is to apply water-based lubricant to the catheter."

   c. "My son may someday learn how to do this for himself."

   d. "We need to soak the catheter in a vinegar and water solution daily."

6. A nurse is caring for a 13-year-old boy with Duchenne muscular dystrophy. He says he feels isolated and that there is no one who understands the challenges of his disease. How should the nurse respond?

   a. "You need to remain as active as possible and have a positive attitude."

   b. "There are many things that you can do like crafts, computers or art."

   c. "There are a lot of kids with the same type of muscular dystrophy you have at the MDA support group."

   d. "You have to go to a support group; it will be very helpful."

7. The nurse is conducting a physical examination of a 10-year-old boy with a suspected neuromuscular disorder. Which of the following is a sign of Duchenne muscular dystrophy?

   a. Walking on the toes or balls of the feet with a rolling or waddling gait

   b. Appearance of smaller than normal calf muscles

   c. Signs of hydrocephalus

   d. Lordosis

8. A nurse is caring for a 2-year-old girl with cerebral palsy. The child is having difficulty with proper nutrition and is not gaining adequate weight. How can the nurse elicit additional information to establish a diagnosis?

   a. "Let's see if she is dehydrated and we'll assess her respiratory system."

   b. "Does she have difficulty swallowing or chewing?"

   c. "Does she like to feed herself or do you feed her?"

   d. "Let's offer her a snack now and you can tell me about her diet on a typical day."

9. The nurse is caring for a 5-year-old child with Guillain–Barré syndrome. Which of the following would be the best way to assess the level of paralysis?

   a. Gentle tickling

   b. Observe for symmetrical flaccid weakness

   c. Monitor for ataxia

   d. Inquire about sensory disturbances

10. The nurse is providing presurgical care for a newborn with myelomeningocele. Which of the following is the central nursing priority?

    a. Maintain infant's body temperature

    b. Prevent rupture or leaking of cerebrospinal fluid

    c. Maintain infant in prone position

    d. Keep lesion free from fecal matter or urine

11. The child has a meningocele and a neurogenic bladder. Which of the following topics should the nurse include in the teaching plan when educating the child and the child's caregivers? Select all that apply.

    a. How and when to administer oxybutynin chloride

    b. The importance of antibiotic use to prevent urinary tract infections from occurring

    c. How and when to perform clean intermittent urinary catheterization

    d. Signs and symptoms of a urinary tract infection

    e. Different types of surgeries used to treat this condition

12. The nurse is assessing a young boy who has been brought to the physician for mobility and balance issues by his parents. Which of the following findings is positively associated with the presence of Duchenne muscular dystrophy? Select all that apply.

    a. Serum creatine kinase levels are elevated

    b. An electromyogram demonstrates the problem is within the nerves, not the muscles

    c. A muscle biopsy shows an absence of dystrophin

    d. The child is unable to rise easily into a standing position when placed on the floor

    e. Genetic testing indicates the presence of a gene associated with spinal muscular atrophy

13. The nurse learns that the child has been admitted with clinical manifestations associated with cholinergic crisis. Which of the following findings is associated with this condition? Select all that apply.

    a. The child exhibits diaphoresis

    b. The child's apical heart rate is 52 beats per minute

    c. The child's blood pressure is 172/94

    d. The child is complaining that his muscles are very weak

    e. The child is drooling excessively

14. The young girl has been prescribed corticosteroids for dermatomyositis. Which of the following statements by her mother indicates the need for further education? Select all that apply.

    a. "I give it to her first thing in the morning before breakfast."

    b. "We are taking her to Disney in the summer."

    c. "The physician said when it's time for her to stop taking this medication; he will gradually start reducing her dose."

    d. "She's got to take this medication to help with the calcium deposits that can form."

    e. "She might recover completely from this condition."

15. The young child has been diagnosed with Guillain–Barré syndrome and it is progressing in a classic manner. Rank the following sequence of events in the order that they typically occur.

    a. The child states that it is difficult to move his arms

    b. The child states that it is difficult to move his legs

    c. The child is having difficulty producing facial expressions

    d. The child complains of numbness and tingling in his toes

CHAPTER 45

Nursing Care of the Child with a Musculoskeletal Disorder

Learning Objectives

- Compare the anatomy and physiology of the musculoskeletal system in children and adults.
- Identify nursing interventions related to common laboratory and diagnostic tests used in the diagnosis and management of musculoskeletal disorders.
- Identify appropriate nursing assessments and interventions related to medications and treatments for common childhood musculoskeletal disorders.
- Distinguish various musculoskeletal disorders occurring in childhood.
- Devise an individualized nursing care plan for the child with a musculoskeletal disorder.
- Develop child/family teaching plans for the child with a musculoskeletal disorder.
- Describe the impact of chronic musculoskeletal disorders on the growth and development of children.

SECTION I: ASSESSING YOUR UNDERSTANDING

Activity A FILL IN THE BLANKS

1. Kyphosis refers to excessive _____ curvature of the spine resulting in a humpback appearance.

2. The _____ is where ossification of new bone occurs.

3. An external _____ is a device that holds bones together externally.

4. Transient _____ of the hip is the most common cause of hip pain in children.

5. Osteomyelitis is a _____ infection of the bone and soft tissue surrounding the bone.

6. _____, the conversion of cartilage to bone, continues throughout childhood and is complete at adolescence.

7. The newborn's feet may display in-toeing, also known as metatarsus _____ as a result of in utero positioning.

Activity B **LABELING**

Label the types of traction.

1. _____
2. _____
3. _____
4. _____
5. _____

6. _____
7. _____
8. _____
9. _____
10. _____

1.

Knees slightly flexed

Buttocks slightly elevated and clear of bed

2.

3.

4.

5.

6.

7.

8.

9.

10.

Activity C MATCHING

Match the medication in Column A with the appropriate indication in Column B.

Column A	Column B
____ 1. Bisphosphonate-IV	a. Relief of mild pain if used alone
____ 2. Narcotic analgesics	b. Treatment of muscle spasms
____ 3. Nonsteroidal anti-inflammatory drugs	c. Relief of moderate to severe pain
	d. Decrease incidence of fractures
____ 4. Benzodiazepines	e. Relief of mild to moderate pain
____ 5. Acetaminophen	

Activity D SEQUENCING

Place the following parts of a physical examination of a child with a suspected clavicle injury in the proper sequence

1. Gently palpate clavicles

2. Observe for any noticeable deformity

3. Palpate neurovascular status of fingers

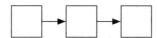

Activity E SHORT ANSWERS

Briefly answer the following.

1. Explain the difference between dislocation, subluxation, and frank dislocation in relation to developmental dysplasia of the hip (DDH).

   _____

   _____

   _____

2. List and explain the four types of fractures seen in children.

   _____

   _____

   _____

3. What should be included in the teaching guidelines for a parent with a child with osteogenesis imperfecta?

   _____

   _____

   _____

4. You are the nurse providing instructions to a 10-year-old boy, and his parents, who has just had an arm cast removed following a fracture. What are important instructions for his care?

   _____

   _____

   _____

5. What is torticollis and what type of exercises are necessary to treat the disorder?

   _____

   _____

   _____

SECTION II: APPLYING YOUR KNOWLEDGE

Activity F CASE STUDY

You are caring for a 2-year-old boy who was brought to the clinic by his mother. He presented with right arm bruising, swelling, and wrist point tenderness. An X-ray confirmed he had a right wrist fracture. The doctor decided he needed a cast.

1. What assessments and interventions should you perform before application of the cast?

_____

_____

_____

2. What assessments and interventions should you perform after application of the cast?

_____

_____

_____

3. What education will the family need for home care of their son?

_____

_____

_____

SECTION III: PRACTICING FOR NCLEX

Activity G NCLEX-STYLE QUESTIONS

Answer the following questions.

1. A nurse is assisting the parents of a child who requires a Pavlik harness. The parents are apprehensive about how to care for their baby. The nurse should stress which of the following teaching points?
   a. "The baby needs the harness only for 2 to 3 weeks."
   b. "It is important that the harness be worn continuously."
   c. "The harness does not hurt the baby."
   d. "Let me teach you how to make appropriate adjustments to the harness."

2. The nurse is conducting a routine physical examination of a newborn to screen for developmental DDH. The nurse correctly assesses the infant by placing the infant:
   a. In a prone position, noting asymmetry of the thigh or gluteal folds.
   b. With both legs extended and observes the hip and knee joint relationship.
   c. With both legs extended and observes the feet.
   d. In a supine position with both legs extended and observes the tibia/fibula.

3. A 5-year-old child is in traction and at risk for impaired skin integrity due to pressure. Which of the following is the most effective intervention?
   a. Inspect the child's skin for rashes, redness, irritation, or pressure sores.
   b. Apply lotion to dry skin.
   c. Gently massage the child's back to stimulate circulation.
   d. Keep the child's skin clean and dry.

4. A nurse is conducting a physical examination of an infant with suspected metatarsus adductus. Which of the following findings would indicate Type II metatarsus adductus? The forefoot is:
   a. Inverted and turned slightly upward
   b. Flexible past neutral actively and passively
   c. Flexible passively past neutral, but only to midline actively
   d. Rigid, does not correct to midline even with passive stretching

5. A nurse is providing instructions for home cast care. Which of the following responses by the parent indicates a need for further teaching?
   a. "We must avoid causing depressions in the cast."
   b. "Pale, cool, or blue skin coloration is to be expected."
   c. "The casted arm must be kept still."
   d. "We need be aware of odor or drainage from the cast."

6. A nurse is caring for a 6-year-old boy with a fractured ulna. He is fearful about the casting process and is resisting treatment. How should the nurse respond?

   a. "The application of the cast will not hurt."

   b. "Would you like to pick out your favorite color?"

   c. "Look over there at the neon fish in our aquarium."

   d. "Will you please take this medicine for pain?"

7. The nurse is providing postoperative care for a boy who has undergone surgical correction for pectus excavatum. The nurse should emphasize which of the following to the child and his parents?

   a. "Please watch for signs of infection."

   b. "Be sure to monitor his vital capacity."

   c. "Do not allow him to lie on either side."

   d. "Do not allow him to lie on his stomach."

8. A nurse is caring for an 11-year-old with an Ilizarov fixator and is providing teaching regarding pin care. The nurse should provide which of the following instructions?

   a. "Cleansing by showering should be sufficient."

   b. "You must clean the pin sites with saline."

   c. "The pin site should be cleaned with anti-bacterial solution."

   d. "Please make sure that the pin site is cleansed with Betadine swabs after showering."

9. The nurse is caring for an infant girl in an outpatient setting. The infant has just been diagnosed with DDH. The mother is very upset about the diagnosis and blames herself for her daughter's condition. Which of the following would best address the mother's concerns?

   a. "There are simple noninvasive treatment options."

   b. "Your daughter will likely wear a Pavlik harness."

   c. "Don't worry; this is a relatively common diagnosis."

   d. "This is not your fault and we will help you with her care and treatment."

10. The nurse is conducting a physical examination of a newborn with suspected osteogenesis imperfecta. Which of the following is a common finding?

    a. Foot is drawn up and inward

    b. Sole of foot faces backwards

    c. Dimpled skin, hair in lumbar region

    d. Blue sclera

11. The young child is experiencing muscle spasms and has been given lorazepam. Which of the following statements by the child indicate that the child may be experiencing some common side effects? Select all that apply.

    a. "I feel sort of dizzy."

    b. "I need to take a nap."

    c. "My muscle cramps are getting worse."

    d. "I think I'm going to throw up."

    e. "My belly hurts."

12. The young boy has fractured his left leg and has had a cast applied. The nurse educates the boy and his parents prior to discharge from the hospital. The parents should call the physician when which of the following occurs? Select all that apply.

    a. The boy experiences mild pain when wiggling his toes.

    b. The boy has had a fever of greater than 102 F for the last 36 hours.

    c. New drainage is seeping out from under the cast.

    d. The outside of the boy's cast got wet and had to be dried using a hair dryer.

    e. The boy's toes are light blue and very swollen.

13. The child has been diagnosed with rickets. The child's mother is educated about the importance of providing the child with 10 μg micrograms (400 International Units) of an oral vitamin D supplement each day. The child's mother purchases over-the-counter vitamin D drops. The supplement is noted to contain 5 μg of vitamin D in each 0.5 mL. How much of the supplement should the mother administer to the child each day?

14. The child has been diagnosed with slipped capital femoral epiphysis. Which of the following characteristics about the patient is risk factor associated with the development of this condition? Select all that apply.

    a. The child is noted to be underweight by the nurse.

    b. The child is 13 years old.

    c. The child is African American.

    d. The child's parents state that the child has recently experienced a "growth spurt."

    e. The child is male.

15. Identify which of the following images is a greenstick fracture.

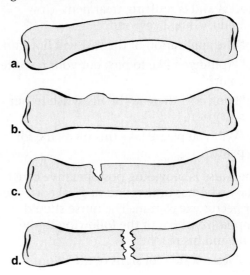

a.

b.

c.

d.

Nursing Care of the Child with an Integumentary Disorder

Learning Objectives

■ Compare anatomic and physiologic differences of the integumentary system in infants and children versus adults.
■ Describe nursing care related to common laboratory and diagnostic tests used in the medical diagnosis of integumentary disorders in infants, children, and adolescents.
■ Distinguish integumentary disorders common in infants, children, and adolescents.
■ Identify appropriate nursing assessments and interventions related to pediatric integumentary disorders.
■ Develop an individualized nursing care plan for the child with an integumentary disorder.
■ Describe the psychosocial impact of a chronic integumentary disorder on children or adolescents.
■ Develop patient/family teaching plans for the child with an integumentary disorder.

SECTION I: ASSESSING YOUR UNDERSTANDING

Activity A FILL IN THE BLANKS

1. Diaper wearing _____ the skin's pH, activating fecal enzymes that further contribute to skin maceration.

2. Serum _____ may be elevated in the child with atopic dermatitis.

3. Urticaria is a type I _____ reaction.

4. Seborrhea in infants is commonly referred to as _____.

5. Acne neonatorum occurs as a response to the presence of maternal _____.

Activity B MATCHING

Match the term in Column A with the correct definition in Column B.

Column A

___ 1. Annular
___ 2. Papule
___ 3. Vesicle
___ 4. Macule
___ 5. Scaling

Column B

a. A flat discolored area on the skin
b. In a circle or ring shape
c. Small raised bump on the skin
d. A fluid-filled bump on the skin
e. Flaking of the skin

Match the medication in Column A with the appropriate indication in Column B.

Column A

___ **1.** Silver sulfadiazine 1%

___ **2.** Isotretinoin

___ **3.** Coal tar preparations

___ **4.** Benzoyl peroxide

Column B

a. Psoriasis, atopic dermatitis

b. Mild acne vulgaris

c. Cystic acne

d. Burns

Activity C SEQUENCING

List in order the stages in the progression of an impetigo lesion.

1. Formation of a crust on an ulcer-like base

2. Papules

3. Painless pustules with an erythematous border

4. Honey-colored exudate

5. Vesicles

☐ → ☐ → ☐ → ☐ → ☐

Activity D SHORT ANSWERS

Briefly answer the following.

1. Review the different cutaneous reactions commonly found in dark-skinned children compared to children with lighter skin.

_____

_____

_____

2. According to the text, what are the four criteria used to describe lesions?

_____

_____

_____

3. What are the differences between bullous impetigo and non-bullous impetigo?

_____

_____

_____

4. List the risk factors that are associated with the development of pressure ulcers. What sites are more prone for pressure ulcer development?

_____

_____

_____

5. Explain the relationship between puberty and acne vulgaris.

_____

_____

_____

SECTION II: APPLYING YOUR KNOWLEDGE

Activity E CASE STUDY

Eva Lopez is a 1-year-old child. She has presented at the ambulatory care clinic with reports of itching and scratching that is worse at night. The assessment reveals dry patches of skin. She has evidence of bleeding at the wrists from scratching. A diagnosis of atopic dermatitis (eczema) is made.

1. The mother states, "I do not understand why the rash comes and goes and only seems to appear after Eva has been scratching?" Address the mother's concerns.

_____

_____

_____

2. What education will the family need to help manage atopic dermatitis?

_____

_____

_____

SECTION III: PRACTICING FOR NCLEX

Activity F NCLEX-STYLE QUESTIONS

Answer the following questions.

1. The nurse is conducting a primary survey of a child with burns. Which of the following assessment findings points to airway injury from burn or smoke inhalation?
   a. Burns on hands
   b. Cervical spine injury
   c. Stridor
   d. Internal injuries

2. The nurse is conducting a physical examination of a child with severe burns. Which of the following internal physiologic manifestations would the nurse expect to occur first?
   a. Insulin resistance
   b. Hypermetabolic response with increased cardiac output
   c. Decrease in cardiac output
   d. Increased protein catabolism

3. The nurse is caring for a 10-month-old with a rash. The child's mother reports that the onset was abrupt. The nurse assesses diffuse erythema and skin tenderness with, ruptured bullae in the axillary area with red weeping surface. The nurse suspects which of the following bacterial infections?
   a. Folliculitis
   b. Impetigo
   c. Non-bullous impetigo
   d. Scalded skin syndrome

4. A nurse providing teaching on ways to promote skin hydration for the parents of an infant with atopic dermatitis. Which of the following responses indicates a need for further teaching?
   a. "We need to avoid any skin product containing perfumes, dyes, or fragrances."
   b. "We should use a mild soap for sensitive skin."
   c. "We should bathe our child in hot water, twice a day."
   d. "We should use soap to clean only dirty areas."

5. A nurse is caring for a child with tinea pedis. Which of the following assessment findings would the nurse expect to note?
   a. Red scaling rash on soles and between the toes
   b. Patches of scaling in the scalp with central hair loss
   c. Inflamed boggy mass filled with pustules
   d. Erythema, scaling, maceration in the inguinal creases and inner thighs

6. A nurse assessing a 6-month-old girl with an integumentary disorder. The nurse notes three virtually identically sized, round red circles with scaling that are symmetrically spaced on both of the girl's inner thighs. What should the nurse ask the mother?
   a. "Has she been exposed to poison ivy?"
   b. "Does she wear sleepers with metal snaps?"
   c. "Do you change her diapers regularly?"
   d. "Tell me about your family history of allergies."

7. The nurse is conducting a physical examination of a boy with erythema multiforme. Which of the following assessment findings would the nurse expect to note?
   a. Lesions over the hands and feet, and extensor surfaces of the extremities with spread to the trunk
   b. Thick or flaky/greasy yellow scales
   c. Silvery or yellow-white scale plaques and sharply demarcated borders
   d. Superficial tan or hypopigmented oval shaped scaly lesions especially on upper back and chest and proximal arms

8. A nurse is caring for a child with a wasp sting. What is the priority nursing intervention?
   a. Remove jewelry or restrictive clothing
   b. Apply ice intermittently
   c. Administer the diphenhydramine per protocol
   d. Cleanse wound with mild soap and water

9. The nurse is examining a child for indications of frostbite and notes blistering with erythema and edema. The nurse notes which of the following degrees of frostbite?

   a. First degree frostbite

   b. Second degree frostbite

   c. Third degree frostbite

   d. Fourth degree frostbite

10. The nurse is providing teaching on ways to maintaining skin integrity and preventing infection for the parents of a boy with atopic dermatitis. Which of the following responses indicates a need for further teaching?

    a. "We should avoid using petroleum jelly."

    b. "We should keep his fingernails short and clean."

    c. "We should avoid tight clothing and heat."

    d. "We need to develop ways to prevent him from scratching."

11. The nurse is providing education to the parents of a teenaged boy diagnosed with impetigo. Which of the following statements by the boy indicates the need for further education?

    a. "I will need to cover my son's skin lesions with bandages until it has healed."

    b. "It is important to remove the crusts before applying any topical medications."

    c. "This condition is contagious."

    d. "My son can continue to attend school while he is taking the prescribed antibiotics."

12. A 16-year-old male who has diagnosed with tinea pedis questions the nurse about how he may have contracted the condition. What information may be provided to the boy by the nurse?

    a. "It is unlikely you will be able to determine the cause of the infection."

    b. "This condition is common in individuals with lowered immunity."

    c. "You may have gotten the condition from a community shower or gym area."

    d. "You likely had an infection in another area of your body and it has spread."

13. The nurse is discussing the use of over-the-counter ointments to manage a mild case of diaper rash. What ingredients should the nurse instruct the parents to look for in a compound? Select all that apply.

    a. Vitamin A

    b. Zinc

    c. Vitamin D

    d. Vitamin B_6

    e. Vitamin B_{12}

14. The nurse is discussing dietary intake with the parents of a 4-year-old child who has been diagnosed with atopic dermatitis. Later nurse notes the menu selection made by the parents for the child. Which selection indicates the need for further instruction?

    a. Peanut butter and jelly sandwich

    b. Chicken nuggets

    c. Tomato soup

    d. Carrot and celery sticks

15. The nurse is developing the plan of care for a 3-year-old child diagnosed with atopic dermatitis. When reviewing the desired patient outcomes which of the following are common focuses for a child with this diagnosis? Select all that apply.

    a. Pain management

    b. Promotion of skin hydration

    c. Maintenance of skin integrity

    d. Reduction in anxiety

    e. Prevention of infection

CHAPTER 47

Nursing Care of the Child with a Hematologic Disorder

Learning Objectives

- Identify major hematologic disorders that affect children.
- Determine priority assessment information for children with hematologic disorders.
- Analyze laboratory data in relation to normal findings and report abnormal findings.
- Provide nursing diagnoses appropriate for the child and family with hematologic disorders.
- Identify priority interventions for children with hematologic disorders.
- Develop a teaching plan for the family of children with hematologic disorders.
- Identify resources for children and families with hematologic disorders or nutrition deficits.

SECTION I: ASSESSING YOUR UNDERSTANDING

Activity A FILL IN THE BLANKS

1. The complete blood count is also called the CBC or _____.

2. Anemia is the reduction of red blood cells or hemoglobin in the total blood _____.

3. Erythropoietin is a hormone produced by the _____ that stimulates the production of red blood cells.

4. Mean corpuscular volume (MCV) is a measure of the average _____ of the RBC.

5. Heme is iron surrounded by _____.

6. _____ is the measurement of the size of the platelets.

7. If the levels of RBCs and Hgb are lower than normal _____ is present.

Activity B LABELING

Place the following labels in the appropriate location on the diagram.

1. _____
2. _____
3. _____
4. _____
5. _____
6. _____

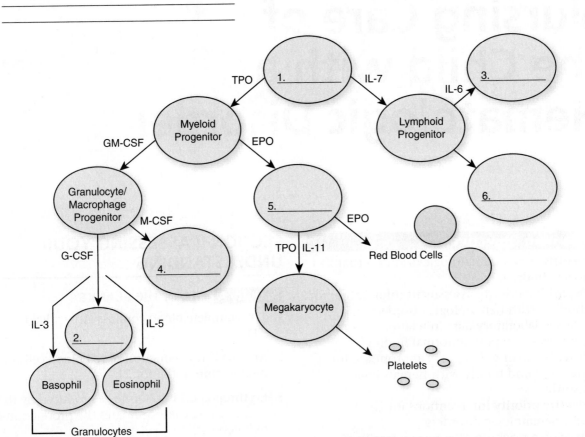

Activity C MATCHING

Match the medication in Column A with the appropriate indication in Column B.

Column A

____ **1.** Factor VII

____ **2.** Deferoxamine

____ **3.** Intravenous immune globulin (IVIG)

____ **4.** Penicillin

____ **5.** Chelating agents

Column B

a. Blood lead levels greater than 45 μg/dL

b. Prophylaxis of infection in asplenia

c. Iron toxicity

d. Idiopathic thrombocytopenic purpura

e. Hemophilia

Activity D SHORT ANSWERS

Briefly answer the following.

1. Explain the difference between folic acid deficiency and pernicious anemia. What is the appropriate management for each?

   _____

   _____

   _____

2. According to the American Academy of Pediatrics, what is the recommended action for a blood lead level of 20 to 44 µg/dL?

_____

_____

_____

3. Signs of changes in the hematologic system are often subtle and overlooked. What are some of the first signs of a problem developing?

_____

_____

_____

4. Discuss the incidence of sickle cell anemia.

_____

_____

_____

5. Discuss how iron deficiency anemia occurs and which age groups it is most prevalent in.

_____

_____

_____

SECTION II: APPLYING YOUR KNOWLEDGE

Activity E CASE STUDY

Jayda Johnson, 15-months-old, is brought to the clinic for a routine exam. Her parents state she has been irritable lately. Assessment findings reveal pallor of the mucous membranes and conjunctivae, heart rate of 120 and a heart murmur heard upon auscultation.

1. What other assessment information about the home environment is important for the nurse to gather.

_____

_____

_____

2. Lab results revealed hemoglobin of 10 g/dL and hematocrit of 29%. The physician decides to start Jayda on a daily dose of ferrous sulfate. What instructions should be given to the child's parents?

_____

_____

_____

3. What sociocultural influences may be related to the child's condition?

_____

_____

_____

SECTION III: PRACTICING FOR NCLEX

Activity F NCLEX-STYLE QUESTIONS

Answer the following questions.

1. The nurse is caring for a child with DIC. The nurse notices signs of neurological deficit. The appropriate nursing action is to:

  a. Continue to monitor neurological signs

  b. Notify the physician

  c. Evaluate respiratory status

  d. Inspect for signs of bleeding

2. The nurse is examining the hands of a child with suspected iron deficiency anemia. Which of the following would the nurse expect to find?

  a. Capillary refill in less than 2 seconds

  b. Pink palms and nail beds

  c. Absence of bruising

  d. Spooning of nails

3. The nurse is evaluating the complete blood count of a 7-year-old child with a suspected hematological disorder. Which of the following findings would be associated with an elevated mean corpuscular volume (MCV)?

   a. Macrocytic RBCs
   b. Decreased WBCs
   c. Platelet count of 250,000
   d. Hgb of 11.2 g/dL

4. A nurse is caring for a newborn whose screening test result indicates the possibility of SCA or sickle cell trait. The nurse would expect the test result to be confirmed by which of the following lab tests:

   a. Reticulocyte count
   b. Peripheral blood smear
   c. Erythrocyte sedimentation rate
   d. Hemoglobin electrophoresis

5. A nurse is providing dietary interventions for a 5-year-old with an iron deficiency. Which of the following responses indicates a need for further teaching?

   a. "Red meat is a good option; he loves the hamburgers from the drive-thru."
   b. "He will enjoy tuna casserole and eggs"
   c. "There are many iron fortified cereals that he likes"
   d. "I must encourage a variety of iron-rich foods that he likes"

6. A nurse is caring for a 7-year-old boy with hemophilia who requires an infusion of factor VIII. He is fearful about the process and is resisting treatment. How should the nurse respond?

   a. "Would you like to administer the infusion?"
   b. "Would you help me dilute this and mix it up?"
   c. "Will you help me apply this band-aid?"
   d. "Please be brave; we need to stop the bleeding"

7. The nurse is providing teaching about iron supplement administration to the parents of a 10-month-old child. It is critical that the nurse emphasize which of the following teaching points to the parents?

   a. "You must precisely measure the amount of iron"
   b. "Your child may become constipated from the iron"
   c. "Please give him plenty of fluids and encourage fiber"
   d. "Place the liquid behind the teeth; the pigment can cause staining"

8. A nurse in the emergency department is examining a 6-month-old with symmetrical swelling of the hands and feet. The nurse immediately suspects:

   a. Cooley's anemia
   b. ITP
   c. Sickle cell disease
   d. Hemophilia

9. The nurse is caring for a child with aplastic anemia. The nurse is reviewing the child's blood work and notes the granulocyte count about 500, platelets over 20,000, and the reticulocyte count is over 1%. The parents ask if these values have any significance. The nurse is correct in responding:

   a. "The doctor will discuss these findings with you when he comes to the hospital."
   b. "These values will help us monitor the disease."
   c. "These labs are just common labs for children with this disease."
   d. "I'm really not allowed to discuss these findings with you."

10. The nurse is caring for an 18-month-old with suspected iron deficiency anemia. Which of the following lab results confirms the diagnosis?

    a. Increased hemoglobin and hematocrit, increased reticulocyte count, microcytosis, and hypochromia

    b. Increased serum iron and ferritin levels: decreased FEP level, microcytosis and hypochromia

    c. Decreased hemoglobin and hematocrit, decreased reticulocyte count, microcytosis, and hypochromia, decreased serum iron and ferritin levels and increase FEP level

    d. Increased hemoglobin and hematocrit, increased reticulocyte, microcytosis and hypochromia, increased serum iron and ferritin levels and decreased FEP level

11. The blood cell becomes an erythrocyte. Rank the following steps in the proper order of occurrence.

    a. The myeloid cell becomes a megakaryocyte

    b. Erythropoietin helps the cell turn into a red blood cell

    c. Thrombopoietin acts on the cell

    d. The bone marrow releases a stem cell

12. The young girl has been diagnosed with a hematologic disorder. Her erythrocyte count is below normal. The mean corpuscular volume is below normal. The girl's mean corpuscular hemoglobin concentration is below normal. Which of the following statements by the girl's nurse is true regarding this girl? Select all that apply.

    a. "She's anemic."

    b. "Her red blood cells are macrocytic."

    c. "Her red blood cells are hypochromic."

    d. "The amount of hemoglobin in her red blood cells is very dilute."

    e. "Her red blood cells are smaller than normal."

13. The young boy has had his spleen surgically removed. Which of the following statements by the boy's parents prior to discharge indicates that an adequate amount of learning has occurred?

    a. "If he gets a fever, I'm going to call our physician right away."

    b. "If he does get sick, then we'll need to put on his medic alert bracelet."

    c. "Before he goes to the dentist, we'll make sure he gets antibiotics."

    d. "He's going to need several vaccines."

    e. "He's going to get really good at washing his hands."

14. The child has anemia and iron supplements will be administered by his parents at home. Which of the following statements by the child's parents indicates that further education is required?

    a. "It's better if I give the iron with orange juice."

    b. "I can give the iron mixed with chocolate milk."

    c. "If the iron is mixed in a drink, then he should drink it with a straw."

    d. "He may develop diarrhea."

    e. "His urine may look dark."

15. The child has been diagnosed with severe iron deficiency anemia. The child requires 5 mg/kg of elemental iron per day in three equally divided doses. The child weighs 47.3 pounds. How many milligrams of elemental iron should the child receive with each dose? Round to the nearest whole number.

Nursing Care of the Child with an Immunologic Disorder

Learning Objectives

- Explain anatomic and physiologic differences of the immune system in infants and children versus adults.
- Describe nursing care related to common laboratory and diagnostic testing used in the medical diagnosis of pediatric immune and autoimmune disorders.
- Distinguish immune, autoimmune, and allergic disorders common in infants, children, and adolescents.
- Identify appropriate nursing assessments and interventions related to medications and treatments for pediatric immune, autoimmune, and allergic disorders.
- Develop an individualized nursing care plan for the child with an immune or autoimmune disorder.
- Describe the psychosocial impact of chronic immune disorders on children.
- Devise a nutrition plan for the child with immunodeficiency.
- Develop patient/family teaching plans for the child with an immune or autoimmune disorder.

SECTION I: ASSESSING YOUR UNDERSTANDING

Activity A FILL IN THE BLANKS

1. In systemic lupus erythematosus (SLE), auto-antibodies react with the child's _____ to form immune complexes.

2. _____ is the movement of white blood cells to an inflamed or infected area of the body in response to chemicals released by neutrophils, monocytes, and the suffering tissue.

3. Primary immune deficiencies such as SCID and Wiskott–Aldrich syndrome are cured only by _____ or stem cell transplantation.

4. The malar rash of SLE resembles the shape of a _____.

5. For most children only allergies to fish, shell-fish, tree nuts, and _____ persist into adulthood.

6. A _____ rash is often an early sign of a graft-versus-host disease that is developing in response to a bone marrow or stem cell transplant.

7. HIV infects the CD4 cells, also known as the _____ cells.

Activity B MATCHING

Match the medication in Column A with the appropriate indication in Column B.

Column A

_____ **1.** Cyclophosphamide

_____ **2.** Protease inhibitors

_____ **3.** Cyclosporine A

_____ **4.** Methotrexate

_____ **5.** NSAIDs

Column B

a. Severe polyarticular juvenile idiopathic arthritis (JIA)

b. Prevention of rejection of renal transplants

c. JIA

d. Treatment of HIV as part of 3-drug regimen

e. Severe SLE

Activity C SEQUENCING

Place the following anaphylaxis treatment priorities in the proper sequence.

1. Administration of corticosteroids

2. Injection of intramuscular epinephrine

3. Administration of intravenous diphenhydramine

4. Assessment of airway and support of the airway, breathing, and circulation

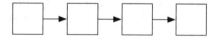

Activity D SHORT ANSWERS

Briefly answer the following.

1. What is the complement in relation to the immune system?

_____

_____

_____

2. Which laboratory test for HIV requires serial testing? Why?

_____

_____

_____

3. Why are skin test responses (such as PPD for tuberculosis detection) diminished until about 1 year of age?

_____

_____

_____

4. Discuss what is meant by the statement, "Children acquire HIV infection either vertically or horizontally."

_____

_____

_____

5. What is avascular necrosis and what group of patients are at an increased risk of developing this complication?

_____

_____

_____

SECTION II: APPLYING YOUR KNOWLEDGE

Activity E CASE STUDY

A 15-year-old female presents with complaints of pain and swelling in her joints, weight gain, and fatigue. After further assessment the physician suspects SLE.

1. What laboratory and diagnostic tests may you expect the physician to order?

_____

_____

2. The mother asks, "Will these tests confirm whether or not my daughter has lupus?" How would you respond?

_____

_____

_____

3. If the diagnosis is confirmed, what education will be necessary for the girl and her mother?

_____

_____

_____

SECTION III: PRACTICING FOR NCLEX

Activity F NCLEX-STYLE QUESTIONS

Answer the following questions.

1. The nurse is caring for a 6-month-old boy with Wiskott–Aldrich syndrome. The nurse teaches the parents which of the following:

  a. "Don't use a tub bath for daily cleansing"

  b. "Don't encourage a pacifier due to possible oral malformation"

  c. "Do not insert anything in the rectum"

  d. "Do not use a sponge bath for light cleaning"

2. The nurse is preparing to administer intravenous immunoglobulin (IVIG) for a child who has not had an IVIG infusion in over 10 weeks. The nurse knows to first:

  a. Begin infusion slowly increasing to prescribed rate

  b. Assess for adverse reaction

  c. Obtain baseline physical assessment

  d. Premedicate with acetaminophen or diphenhydramine

3. The nurse is providing instructions to the parents of a child with a severe peanut allergy. Which of the following statements by the parents indicates a need for further teaching about the use of the EpiPen Jr.®?

  a. "We must massage the area for 10 seconds after administration"

  b. "We must make sure that the black tip is pointed downward"

  c. "The EpiPen Jr.® should be jabbed into the upper arm"

  d. "The EpiPen Jr.® must be held firmly for 10 seconds"

4. A nurse is caring for an infant whose mother is HIV positive. The nurse knows that which of the following diagnostic test results will be positive even if the child is not infected with the virus:

  a. Erythrocyte sedimentation rate

  b. Immunoglobulin electrophoresis

  c. Polymerase chain reaction test

  d. Enzyme-linked immunosorbent assay

5. A nurse is providing dietary interventions for a 12-year-old with a shellfish allergy. Which of the following responses indicates a need for further teaching?

  a. "He will likely outgrow this"

  b. "He must avoid lobster and shrimp"

  c. "We must order carefully when dining out"

  d. "Wheezing is a sign of a severe reaction"

6. A nurse is conducting a physical examination of a 12-year-old girl with suspected SLE. How would the nurse best interview the girl?

  a. "Do you notice any wheezing when you breathe or a runny nose?"

  b. "Do you have any shoulder pain or abdominal tenderness?"

  c. "Tell me if you have noticed any new bruising or different color patterns on your skin"

  d. "Have you noticed any hair loss or redness on your face?"

7. The nurse is providing teaching about food substitutions when cooking for the child with an allergy to eggs. Which of the following responses indicates a need for further teaching?

  a. "I must not feed my child eggs in any form"

  b. "I can use the egg white when baking, but not the yolk"

  c. "1 tsp yeast and ¼ cups warm water is a substitute in baked goods"

  d. "1 teaspoon baking powder equals one egg in a recipe"

8. A nurse in the emergency department is examining an 18-month-old with lip edema, urticaria, stridor, and tachycardia. The nurse immediately suspects:

  a. Severe polyarticular JIA

  b. Anaphylaxis

  c. SLE

  d. SCID

9. The nurse is providing teaching for the parents of a child with a latex allergy. The nurse tells the client to avoid which of the following foods?

    a. Blueberries

    b. Pumpkin

    c. Banana

    d. Pomegranate

10. The nurse is caring for a child with JIA. There is involvement of five or more small joints and it is affecting the body symmetrically. This tells the nurse which of the following?

    a. The child has polyarticular JIA

    b. The child has systemic JIA

    c. The child has pauciarticular JIA

    d. The child is at risk for anaphylaxis

11. The child has a peanut allergy and accidentally ate food that contained peanuts. Which of the following findings are clinical manifestations of anaphylaxis? Select all that apply.

    a. The child's pulse is 52 beats per minute

    b. The child states that his tongue feels "too big" for his mouth

    c. The child has developed hives on his face and trunk

    d. The child states he feels might "throw up"

    e. The child states that he feels like he might faint

12. The nurse is preparing to administer the child's dose of IVIG. Which of the following activities by the nurse indicates the need for further education? Select all that apply.

    a. The nurse is preparing to administer the medication ventrogluteal site as an intramuscular injection

    b. The nurse takes baseline vital signs and will monitor the vital signs during the infusion

    c. The nurse is prepared to give acetaminophen to the child

    d. The nurse is prepared to give diphenhydramine to the child

    e. The nurse has mixed the medication with the child's intravenous antibiotic

13. The nurse is assessing children in a physician's office. Which of the following children may have a primary immunodeficiency?

    a. The child has been diagnosed with six episodes of acute otitis media during the previous year

    b. The child is 3 years old and has oral thrush that is unresolved with treatment

    c. The child has been admitted to the hospital three times within the last year with pneumonia

    d. The child has been diagnosed with a severe case of acute sinusitis during the last year

    e. The child has taken antibiotics for the last 3 months without evidence of clearing of the infection

14. The young child is diagnosed with acute otitis media. The child's mother states that the child had a severe reaction to penicillin in the past. Which of the following statements by the nurse indicates that further education is required? Select all that apply.

    a. "You may want to look into desensitization techniques."

    b. "It is important for you to share this information with any future physician."

    c. "Here is your prescription for cephalexin from the physician."

    d. "Here is your prescription from the physician for penicillin V."

    e. "Desensitization procedures are performed in an acute care setting."

15. The young girl has been diagnosed with JIA and has been prescribed methotrexate. Which of the following statements by the child's parent indicates that adequate learning has occurred?

    a. "We'll need to bring her back in for some lab tests after she starts methotrexate."

    b. "She can take methotrexate with yogurt or chocolate milk."

    c. "She may start feeling better by next week."

    d. "Swimming sounds like a good exercise for her."

    e. "A warm bath before bed might help her sleep better."

CHAPTER 49

Nursing Care of the Child with an Endocrine Disorder

Learning Objectives

- Describe the major components and functions of a child's endocrine system.
- Differentiate between the anatomic and physiologic differences of the endocrine system in children and adults.
- Identify the essential assessment elements, common diagnostic procedures, and laboratory tests associated with the diagnosis of endocrine disorders in children.
- Identify the common medications and treatment modalities used for palliation of endocrine disorders in children.
- Distinguish specific disorders of the endocrine system affecting children.
- Link the clinical manifestations of specific disorders in the endocrine system of a child with the appropriate nursing diagnoses.
- Establish the nursing outcomes, evaluative criteria, and interventions for a child with specific disorders in the endocrine system.
- Develop child/family teaching plans for the child with an endocrine disorder.

SECTION I: ASSESSING YOUR UNDERSTANDING

Activity A FILL IN THE BLANKS

1. Insulin is developed and secreted by beta cells, located in the islets of _____ in the pancreas.

2. Ophthalmic changes, due to hyperthyroidism, include _____, which is less pronounced in children.

3. The most common initial symptoms of diabetes mellitus reported are _____ and polydipsia.

4. Twitching of the extremities, referred to as _____, is related to hypocalcemia in children with hypoparathyroidism.

5. Slow, deep _____ respirations are characteristic of air hunger during metabolic acidosis.

6. Dwarfism is due to a growth hormone _____.

7. The presence of a goiter is typically associated with _____.

Activity B LABELING

Circle the areas on the body corresponding with insulin injection sites.

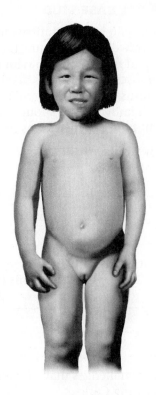 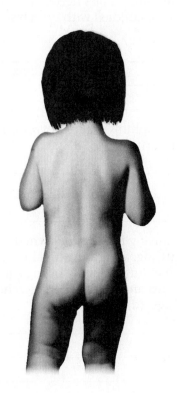

Activity C MATCHING

Match the gland in Column A with the proper word or phrase in Column B.

Column A	Column B
___ **1.** Adrenal gland	**a.** Humoral factors
___ **2.** Pancreas	**b.** Calcium and phosphorus concentration
___ **3.** Parathyroid	
___ **4.** Thymus	**c.** Glucagon and somatostatin
___ **5.** Thyroid	**d.** Calcium and phosphorus homeostasis
	e. Mineralocorticoids

Activity D SEQUENCING

Place the following insulin types in the proper order of their onset times:

1. Lispro

2. NPH

3. Regular

4. Ultralente

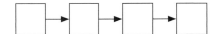

Activity E SHORT ANSWERS

Briefly answer the following.

1. What are the teaching topics needed to educate parents of children with diabetes mellitus?

_____

_____

_____

2. List signs and symptoms of hypothyroidism and hyperthyroidism.

_____

_____

_____

3. What are the nursing implications when teaching, discussing, and caring for children with diabetes mellitus in the following age groups: (a) infants and toddlers, (b) preschoolers, (c) school age, (d) and adolescent?

_____

_____

_____

4. Discuss how *Healthy People 2020* suggests addressing the goal of reducing the annual number of new cases of diagnosed diabetes in the population.

_____

_____

_____

5. What teaching points should the nurse discuss with the parents of a child receiving growth hormone in regards to possible adverse reactions?

_____

_____

_____

SECTION II: APPLYING YOUR KNOWLEDGE

Activity F CASE STUDY

A 12-year-old boy is admitted to the pediatric unit with weakness, fatigue, blurred vision, headaches, and mood and behavior changes. After further assessment he was diagnosed with diabetes mellitus type 2 (DM type 2). His mother states, "I know a little about diabetes and I thought type 2 diabetes was seen only in adults?"

1. How would you address the mother's question?

_____

_____

_____

2. What will be the focus of your nursing management for Carlos and his family?

_____

_____

_____

3. What challenges may you anticipate with educating Carlos?

_____

_____

_____

SECTION III: PRACTICING FOR NCLEX

Activity G NCLEX-STYLE QUESTIONS

Answer the following questions.

1. The nurse is providing acute care for an 11-year-old boy with hypoparathyroidism. Which of the following is the priority intervention?

   a. Providing administration of calcium and vitamin D

   b. Ensuring patency of the IV site to prevent tissue damage

   c. Monitoring fluid intake and urinary calcium output

   d. Administering intravenous calcium gluconate as ordered

2. The nurse is assessing a 4-year-old girl with ambiguous genitalia. Which of the following findings would be consistent with congenital adrenal hyperplasia?

   a. Auscultation reveals irregular heartbeat

   b. Observing pubic hair and hirsutism

   c. Palpation elicits pain from constipation

   d. Observing hyperpigmentation of the skin

3. The nurse is assessing a 7-year-old girl who complains of headache, is irritable, and vomiting. Her health history reveals she has had meningitis. Which of the following is the priority intervention?

   a. Notifying the physician of the neurologic findings

   b. Setting up safety precautions to prevent injury

   c. Monitoring urine volume and specific gravity

   d. Restoring fluid balance with IV sodium chloride

4. The nurse is caring for a 4-year-old boy during a growth hormone stimulation test. Which of the following is a priority task for the care of this child?

   a. Providing a wet washcloth to suck on

   b. Educating family about side effects

   c. Monitoring blood glucose levels

   d. Monitoring intake and output

5. The nurse is assessing a 1-month-old girl who, according to the mother, doesn't eat well. Which of the following assessments would suggest the child has congenital hypothyroidism?

   a. Mother reports frequent diarrhea

   b. Observation of an enlarged tongue

   c. Auscultation reveals tachycardia

   d. Palpation reveals warm, moist skin

6. The nurse is caring for an obese 15-year-old girl who missed two periods and is afraid she is pregnant. Which of the following findings would indicate polycystic ovary syndrome?

   a. Observation of acanthosis nigricans

   b. Complains of blurred vision and headaches

   c. Auscultation reveals increased respiratory rate

   d. Palpation reveals hypertrophy and weakness

7. The nurse is assessing a 16-year-old boy who has had long-term corticosteroid therapy. Which of the following findings, along with the use of the corticosteroids, would indicate Cushing's disease?

   a. History of rapid weight gain

   b. Observing a round, child-like face

   c. Observing high weight to height ratio

   d. Observing delayed dentition

8. The nurse is caring for a 10-year-old girl with hyperparathyroidism. Which of the following would be a primary nursing diagnosis for this child?

   a. Disturbed body image related to hormone dysfunction

   b. Imbalanced nutrition: more than body requirements

   c. Deficient fluid volume related to electrolyte imbalance

   d. Deficient knowledge related to treatment of the disease

9. The nurse is teaching an 11-year-old boy and his family how to manage his diabetes. Which of the following does not focus on glucose management?

   a. Teaching that 50% of daily calories should be carbohydrates

   b. Instructing the child to rotate injection sites to decrease scar formation

   c. Encouraging the child to maintain the proper injection schedule

   d. Promoting higher levels of exercise than previously maintained

10. The nurse is caring for a 12-year-old girl with hypothyroidism. Which of the following will be part of the nurse's teaching plan for the child and family?

    a. Educating how to recognize vitamin D toxicity

    b. Teaching how to maintain fluid intake regimens

    c. Teaching to administer methimazole with meals

    d. Instructing to report irritability or anxiety

11. The child has developed hypothyroidism and has been prescribed sodium L-thyroxine. The starting dose is 12 mg/kg of body weight each day. The child weighs 72 pounds. Calculate the child's dose in micrograms and round to the nearest whole number.

12. Rank the different types of insulin based on their duration of action beginning with the shortest to the longest duration.

    a. Humulin N

    b. Lispro

    c. Lantus

    d. Humulin R

13. The young child has been diagnosed with a secondary growth hormone deficiency. The child weighs 58 pounds. The physician orders the child to receive 0.2 mg of growth hormone for each kilogram of body weight per week, divided into daily doses. How many milligrams of growth hormone would the child receive with each dose? Round to the thousandths place.

14. Which of the following male/female may have delayed puberty? Select all that apply.

    a. The 14-year old female has not developed breasts

    b. The 13-year old female has no pubic hair

    c. The 15-year old male has had no changes to the size of testicles

    d. The 14-year old male has no pubic hair

    e. The 13- year old male has no changes in the appearance of his scrotum

15. The child may have developed thyroid storm. Which of the following are clinical manifestations of thyroid storm? Select all that apply.

    a. The child's temperature is 103.2F

    b. The child's linen is wet and the child complains of feeling "sweaty"

    c. The child's apical heart rate is 172 beats per minute

    d. The child states he feels very tired and wants to take a nap

    e. The child has been mild-mannered and compliant

CHAPTER 50

Nursing Care of the Child with a Neoplastic Disorder

Learning Objectives

- Compare childhood and adult cancers.
- Describe nursing care related to common laboratory and diagnostic testing used in the medical diagnosis of pediatric cancer.
- Identify types of cancer common in infants, children, and adolescents.
- Identify appropriate nursing assessments and interventions related to medications and treatments for pediatric cancer.
- Develop an individualized nursing care plan for the child with cancer.
- Describe the psychosocial impact of cancer on children and their families.
- Devise a nutrition plan for the child with cancer.
- Develop child/family teaching plans for the child with cancer.

SECTION I: ASSESSING YOUR UNDERSTANDING

Activity A FILL IN THE BLANKS

1. Presence of a tumor in the _____ region can cause a child with cancer to complain of chest pain or shortness of breath.

2. Retinoblastoma may be identified by the presence of _____ in one or both eyes

3. Untreated, neutropenia can lead to _____ and should be treated with IV antibiotics immediately.

4. Nursing care for a child receiving treatment for cancer focuses on _____ and palliation of side effects.

5. Bone cancer may be treated with a combination of _____ procedure, radiation, and chemotherapy.

6. _____ is the most frequently occurring type of childhood cancer.

7. A _____ is a carefully designed research study that assesses the effectiveness of a treatment as well as its acute and long-term effects on the patient.

Activity B LABELING

Place an X on the most common locations where rhabdomyosarcoma occurs.

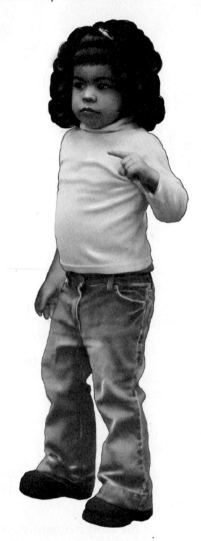

Activity C MATCHING

Match the medical treatment in Column A with the proper word or phrase in Column B.

Column A

___ **1.** Biopsy

___ **2.** Central venous catheter

___ **3.** Implanted port

___ **4.** Leukapheresis

___ **5.** Radiation therapy

Column B

a. High-energy X-ray

b. Long-term IV medication

c. May be done with needle

d. Vena cava or subclavian vein

e. White blood cell extraction

Activity D SEQUENCING

Place the following phases of the cell cycle in the proper order:

1. G0

2. G1

3. G2

4. M

5. S

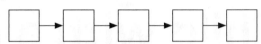

Activity E SHORT ANSWERS

Briefly answer the following.

1. Describe the signs and symptoms of rhabdomyosarcoma based on the location of the tumor.

_____

_____

_____

2. Name the eight drugs discussed in this chapter that help prevent or palliate the effects of chemotherapy and other tests and therapies.

_____

_____

_____

3. Name the five kinds of imaging used to diagnose cancer. Briefly describe how they work, what information they provide, and what the nursing implications are.

_____

_____

_____

4. Discuss three ways how childhood cancer differs from adult cancer.

_____

_____

_____

5. Discuss how chemotherapy agents work in relation to the cell cycle.

_____

_____

_____

SECTION II: APPLYING YOUR KNOWLEDGE

Activity F CASE STUDY

A 4-year-old boy is brought to the clinic by his parents due to fever. After further assessment the diagnosis of acute lymphoblastic leukemia (ALL) was confirmed. The child was admitted to your unit and started on treatment immediately. Upon assessment and review of his lab work today you find his temperature to be 101.2°F, HR 100, RR 24. His absolute neutrophil count (ANC) is <500.

1. What will be your priority nursing interventions?

_____

_____

_____

2. One week later, John is ready to be discharged home and will receive his treatment in the outpatient setting. What education will you review with the family regarding preventing infection?

_____

_____

_____

3. The mother asks, "How can we help John's development not fall behind other children his age?"

_____

_____

_____

SECTION III: PRACTICING FOR NCLEX

Activity G NCLEX-STYLE QUESTIONS

Answer the following questions.

1. The nurse is teaching the parents of a 15-year-old boy who is being treated for acute myelogenous leukemia about the side effects of chemotherapy. For which of the following symptoms should the parents seek medical care immediately?

   a. Earache, stiff neck, or sore throat

   b. Blisters, ulcers, or a rash appear

   c. A temperature of 101°F or greater

   d. Difficulty or pain when swallowing

2. The nurse is assessing a 2-year-old girl whose parents noticed that one of her pupils appeared to be white. Which of the following findings is typical of retinoblastoma? (Select all that apply)

   a. Observation of eyes reveals yellow discharge

   b. Parents report that the child has headaches

   c. Observation confirms cat's eye reflex in pupil

   d. Assessment discloses hyphema in one eye

   e. Usually diagnosed when the child is over the age of 7 years

3. The nurse is providing preoperative care for a 7-year-old boy with a brain tumor and his parents. Which of the following is the priority intervention?

   a. Assessing the child's level of consciousness

   b. Providing a tour of the intensive care unit

   c. Educating the child and parents about shunts

   d. Having him talk to a child who has had this surgery

4. The nurse is assessing a 14-year-old girl with a tumor. Which of the following findings would indicate Ewing's sarcoma?

   a. Child complains of dull bone pain just below her knee

   b. Palpation reveals swelling and redness on the right ribs

   c. Child complains of persistent pain from minor ankle injury

   d. Palpation discloses asymptomatic mass on the upper back

5. The nurse is teaching a group of 13-year-old boys and girls about screening and prevention of reproductive cancers. Which of the following subjects would not be included in the nurse's teaching plan? (Select all that apply)

   a. Self-examination is an effective screening method for testicular cancer

   b. Testicular cancer is one of the most difficult cancers to cure

   c. A Papanicolaou smear does not require parent consent in most states

   d. Sexually transmitted disease is a risk factor for cervical cancer

   e. Provide information regarding the benefits of receiving the HPV vaccine

6. The nurse is caring for a 4-year-old boy following surgical removal of a stage I neuroblastoma. Which of the following interventions will be most appropriate for this child?

   a. Applying aloe vera lotion to irradiated areas of skin

   b. Administering antiemetics as prescribed for nausea

   c. Giving medications as ordered via least invasive route

   d. Maintaining isolation as prescribed to avoid infection

7. The nurse is caring for a 6-year-old girl with leukemia who is having an oncological emergency. Which of the following signs and symptoms would indicate hyperleukocytosis?

   a. Bradycardia and distinct S1 and S2 sounds

   b. Wheezing and diminished breath sounds

   c. Respiratory distress and poor perfusion

   d. Tachycardia and respiratory distress

8. The nurse is assessing a 3-year-old boy whose mother complains that he is listless and has been having trouble swallowing. Which of the following findings would suggest the child has a brain tumor?

   a. Observation reveals nystagmus and head tilt

   b. Vital signs show blood pressure measures 120/80

   c. Examination shows temperature of 38.5°C and headache

   d. Observation reveals a cough and labored breathing

9. The nurse is assessing a 4-year-old girl whose mother complains that she is not eating well, is losing weight, and has started vomiting after eating. Which of the following risk factors from the health history would suggest the child may have a Wilms tumor?

   a. The child has Down syndrome

   b. The child has Beckwith–Wiedemann syndrome

   c. The child has Shwachman syndrome

   d. There is a family history of neurofibromatosis

10. The nurse is educating the parents of a 16-year-old boy who has just been diagnosed with Hodgkin's disease. Which of the following subjects would be most appropriate at this time?

   a. Describing the two ways of staging the disease

   b. Telling about the drugs and side effects of chemotherapy

   c. Informing the parents about postoperative care

   d. Explaining how to care for skin after radiation therapy

11. The child has been diagnosed with cancer and is being treated with chemotherapy. Which of the following findings are most likely common side effects of this type of treatment? Select all that apply.

    a. The child's mother states, "It seems like he catches every bug that comes along."

    b. The child's teeth are enlarged

    c. The child has no hair on his head

    d. The child's mother states that she often has to repeat herself because he can't hear very well

    e. The child is complaining of feeling nauseated

12. The child has been prescribed chemotherapy. In order to properly calculate the child's dose, the nurse must first figure the child's body surface area (BSA). The child is 130 cm tall and weighs 27 kg. Calculate the child's BSA and round to the hundredths place.

13. The child has been diagnosed with leukemia. Rank the following medications used to treat leukemia in order based on the stage of treatment.

    a. The child is receiving chemotherapy through an intrathecal catheter

    b. The child is receiving high doses of mercaptopurine and methotrexate

    c. The child is receiving low doses of mercaptopurine and methotrexate

    d. The child is receiving vincristine through an intravenous line and oral steroids

14. The physician requests the nurse to calculate the child's ANC. The complete blood count indicates that the child's "segs" are 14%, bands are 9%, and white blood cells (WBC) are 15,000. Calculate the child's absolute neutrophil count.

15. The child has been admitted to the hospital. Her absolute neutrophil count is 450 and the child has been placed in neutropenic precautions. Which of the following nursing interventions indicates that the nurse requires further education? Select all that apply.

    a. The child has been placed in a semiprivate room

    b. The child is being transported to radiology for an X-ray and the nurse places gloves on the child's hands

    c. The nurse monitors the child's vital signs every 2 to 4 hours

    d. The nurse assesses the child for clinical manifestations of an infection every 4 to 8 hours

    e. The nurse carefully washes his hands before and after providing care for the child

Nursing Care of the Child with a Genetic Disorder

Learning Objectives

- Discuss various inheritance patterns, including nontraditional patterns of inheritance.
- Discuss ethical and legal issues associated with genetic testing.
- Discuss genetic counseling and the role of the nurse.
- Discuss the nurse's role and responsibilities when caring for a child diagnosed with a genetic disorder and his/her family.
- Identify nursing interventions related to common laboratory and diagnostic tests used in the diagnosis and management of genetic conditions.
- Distinguish various genetic disorders occurring in childhood.
- Devise an individualized nursing care plan for the child with a genetic disorder.
- Develop child/family teaching plans for the child with a genetic disorder.

SECTION I: ASSESSING YOUR UNDERSTANDING

Activity A FILL IN THE BLANKS

1. Many time genes for the same trait have two or more _____ or versions that may be expressed.

2. Close blood relationship, referred to as _____, is a risk factor for genetic disorders.

3. The physical appearance, or _____, is the expression of a dominant gene or two recessive genes.

4. When a child receives different genes from the mother and father for the same trait, the child's genes are _____, and usually the dominant gene will be expressed.

5. Trisomy 21 is a disorder caused by _____ or an error in cell division during meiosis.

6. The _____ of an organism is its entire hereditary information encoded in the DNA.

7. A _____ is a long, continuous strand of DNA that carries genetic information.

Activity B MATCHING

Match the disorder in Column A with the phrase in Column B.

Column A

___ 1. Achondroplasia

___ 2. Apert syndrome

___ 3. CHARGE syndrome

___ 4. Marfan syndrome

___ 5. VATER association

Column B

a. No single feature present in all individuals

b. Not a diagnosis

c. Disorder of connective tissue

d. Disordered growth

e. Older paternal age

Activity C SHORT ANSWERS

Briefly answer the following.

1. Describe at least five major complications a child with Down syndrome can experience.

2. Summarize the guiding principles for nurses providing support and education to families of children with genetic abnormalities.

3. Briefly describe how the four errors of metabolism disorders are associated with specific odors of a child's excretions.

4. Discuss the incidence of Trisomy 21.

5. What are the common clinical manifestations that would alert the nurse to the likelihood that an infant has Trisomy 13?

SECTION II: APPLYING YOUR KNOWLEDGE

Activity D CASE STUDY

A 1-week-old baby girl named Chloe is seen in your clinic secondary to abnormal newborn screening results. Her mother states, "Chloe has been doing great. She eats well, every 2 to 3 hours. I do not understand why we are here today. The nurse called and mentioned something about an inborn error of metabolism. I do not understand what that is and how Chloe could have that? She is not even sick."

1. How would you address the mother's concerns?

2. The newborn screen came back positive for a fatty acid oxidation disorder, medium-chain acyl-CoA dehydrogenase deficiency. After further testing the diagnosis was confirmed. What education and nursing management will you provide?

SECTION III: PRACTICING FOR NCLEX

Activity E NCLEX-STYLE QUESTIONS

Answer the following questions.

1. The nurse is assessing a newborn boy. Which of the following findings would indicate the possibility of the disorder neurofibromatosis? (Select all that apply)
   a. History shows a grandparent had neurofibromatosis
   b. Measurement shows a slightly larger head size
   c. Inspection discloses several café au lait spots on the trunk
   d. Observation reveals freckles on the lower extremities
   e. Abnormal curvature of the spine

2. The nurse is caring for a 9-year-old girl with Marfan syndrome. Which of the following interventions would be part of the nursing plan of care for this child? (Select all that apply)
   a. Arranging for respiratory therapy at home
   b. Promoting annual ophthalmology examinations
   c. Monitoring for bone and joint problems
   d. Encourage use of antibiotics before dentistry
   e. Including in home physical therapy

3. The nurse is examining an 8-year-old boy with chromosomal abnormalities. Which of the following signs and symptoms suggest the boy has Angelman syndrome?
   a. Palpation discloses reduced muscular tonicity
   b. Observation reveals moonlike round face
   c. History shows surgery for cleft palate repair
   d. Observation shows jerky ataxic movement

4. The nurse is counseling a couple who are concerned that the woman has achondroplasia in her family. The woman is not affected. Which of the following statements by the couple indicates the need for more teaching?
   a. "If the mother has the gene, then there is a 50% chance of passing it on."
   b. "If the father doesn't have the gene, then his son won't have achondroplasia."
   c. "If the father has the gene, then there is a 50% chance of passing it on."
   d. "Since neither one of us has the disorder, we won't pass it on."

5. The nurse is caring for an 8-year-old girl who has just been diagnosed with fragile X syndrome. Which of the following interventions would be the priority?
   a. Explain care required due to the disorder
   b. Assess family's ability to learn about the disorder
   c. Educate the family about available resources
   d. Screen to determine current level of functioning

6. The nurse is assessing a 2-week-old boy who was born at home and has not had metabolic screening. Which of the following signs or symptoms would indicate phenylketonuria?
   a. Palpation reveals increased reflex action
   b. Observation shows signs of jaundice
   c. Detection of a musty odor to the urine
   d. The parents report the child has seizures

7. The nurse is examining a 2-year-old girl with Vater association. Which of the following signs or symptoms would be noted?
   a. Observation that the child has a hearing aid
   b. Inspection reveals underdeveloped labia
   c. Assessment of the eye reveals a cleft in the iris
   d. History of corrective surgery for anal atresia

8. The nurse is assessing infants in the newborn nursery. Which of the following assessments would be indicative of a major anomaly?

   a. A 12-hour Caucasian male with café au lait macules on his trunk

   b. A 16-hour African American male with polydactyly

   c. A set of Indian identical twin females with syndactyly

   d. A 4-hour Asian female with protruding ears

9. The nurse is caring for a newborn girl with galactosemia. Which of the following interventions will be necessary for her health?

   a. Adhering to a low phenylalanine diet

   b. Eliminating dairy products from her diet

   c. Eating frequent meals and never fasting

   d. Lifetime supplementation with thiamine

10. The nurse is assessing a 3-year-old boy with Sturge–Weber syndrome. Which of the following findings is most indicative of the disorder?

    a. Record shows the boy has seizures

    b. Observation shows behavior problems

    c. Inspection reveals a port wine stain

    d. Observation indicates mild retardation

11. The nurse is interviewing parents after their newborn was diagnosed with a genetic disorder. Which of the following statements by the mother is associated with risk factors of genetic disorders? (Select all that apply)

    a. "Our obstetrician told us that I wasn't making enough amniotic fluid during this pregnancy."

    b. "My husband is 55 years old."

    c. "Our alpha-fetoprotein came back negative when I was 18 weeks pregnant."

    d. "My sister's baby was born with trisomy 18."

    e. "He is our first child."

12. The 14-year-old boy may have Klinefelter syndrome. Which of the following findings is associated with this genetic disorder? (Select all that apply)

    a. He has a long trunk and short legs

    b. He is shorter than average for his age

    c. He has been diagnosed with dyslexia

    d. His scrotum is smaller than normal

    e. He has developed a significant amount of breast tissue

13. The experienced pediatric nurse is quizzing a student nurse regarding the appearance of a newborn with trisomy 18. Which of the following statements by the student nurse indicates the need for further education? (Select all that apply)

    a. "This newborn may have a very small head."

    b. "This newborn may have extra fingers or toes."

    c. "This newborn may have a major heart problem."

    d. "This newborn may have webbed fingers and toes."

    e. "This newborn may have ears that look like they are placed low."

14. The nursing student is studying patterns of inheritance regarding genetic disorders. The student demonstrates understanding when recognizing that monogenic disorders include which of the following? (Select all that apply)

    a. Autosomal dominant

    b. Autosomal recessive

    c. X-linked dominant

    d. Mitochondrial inheritance

    e. Genomic imprinting

15. The experienced nurse works for an obstetrician. Which of the following couples may benefit from genetic counseling? (Select all that apply)

    a. The mother-to-be is 29 years old

    b. The father-to-be is 58 years old

    c. The parents-to-be are cousins

    d. The parents-to-be are African American

    e. The parents-to-be have a child who was born blind and deaf

Nursing Care of the Child with a Cognitive or Mental Health Disorder

- Discuss the impact of alterations in mental health upon the growth and development of infants, children, and adolescents.
- Describe the techniques used to evaluate the status of mental health in children.
- Identify appropriate nursing assessments and interventions related to therapy and medications for the treatment of childhood and adolescent mental health disorders.
- Distinguish mental health disorders common in infants, children, and adolescents.
- Develop an individualized nursing care plan for the child with a mental health disorder.
- Develop child/family teaching plans for the child with a mental health disorder.

SECTION I: ASSESSING YOUR UNDERSTANDING

Activity A FILL IN THE BLANKS

1. Purging is self-induced vomiting or evacuation of the _____.

2. For a diagnosis of attention-deficit/hyperactivity disorder (ADHD), the symptoms of impulsivity and hyperactivity begin before 7 years of age and must persist longer than _____ months.

3. Children with _____ experience difficulty with reading, writing, and spelling.

4. Burns that appear in a _____ or glove pattern are highly suspicious of inflicted burns.

5. _____ is defined as failure to provide a child with appropriate food, clothing, shelter, medical care, and schooling.

6. A disorder in which an adult meets her own psychological needs by having an ill child is known as _____.

7. Pervasive developmental disorder is another name for _____.

Activity B LABELING

Mark an X on all of the areas that indicate injury sites that are suspicious for abuse.

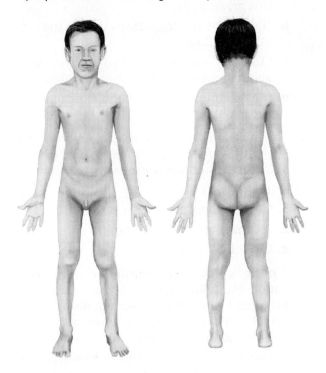

Activity C MATCHING

Match the term in Column A with the proper definition in Column B.

Column A

____ **1.** Affect

____ **2.** Anxiety

____ **3.** Binging

____ **4.** Dysgraphia

____ **5.** Dyscalculia

Column B

a. Feelings of dread, worry, discomfort

b. Emotional reaction associated with an experience

c. Problems with math and computation

d. Rapid excessive consumption of food or drink

e. Difficulty producing the written word

Activity D SHORT ANSWERS

Briefly answer the following.

1. What are some common behavior management techniques that can be utilized in the hospital, clinic, classroom, or home setting?

_____

_____

_____

2. According to the text, what common laboratory and diagnostic studies are ordered for the assessment of abuse?

_____

_____

_____

3. What is generalized anxiety disorder?

_____

_____

_____

4. Discuss the data that should be collected if the nurse suspects an adolescent patient is suffering from depression.

_____

_____

_____

5. What are the common classifications of medications used to treat ADHD and what is the intended goal of medication treatment?

_____

_____

_____

SECTION II: APPLYING YOUR KNOWLEDGE

Activity E   CASE STUDY

Elisa, a 6-month-old female is seen in your clinic for her wellness check-up. Her mother states "I have seen so much about autism in the news lately. What is autism and how would I know if Elisa has this disorder?"

1. How would you explain autism to Elisa's mother?

   _____

   _____

   _____

2. What signs and symptoms would be exhibited by an infant or toddler who has autism?

   _____

   _____

   _____

SECTION III: PRACTICING FOR NCLEX

Activity F   NCLEX-STYLE QUESTIONS

Answer the following questions.

1. The nurse is conducting a well-child assessment of a 3-year-old. Which of the following statements by the parents would warrant further investigation?
   a. "He spends a lot of time playing with his little cars"
   b. "He spends hours repeatedly lining up his cars"
   c. "He is very active and keeps very busy"
   d. "He would rather run around than sit on my lap and read a book"

2. The mother of a 10-year-old boy with attention deficit/hyperactivity disorder contacts the school nurse. She is upset because her son has been made to feel different by his peers because he has to visit the nurse's office for a lunch time dose of medication. The boy is threatening to stop taking his medication. How should the nurse respond?
   a. "He should ignore the children, he needs this medication"
   b. "I can have the teacher speak with the other children"
   c. "You may want to talk to your physician about an extended release medication"
   d. "Remind him that his schoolwork may deteriorate"

3. The nurse is conducting an examination of a boy with Tourette's syndrome. Which of the following would the nurse expect to observe?
   a. Toe walking
   b. Sudden, rapid stereotypical sounds
   c. Spinning and hand flapping
   d. Lack of eye contact

4. A nurse is providing a routine wellness examination and follow-up for a 3-year-old recently diagnosed with autism spectrum disorder. Which of the following responses indicates a need for additional referral or follow-up?
   a. "We have recently completed his individualized education plan"
   b. "We really like the treatment plan that has been created by his school"
   c. "We try to be flexible and change his routine from day to day"
   d. "We have a couple of baby sitters who know how to handle his needs"

5. A nurse is caring for a child with intellectual disability. The medical chart indicates an IQ of 37. The nurse understands that the degree of disability is classified as which of the following?
   a. Mild
   b. Moderate
   c. Severe
   d. Profound

6. A nurse is caring for a 10-year-old intellectually disabled girl hospitalized for a scheduled cholecystectomy. The girl expresses fear related to her hospitalization and unfamiliar surroundings. How should the nurse respond?

    a. "Don't worry, you will be going home soon"

    b. "Tell me about a typical day at home"

    c. "Have you talked to your parents about this?"

    d. "Do you want some art supplies?"

7. The nurse is caring for a girl with anorexia who has been hospitalized with unstable vital signs and food refusal. The girl requires enteral nutrition. The nurse is alert for which of the complications that signal re-feeding syndrome?

    a. Cardiac arrhythmias, confusion, seizures

    b. Orthostatic hypotension

    c. Hypothermia and irregular pulse

    d. Bradycardia with ectopy

8. A nurse is conducting a physical examination of an adolescent girl with suspected bulimia. Which of the following assessment findings would the nurse expect to note?

    a. Eroded dental enamel

    b. Dry sallow skin

    c. Soft sparse body hair

    d. Thinning scalp hair

9. The nurse is examining a child with fetal alcohol syndrome. Which of the following assessment findings would the nurse expect to note?

    a. Macrocephaly

    b. Low nasal bridge with short upturned nose

    c. Clubbing of fingers

    d. Short filtrum with thick upper lip

10. The nurse is providing teaching about medication management of attention deficit hyperactivity disorder. Which of the following responses indicates a need for further teaching?

    a. "We should give it to him after he eats breakfast"

    b. "This may cause him to have difficulty sleeping"

    c. "If he takes this medicine he will no longer have ADHD"

    d. "We should see an improvement in his schoolwork"

11. The school-aged child has been diagnosed with dysgraphia and dyslexia. Which of the following findings may be present? Select all that apply.

    a. The child experiences difficulty when asked to hop on one foot

    b. The child experiences difficulty when asked to add and subtract numbers

    c. The child experiences difficulty when asked to jump rope

    d. The child experiences difficulty when asked to write words

    e. The child experiences difficulty when asked to spell his name

12. The 18-month-old toddler has been brought into the pediatrician's office by his parents. Which of the following findings are warning signs that the toddler may be autistic based on what he should be able to do according to his age? Select all that apply.

    a. The parents stated that the toddler has never "babbled"

    b. The toddler does not exhibit attempts to communicate by pointing to objects

    c. The child does not use any words

    d. The child does not speak in short sentences

    e. The child cannot jump rope

13. The child has been diagnosed with attention deficit hyperactivity disorder and has been prescribed Ritalin (methylphenidate). Which of the following findings are most likely adverse effects related to this type of medication? Select all that apply.

    a. The child has gained weight since beginning Ritalin

    b. The child complains that his head hurts at times

    c. The child's parents state that he sleeps much longer than he used to

    d. The child has been more irritable since beginning Ritalin

    e. The child complains that he has developed abdominal pain

14. The child has been diagnosed with a mental health disorder and the child's parents are beginning to incorporate behavior management techniques. Which of the following statements by the child's parent indicates the need for further education? Select all that apply.

    a. "I use a higher pitched voice when I communicate with her."

    b. "I am quick to point out the things that she does that make me crazy."

    c. "We have set some boundaries that are nonnegotiable."

    d. "We tell her when she is doing something well."

    e. "We're trying to make her accountable and responsible for her own behavior."

15. The parents of an adolescent are concerned about his mental health and have brought the adolescent into the physician's office for an evaluation. Which of the following statements by the child's parents indicates that the child may have a mental health disorder? Select all that apply.

    a. "He has started sleeping for only 3 hours each night."

    b. "He has lost 10 pounds over the last 4 months."

    c. "He hangs out with the same kids he always has."

    d. "He used to be a straight-A student and now he's bringing home Cs and Ds."

    e. "He still enjoys playing a lot of baseball."

Nursing Care during a Pediatric Emergency

- Identify various factors contributing to emergency situations among infants and children.
- Discuss common treatments and medications used during pediatric emergencies.
- Conduct a health history of a child in an emergency situation, specific to the emergency.
- Perform a rapid cardiopulmonary assessment.
- Discuss common laboratory and other diagnostic tests used during pediatric emergencies.
- Integrate the principles of the American Heart Association (AHA) and Pediatric Advanced Life Support (PALS) in the comprehensive management of pediatric emergencies, such as respiratory arrest, shock, cardiac arrest, near drowning, poisoning, and trauma.

SECTION I: ASSESSING YOUR UNDERSTANDING

Activity A FILL IN THE BLANKS

1. Children as old as 18 years of age should be managed using the _____ advanced life support guidelines.

2. Use the mnemonic _____ to remember which drugs may be given via the tracheal route

3. The assessment and management of the _____ of a prearresting or arresting child is always the first intervention in a pediatric emergency situation.

4. A nonreactive _____ indicates the need for immediate relief of increased intracranial pressure.

5. Circumoral pallor or _____ is a late and often ominous sign of respiratory distress.

6. To open the airway of a victim suspected of having a neck injury the rescuer should utilize the _____ technique.

7. The best place to check the pulse in a child is either at the _____ or carotid site.

Activity B **LABELING**

Identify the arrhythmia by placing the proper arrhythmia type under the appropriate illustration.

1. Supraventricular tachycardia
2. Ventricular tachycardia
3. Sinus tachycardia
4. Coarse ventricular fibrillation

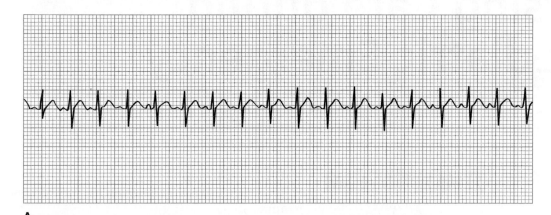

A _____

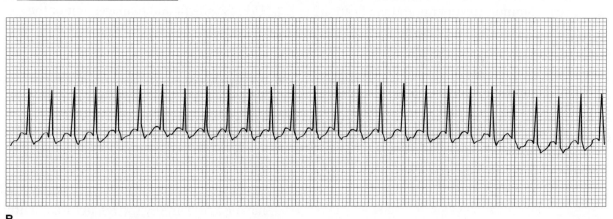

B _____

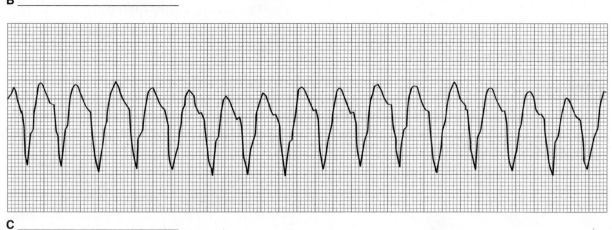

C _____

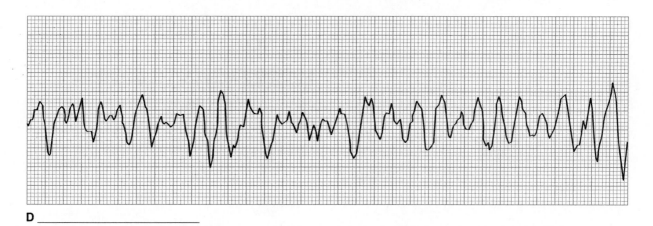

D _____

1. Supraventricular tachycardia (SVT): note rate above 220, abnormal P waves, no beat-to-beat variability.
2. Ventricular tachycardia: rapid and regular rhythm, wide QRS without P waves.
3. Sinus tachycardia: normal QRS and P waves, mild beat-to-beat variability.
4. Coarse ventricular fibrillation: chaotic electrical activity.

Activity C MATCHING

Match the test in Column A with the correct statement in Column B.

Column A

___ **1.** Arterial blood gas

___ **2.** Chest X-ray

___ **3.** Computerized tomography

___ **4.** Toxicology panel

___ **5.** Urinalysis

Column B

a. Usually available in emergency department

b. Accompany the child to observe and manage

c. Never delay resuscitation efforts pending results

d. Notify lab of drugs the child is taking

e. Standards vary with agency used

Activity D SEQUENCING

Place the following CPR steps in the proper order.

1. Administer 100% oxygen
2. Evaluate heart rate and pulses
3. Look, listen, feel for respirations
4. Position to open airway
5. Suction

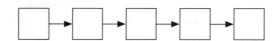

Activity E SHORT ANSWERS

Briefly answer the following.

1. Describe rates of compression to breaths and the hand positions used with CPR for infants and children for both one-person and two-person CPR.

   _____

   _____

   _____

2. Describe how to distinguish SVT from sinus tachycardia.

   _____

   _____

   _____

3. Describe the proper procedure for one person to ventilate a child with a bag valve mask.

   _____

   _____

   _____

4. What is the purpose of using cricoid pressure during resuscitation?

_____

_____

_____

5. Discuss the mnemonic "DOPE" in regards to a child who is intubated.

_____

_____

_____

SECTION II: APPLYING YOUR KNOWLEDGE

Activity F   **CASE STUDY**

A nurse is providing training for pediatric emergencies to a day care staff, including CPR, use of a defibrillator, poisonings, and near-drowning interventions. One of the day care providers states that she didn't think automatic external defibrillators (AEDs) were used for children. Another day care provider questions how the chain of survival is different for children compared to adults since she was certified in adult CPR several months ago.

1. How would you respond to the question regarding the use of AEDs with children?

_____

_____

_____

2. How does the chain of survival for children differ from the chain of survival for adults?

_____

_____

_____

SECTION III: PRACTICING FOR NCLEX

Activity G   **NCLEX-STYLE QUESTIONS**

Answer the following questions.

1. A 6-year-old girl who is being treated for shock is pulseless with an irregular heart rate of 32 BPM. Choose the priority intervention:

    a. Give three doses of epinephrine

    b. Administer doses defibrillator shocks in a row

    c. Initiate cardiac compressions

    d. Defibrillate once followed by three cycles of CPR

2. The parents of a 7-month-old boy with a broken arm agree on how the accident happened. Which account would lead the nurse to suspect child abuse?

    a. "He was climbing out of his crib and fell."

    b. "He fell out of a shopping cart in the store."

    c. "Mom turned and he fell from changing table."

    d. "The gate was open and he fell down three steps."

3. A 3-year-old girl had a near-drowning incident when she fell into a wading pool. Which intervention would be of the highest priority?

    a. Suctioning the upper airway to ensure airway patency

    b. Inserting a nasogastric tube to decompress stomach

    c. Covering the child with warming blankets

    d. Assuring the child stays still during an X-ray

4. A 2-year-old boy is in respiratory distress. Which nursing assessment finding would suggest the child aspirated a foreign body?

    a. Hearing dullness when percussing the lungs

    b. Noting absent breath sounds in one lung

    c. Auscultating a low-pitched, grating breath sound

    d. Hearing a hyperresonant sound on percussion

5. The nurse is ventilating a 9-year-old girl with a bag valve mask. Which action would most likely reduce the effectiveness of ventilation?

   a. Checking the tail for free flow of oxygen

   b. Setting the oxygen flow rate at 15 L/minute

   c. Pressing down on the mask below the mouth

   d. Referring to Broselow tape for bag size

6. The nurse is examining a 10-year-old boy with tachypnea and increased work of breathing. Which finding is a late sign that the child is in shock?

   a. Blood pressure slightly less than normal

   b. Equally strong central and distal pulses

   c. Significantly decreased skin elasticity

   d. Delayed capillary refill with cool extremities

7. The nurse is examining a 10-month-old girl who has fallen from the back porch. Which assessment will directly follow evaluation of the "ABCs?"

   a. Observing skin color and perfusion

   b. Palpating the abdomen for soreness

   c. Auscultating for bowel sounds

   d. Palpating the anterior fontanel

8. The nurse is caring for a 10-month-old infant with signs of respiratory distress. Which is the best way to maintain this child's airway?

   a. Placing the hand under the neck

   b. Inserting a small towel under shoulders

   c. Using the head tilt chin lift technique

   d. Employing the jaw-thrust maneuver

9. The nurse is caring for a 4-year-old boy who is receiving mechanical ventilation. Which is the priority intervention when moving this child?

   a. Auscultating the lungs for equal air entry

   b. Checking the CO_2 monitor for a yellow display

   c. Watching for disconnections in the breathing circuit

   d. Monitoring the pulse oximeter for oxygen saturation

10. CPR is in progress on an 8-year-old boy who is in shock. Which is the priority nursing intervention?

    a. Using a large bore catheter for peripheral venous access

    b. Inserting an indwelling urinary catheter to measure urine output

    c. Attaining central venous access via the femoral route

    d. Drawing a blood sample for arterial blood gas analysis

11. The child needs a tracheal tube placed. The child is 8 years old. Calculate the size of the tracheal tube that should be used for this child.

12. The nurse must calculate the adolescent's cardiac output. The child's heart rate is 76 beats per minute and the stroke volume is 75 mL. Calculate the child's cardiac output.

13. The child's physician requests that the nurse should notify her if the child's urine output is less than 1 mL/kg of body weight each hour. The child weighs 56 pounds. Calculate the minimum amount of urine output the child should produce each hour. Round to the nearest whole number.

14. The child's ability to perfuse well is poor due to inadequate circulation. The physician writes an order for the child to receive 20 mL of normal saline for each kilogram of body weight. The child will receive the normal saline as a bolus through a central intravenous line. The child weighs 78 pounds. Calculate the amount of normal saline the nurse should administer as a bolus. Round to the nearest whole number.

15. The nurse has been monitoring the child's vital signs. The child is 7 years old. Calculate the child's minimum acceptable systolic blood pressure.

CHAPTER 1

SECTION I: ASSESSING YOUR UNDERSTANDING

Activity A FILL IN THE BLANKS

1. Doula
2. Family
3. Emancipated
4. Competence
5. Morbidity
6. Unintentional
7. Guardians
8. Protective
9. Spirituality
10. Easy

Activity B MATCHING

1. d   2. e   3. c   4. a   5. b

Activity C SEQUENCING

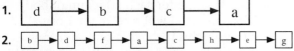

1. d → b → c → a
2. b → d → f → a → c → h → e → g

Activity D SHORT ANSWERS

1. Nurses need to look beyond the obvious "crushing chest pain" textbook symptom that heralds a heart attack in men. Risk factors of heart disease differ between men and women in several other ways—for example, menopause (associated with a significant rise in coronary events); diabetes, high cholesterol levels, and left ventricular hypertrophy; and repeated episodes of weight loss and gain (increased coronary morbidity and mortality).

2. A positive family history of breast cancer, aging, and irregularities in the menstrual cycle at an early age are major risk factors. Other risk factors include excess weight, not having children, oral contraceptive use, excessive alcohol consumption, a high-fat diet, and long-term use of hormone replacement therapy.

3. The maternal mortality rate is the annual number of deaths from any cause related to or aggravated by pregnancy or its management (excluding accidental or incidental causes) during pregnancy and childbirth or within 42 days of termination of pregnancy, irrespective of the duration and site of the pregnancy, per 100,000 live births, for a specified year.

4. Congenital anomalies remain the leading cause of infant mortality in the United States. In addition, low birth weight and prematurity are major indicators of infant health and significant predictors of infant mortality.

5. The Women, Infants, Children program provides nutritional supplementation and education to low-income families, women who are pregnant, postpartum or lactating, and infants and children up to age 5.

6. For positive reinforcement to be effective, feedback must be immediate, consistent, and frequent.

SECTION II: APPLYING YOUR KNOWLEDGE

Activity E CASE STUDY

1. Barriers may include: Financial barriers such as lack of insurance, not enough insurance, or inability to pay for services; sociocultural and ethnic factors such as lack of transportation and the need for both parents to work; knowledge barriers (eg, lack of understanding of the importance of preventive health care), language barriers (eg, speaking a different language than the health care providers), or spiritual barriers (eg, religious beliefs discouraging some forms of treatment); health care delivery system barriers, such as the cost containment movement and possible limited access to specialty care—which greatly affects clients with chronic or long-term illnesses, facility hours of operation and inability to meet the needs of the clients and the possible negative attitudes of health care workers.

2. As the family is Hispanic, you need to remember that the father is viewed as the source of strength, wisdom, and self-confidence and the mother is the caretaker and decision-maker for health. Children are viewed as people to continue the family and culture. This family would also view health as God's will and may use folk medicine practices and payers, herbal teas and poultices for illness treatment.

SECTION III: PRACTICING FOR NCLEX
Activity F NCLEX-STYLE QUESTIONS

1. **Answer: b**
   RATIONALE: Breastfeeding reduces the rates of infection in infants and helps to improve long-term maternal health. Placing the infant on his or her back to sleep prevents sudden infant death syndrome (SIDS) but does not prevent infections in the infant. Feeding foods high in starch or feeding liquids frequently will not prevent infections either.

2. **Answer: a**
   RATIONALE: The nurses should advocate adequate intake of folic acid supplements during pregnancy to reduce the prevalence of neural defects in infants. Taking vitamin E supplements, engaging in mild exercises during pregnancy, and regularly consuming citrus fruits are healthy habits for the mother and infant, but they do not reduce the risk of developing neural defects among infants.

3. **Answer: d**
   RATIONALE: According to the ANA's code of ethics, the nurse could make arrangements for alternate care providers for a client undergoing an abortion, if the nurse ethically opposes the procedure. Nurses need to make their values and beliefs known to their managers before the situation occurs so that alternate staffing arrangement can be made. Under the ANA's code of ethics for nurses, the nurse need not provide emotional support to the client nor should he or she involve the client's family in convincing the client against an abortion.

4. **Answer: d**
   RATIONALE: The nurse should instruct the client to place her infant on his or her back to sleep to prevent SIDS. Draping the infant in warm clothes, providing very soft bedding, or feeding a mixture of salts, sugar, and water will not prevent SIDS in the infant.

5. **Answer: b**
   RATIONALE: Lung cancer has no early symptoms, making its early detection almost impossible. It is equally fatal for both men and women; it is not more deadly in men. Women do not have a stronger resistance to lung cancer. It is the most common cancer in women due to the increasing frequency of smoking. Although the early detection of lung cancer is very difficult, its diagnosis is not more challenging in women than in men.

6. **Answer: c**
   RATIONALE: A traditional method used in this country to measure health is to examine mortality and morbidity data. Information is collected and analyzed to provide an objective description of the nation's health. Tracking the incidence of violent crime does not give information on the health status of this country; neither does examining health disparities between ethnic groups or identifying specific national goals related to maternal and infant care without acting on the information.

7. **Answer: c**
   RATIONALE: In the Arab-American culture, women are viewed as subordinate to men. The nurse would deal directly and exclusively with the husband. This family would not place much emphasis on preventive care either. Inquiring about folk remedies used may be appropriate with African American families. Coordinating care through the client's mother might be appropriate with a Hispanic family.

8. **Answer: b**
   RATIONALE: Clients have the right to refuse medical treatment, based on the American Hospital Association's Bill of Rights. The nurse needs to heed the client's wishes and not give the medication.

9. **Answer: a**
   RATIONALE: Reminding the mother that the child will imitate her parents may prevent the child from imitating dangerous behavior, but this is less likely to be a danger. Explaining how to toddler proof the house helps prevent injury to the child. Explaining how to teach self hand washing helps prevent infection. Describing self care for brushing teeth helps prevent dental caries. These interventions help avoid common health problems.

10. **Answer: b**
    RATIONALE: It is important to log-off whenever leaving the computer. The person who shares the nurse's log-on session may get called away from the computer leaving the nurse responsible for any breech in security. Keeping IDs and passwords confidential is basic computer security. Email is not a safe way to transmit confidential information for transmittal. Printing is safer. Closing client files before stepping away from the computer helps ensure privacy.

11. **Answer: b**
    RATIONALE: One of the factors associated with childhood injuries is parental drug or alcohol abuse. This is the leading cause for child mortality. Low-birth weight babies are at higher risk for infant mortality. Foreign-born adoption is a factor for childhood morbidity. The child's hostility toward other children may be an environmental or psychosocial factor for childhood morbidity.

12. **Answer: d**
    RATIONALE: One trend in the United States is the increasing number of children with mental health disorders and related emotional, social, or behavioral problems. The best way to determine the reliability of the teacher's concerns would be to determine the behaviors being noticed.

13. **Answer: d**
    RATIONALE: Requests of the parents and child must be documented. The surgeon does not have the automatic authority to override the parents' wishes. The child is under age and does not have decision-making authority.

14. **Answer: c**
    RATIONALE: In cases of abuse and violence, nurses can serve their clients best by not trying to rescue them but by helping them build on their strengths, providing support, and empowering them to help themselves. Counseling the client's partner against abuse, helping her know the legal impact of her situation, and introducing the client to a women's rights group to garner support are not the best ways of serving the client.

15. **Answer: c**
    RATIONALE: Congenital anomalies are the leading cause of infant mortality in the United States. Low birth weight and prematurity are major indicators of infant health and significant predictors of infant mortality. Sudden infant death, cardiac disorders, and respiratory infection are causes of infant mortality but are not the greatest cause.

16. **Answer: c**
    RATIONALE: Cardiovascular disease is the leading cause of death of women in the United States. Elevations in death rates are in part to the difficulty recognizing cardiovascular concerns in women. The second leading cause of death in women is cancer. Lung cancer exceeds other types of cancer in women. HIV infection, while impacting the mortality rates of women, is not the greatest cause of death.

17. **Answer: a, c, & e**
    RATIONALE: Culture is a view of the world and a set of traditions that are used by a specific social group and are transmitted to the next generation. Culture is a complex phenomenon involving many components, such as beliefs, values, language, time, personal space, and view of the world, all of which shape a person's actions and behavior. Race refers to ethnicity of an individual. The level of education provides information on an individual's socioeconomic status.

18. **Answer: d**
    RATIONALE: Extended families consist of parents, children, and aunts, uncles, and/or grandparents. Blended families consist of parents who have children from previous marriages and potentially children from the new marriage. Groups of individuals who are not necessarily related by blood ties but who are living together to raise their families are referred to as communal families. In the binuclear family, children are members of two families as a result of custody or "joint parenting" arrangements.

Answers

CHAPTER 2

SECTION I: ASSESSING YOUR UNDERSTANDING

Activity A FILL IN THE BLANKS

1. Case management
2. Nonverbal
3. Community
4. Primary
5. Encounters
6. Health

Activity B MATCHING

1. d   2. c   3. b   4. a

Activity C SEQUENCING

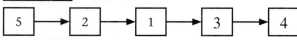

Activity D SHORT ANSWERS

1. Maternal and pediatric nurses provide care at the primary, secondary, and tertiary levels of prevention. The concept of primary prevention involves preventing the disease or condition before it occurs through health promotion activities, environmental protection, and specific protection against disease or injury. Its focus is on health promotion to reduce the person's vulnerability to any illness by strengthening the person's capacity to withstand physical, emotional, and environmental stressors. Secondary prevention is the early detection and treatment of adverse health conditions. This level of prevention is aimed at halting the disease, thus shortening its duration and severity to get the person back to a normal state of functioning. Tertiary prevention is designed to reduce or limit the progression of a permanent, irreversible disease or disability. The purpose of tertiary prevention is to restore individuals to their maximum potential.

2. Case management involves: advocacy, communication, and resource management; client-focused comprehensive care across a continuum; and coordinated care with an interdisciplinary approach.

3. Some of the techniques that the nurse can use to enhance learning include:
   - Slowing down and repeating information often
   - Speaking in conversational style using plain, nonmedical language
   - "Chunking" information and teaching it in small bites using logical steps
   - Prioritizing information and teaching "survival skills" first
   - Using visuals, such as pictures, videos, and models
   - Teaching using an interactive, "hands-on" approach

4. The four main purposes of nursing documentation are: the client's medical record serves as a communication tool that the entire interdisciplinary team can use to keep track of what the client and family has learned already and what learning still needs to occur. Next, it serves to testify to the education the family has received if and when legal matters arise. Thirdly, it verifies standards set by the Joint Commission on Accreditation of Healthcare Organizations, Centers for Medicare and Medicaid Services (CMS), and other accrediting bodies that hold health care providers accountable for client and family education activities. And lastly, it informs third-party payers of goods and services provided for reimbursement purposes.

5. Both contribute to improved transition from the hospital to the community for women, children, their families, and the health care team.

6. Community health nursing focuses on prevention and improvement of the health of populations and communities, addressing current and potential health needs of the population or community, promoting and preserving the health of a population regardless of a particular age group or diagnosis.

7. A birthing center provides a cross between a home birth and a hospital birth. Birthing centers offer a homelike setting with close proximity to a hospital in case of complications. Midwives are often the sole care providers in freestanding birthing centers, with obstetricians as backups in case of emergencies.

Birthing centers usually have fewer restrictions and guidelines for families to follow and allow for more freedom in making laboring decisions. Birthing centers aim to provide a relaxing home environment and promote a culture of normalcy.

SECTION II: APPLYING YOUR KNOWLEDGE
Activity E **CASE STUDY**

1. Our hospital defines "family-centered care" as the delivery of safe, satisfying, high-quality health care that focuses on and adapts to the physical and psychosocial needs of the family. It is a cooperative effort of families and other caregivers that recognizes the strength and integrity of the family. What that really means is that when you come in to have your baby, we will not only take care of you and your newborn, we will also include your husband as part of your family unit. We will listen to what you and your husband want and include it in your plan of care as best we can.

2. "Evidence-based nursing practice" involves the use of research or evidence in establishing a plan of care and implementing that care. It is a clinical decision making approach involving the integration of the best scientific evidence, client values and preferences, clinical circumstances, and clinical expertise to promote best outcomes.

SECTION III: PRACTICING FOR NCLEX
Activity F **NCLEX-STYLE QUESTIONS**

1. **Answer: d**
   RATIONALE: Case management focuses on coordinating health care services while balancing quality and cost outcomes. The nurse would be most likely involved with scheduling speech and respiratory services, ensuring these services are integrated into the client's plan of care in a coordinated manner. Helping a person learn a procedure or assessing the sanitary conditions of the home and establishing eligibility are not activities associated with case management.

2. **Answer: a**
   RATIONALE: With family-centered care, support and respect for the uniqueness and diversity of families are essential, along with encouragement and enhancement of the family's strengths and competencies. It is important for nurses to remain neutral to all they hear and see in order to enhance trust and maintain open communication lines with all family members. Nurses need to remember that the client is an expert of their own health, thus nurses should work within the client's framework when planning health promotion interventions. The client and family are in control. The nurse provides them with information that they need, not that which is only absolutely necessary. The nurse also integrates an understanding of the family's culture to foster empowerment.

3. **Answer: c**
   RATIONALE: When working with an interpreter, avoid side conversations during sessions. These can be uncomfortable for the family and jeopardize client–provider relationships and trust. It is important to provide ample time for the interpretation because it often takes longer to say in some languages what has already been said in English. It is recommended that the interpreter have some medical background so that the message is interpreted correctly.

4. **Answer: d**
   RATIONALE: Regardless of the setting, the common goal is to ensure the health and well-being of the clients and their families. Certain settings may have individual goals and focus on removing barriers or promoting the health of specific client group.

5. **Answer: d**
   RATIONALE: Trust, respect, and empathy are three factors needed to create and foster effective therapeutic communication between people. Literacy would be important for education.

6. **Answers: b, c, & e**
   RATIONALE: To enhance learning, the nurse should speak in a conversational style using plain, nonmedical language, chunk information with breaks every 10–15 minutes, prioritize and teach the "survival skills" or need-to-know information first, repeating information at least 4–5 times, and use visuals such as pictures, videos, and models to facilitate learning.

7. **Answer: a, b, & c**
   RATIONALE: Primary prevention activities would include drug education programs for schools, smoking cessation programs, and poison prevention educational programs. Cholesterol monitoring and fecal occult blood testing are examples of secondary prevention activities.

8. **Answer: b**
   RATIONALE: Feng shui is the Chinese art of placement in which objects in the environment are position to induce harmony with chi. Reflexology is the use of deep massage on identified points of the foot and hand to scan and rebalance body parts that correspond to each point. Therapeutic touch involves the balancing of energy by centering. Aromatherapy involves the use of essential oils to stimulate the sense of smell for balancing mind, body, and spirit.

9. **Answer: c**
   RATIONALE: When working with an interpreter, it is important to allow additional times because if often takes longer to say in some languages what has already been said in English. You should place yourself so that you are facing the family and the family is facing you. The y interpreter is the communication bridge, not the content expert. You should talk directly to the family, not to the interpreter.

10. **Answer: a**
RATIONALE: Adults are self-directed and value independence and want to learn on their own terms. They are problem-focused and task-oriented, valuing past experiences and beliefs and wanting immediate need satisfaction.

11. **Answer: a**
RATIONALE: The first step to cultural competence is cultural awareness in which the person becomes aware of, appreciates, and becomes sensitive to the values, beliefs, customs, and behaviors that have shaped one's culture. Next, the nurse would obtain knowledge about various worldviews and then assess each client's unique cultural beliefs, values and practices, ultimately engaging in cross-cultural interactions with people from culturally diverse backgrounds.

12. **Answer: d**
RATIONALE: Atraumatic care refers to the delivery of care that minimizes or eliminates the psychological and physical distress experienced by children and their families in the health care system. The key principles of atraumatic care include preventing or minimizing physical stressors, preventing or minimizing separation of the child from the family, and promoting a sense of control. Allowing the parents to stay, allowing the child to touch the stethoscope, and explaining that the stethoscope may feel cold are appropriate. Wrapping the child so that he cannot move would be stressful and traumatic.

CHAPTER 3

SECTION I: ASSESSING YOUR UNDERSTANDING

Activity A FILL IN THE BLANKS

1. rugae
2. Prolactin
3. epididymis
4. urethra
5. endometrium
6. Skene
7. episiotomy
8. prostate
9. uterus
10. scrotum

Activity B MATCHING

1. e   **2.** c   **3.** b   **4.** d   **5.** a

Activity C SEQUENCING

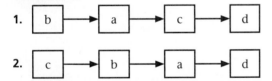

1. b → a → c → d

2. c → b → a → d

Activity D SHORT ANSWERS

1. The external female reproductive organs collectively are called the vulva. The vulva serves to protect the urethral and vaginal openings. The structures that make up the vulva include the mons pubis, the labia majora and minora, the clitoris, the structures within the vestibule, and the perineum.

2. Colostrum is a dark yellow fluid that contains more minerals and protein, but less sugar and fat, than mature breast milk. It is initially produced during pregnancy. After childbirth, colostrum is secreted for approximately a week, with a gradual conversion to mature breast milk. Colostrum is rich in maternal antibodies, especially immunoglobulin A, which offers protection for the newborn against enteric pathogens.

3. During the perimenopausal years, women may experience physical changes associated with decreasing estrogen levels, which may include vasomotor symptoms of hot flashes, irregular menstrual cycles, sleep disruptions, forgetfulness, irritability, mood disturbances, decreased vaginal lubrication, fatigue, vaginal atrophy, and depression.

4. Nurses can play a major role in assisting menopausal women by educating and counseling them about the multitude of options available for disease prevention, treatment for menopausal symptoms, and health promotion during this time of change in their lives.

5. The testes produce sperm and synthesize testosterone, which is the primary male sex hormone. Sperm is produced in the seminiferous tubules of the testes.

6. The bulbourethral (Cowper) glands are two small structures about the size of peas, located inferior to the prostate gland. They are composed of several tubes whose epithelial linings secrete a mucus-like fluid. It is released in response to sexual stimulation and lubricates the head of the penis in preparation for sexual intercourse. They gradually diminish in size with advancing age.

SECTION II: APPLYING YOUR KNOWLEDGE

Activity E CASE STUDY

1. The nurse should inform Susan about the following: the main function of the reproductive cycle is to stimulate growth of a follicle to release an egg and prepare a site for implantation if fertilization occurs; menstruation, the monthly shedding of the uterine lining, marks the beginning of a new cycle; the menstrual cycle involves a complex interaction of hormones; the ovarian cycle is the series of events associated with a developing oocyte (ovum or egg) within the ovaries; at ovulation, a mature follicle ruptures in response to a surge of LH, releasing a mature oocyte (ovum); the endometrial cycle is divided into three phases: the follicular or proliferative phase, the luteal or secretory phase, and the menstrual phase; the endometrium, ovaries, pituitary gland, and hypothalamus are all involved in the cyclic changes that help prepare the body for fertilization; the menstrual cycle results from a functional hypothalamic–pituitary–ovarian axis and a precise sequencing of hormones that lead to ovulation; if conception doesn't occur,

menses ensues; and the one thing to remember is that whether a women's cycle is 28 or 120 days, ovulation takes place 14 days before menstruation.

2. The nurse should inform Susan that cycles vary in frequency from 21 to 36 days; bleeding lasts 3 to 8 days; blood loss averages 20 to 80 mL; the average cycle is 28 days long, but this varies; and irregular menses can be associated with irregular ovulation, stress, disease, and hormonal imbalances.

3. The range for the onset of menstruation is between 8 and 18 years. The average age is 12.8 years. There are several factors that influence the age of menstruation onset. Genetics is the most important factor in determining the age at which menarche starts, but geographic location, nutrition, weight, general health, nutrition, and cultural and social practices are also potential variables.

SECTION III: PRACTICING FOR NCLEX

Activity F NCLEX-STYLE QUESTIONS

1. **Answer: b**
   RATIONALE: To increase the chances of conceiving, the best time for intercourse is 1 or 2 days before ovulation. This ensures that the sperm meets the ovum at the right time. The average life of a sperm cell is 2 to 3 days, and the sperm cells will not be able to survive until ovulation if intercourse occurs a week before ovulation. The chances of conception are minimal for intercourse after ovulation.

2. **Answer: d**
   RATIONALE: Bartholin glands, when stimulated, secrete mucus that supplies lubrication for intercourse. Endocrine glands secrete hormones for various bodily functions. The pituitary gland releases FSH to stimulate the ovary to produce follicles. Skene glands secrete a small amount of mucus to keep the opening to the urethra moist and lubricated for the passage of urine.

3. **Answer: a**
   RATIONALE: The endometrium is the mucosal layer that lines the uterine cavity in nonpregnant women. The fundus is the convex portion above the uterine tubes. The mons pubis is the elevated, rounded, fleshy prominence over the symphysis pubis. The clitoris is a small, cylindrical mass of erectile tissue and nerves located at the anterior junction of the labia minora.

4. **Answer: b**
   RATIONALE: The nurse should inform the client that the yellow fluid is called colostrum, and it contains more minerals and protein, but less sugar and fat, than mature breast milk and is also rich in maternal antibodies. The nurse should inform the client that, gradually, the production of colostrum stops and the production of regular breast milk begins, but there is no need to avoid breastfeeding when colostrum is being produced, if the client's culture allows for it. There is no need to modify diet or to feed formula to the infant.

5. **Answer: c**
   RATIONALE: During ovulation, some women can feel a pain around the time the egg is released on one side of the abdomen. Discomfort is referred to as mittelschmerz. The pain is not a sign of pregnancy, as the client experiences this pain regularly during ovulation. The pain is also not related to an irregular menstruation cycle or the client's exercise regimen.

6. **Answer: b**
   RATIONALE: The nurse should inform the client that there will be a significant increase in temperature, usually 0.5° to 1° F, within a day or two after ovulation has occurred. The temperature remains elevated for 12 to 16 days, until menstruation begins. During ovulation, some women can feel a pain on one side of the abdomen around the time the egg is released. There is no significant correlation between ovulation and lack of sleep or feeling uneasiness or sickness.

7. **Answer: b**
   RATIONALE: After menopause, the uterus shrinks and gradually atrophies. A full bladder, not menopause, causes the uterus to tilt backward. Cervical muscle content does not increase during menopause. Menopause has no significant effect on the outer layer of the cervix.

8. **Answer: d**
   RATIONALE: Progesterone is called the hormone of pregnancy because it reduces uterine contractions, thus producing a calming effect on the uterus, allowing pregnancy to be maintained. FSH is primarily responsible for the maturation of the ovarian follicle. LH is required for both the final maturation of preovulatory follicles and the luteinization of the ruptured follicle. Estrogen is crucial for the development and maturation of the follicle.

9. **Answer: c**
   RATIONALE: During cold conditions, the scrotum is pulled closer to the body for warmth or protection. The cremaster muscles in the scrotal wall contract to allow the testes to be pulled closer to the body. Frequency of urination has no significant impact in maintaining the scrotal temperature. Increase in blood flow to the genital area occurs primarily during erection and is not due to climatic conditions.

10. **Answer: a**
    RATIONALE: With age, the prostate gland gradually enlarges, leading to difficulty during urination. Production of semen never stops, even though the quantity of semen produced may decrease. The prostate gland is not associated with painful erection. During the normal aging process, the prostate gland does not stop functioning, even though its capacity may be somewhat diminished.

11. **Answer: b**
    RATIONALE: The epididymis provides the space and environment for sperm to mature. The testes

produce sperm, but they have to mature in the epididymis to become capable of impregnating the ovum. The vas deferens is the organ that transports sperm from the epididymis. The Cowper glands secrete mucus-like fluid for lubrication during sexual intercourse.

12.   Answer: c
RATIONALE: The nurse should inform the client that the duration of the flow is about 3 to 7 days. An average cycle length is about 21 to 36 days, not 15 to 20 days. In the ovary, 2 million oocytes are present at birth, and about 400,000 follicles are still present at puberty. Blood loss averages 20 to 80 mL, not 120 to 150 mL.

13.   Answer: c
RATIONALE: At ovulation, a mature follicle ruptures, releasing a mature oocyte (ovum). Ovulation always takes place 14 days, not 10 days, before menstruation. The lifespan of the ovum is only about 24 hours, not 48 hours;

unless it meets a sperm on its journey within that time, it will die. When ovulation occurs, there is a drop, not a rise, in estrogen levels.

14.   Answer: b
RATIONALE: Gonadotropin-releasing hormone is secreted from the hypothalamus in a pulsatile manner throughout the reproductive cycle. It induces the release of FSH and LH to assist with ovulation, both of which are secreted by the anterior pituitary gland. Estrogen is secreted by the ovaries and is crucial for the development and maturation of the follicle.

15.   Answer: b
RATIONALE: The mature ovum is released from the ovary, resulting in the corpus luteum. Progesterone is produced by the corpus luteum. Estrogen is secreted by the ovaries. Glycogen is secreted by the endometrial glands during the luteal phase. Luteinizing hormone is not a product of the corpus luteum.

Answers

CHAPTER 4

SECTION I: ASSESSING YOUR UNDERSTANDING

Activity A FILL IN THE BLANKS

1. Adenomyosis
2. prostaglandin
3. Laparoscopy
4. perimenopause
5. vasectomy
6. medical
7. Osteoporosis
8. spinnbarkeit
9. basal
10. minipills

Activity B MATCHING

1. c **2.** d **3.** a **4.** e **5.** b

Activity C SEQUENCING

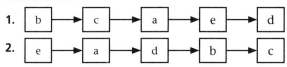

1. b → c → a → e → d
2. e → a → d → b → c

Activity D SHORT ANSWERS

1. Common laboratory tests ordered to determine the cause of amenorrhea are karyotype, ultrasound to detect ovarian cysts, pregnancy test, thyroid function studies, prolactin level, FSH level, LH level, 17-ketosteroids tests, laparoscopy, and CT scan of head.
2. Menopause refers to the cessation of regular menstrual cycles. It is the end of menstruation and childbearing capacity. Natural menopause is defined as 1 year without a menstrual period. The average age at which it occurs is 51 years.
3. The risk factors associated with endometriosis are increasing age, family history of endometriosis, short menstrual cycle, long menstrual flow, young age at menarche, and few or no pregnancies.
4. Infertility refers to the inability to conceive a child after a year of regular sexual intercourse unprotected by contraception, or the inability to carry a pregnancy to term. Secondary infertility results when an individual is unable to conceive after having done so in the past.
5. In the Two-Day Method, women observe the presence or absence of cervical secretions by examining toilet paper or underwear or by monitoring their physical sensations. Every day, the woman asks two simple questions: "Did I note any secretions yesterday?" and "Did I note any secretions today?" If the answer to either question is yes, she considers herself fertile and avoids unprotected intercourse. If the answers are no, she is unlikely to become pregnant from unprotected intercourse on that day.
6. Intrauterine systems (IUSs) are small, plastic, T-shaped objects that are placed inside the uterus to provide contraception. They prevent pregnancy by making the endometrium of the uterus hostile to implantation of a fertilized ovum, by causing a nonspecific inflammatory reaction.

SECTION II: APPLYING YOUR KNOWLEDGE

Activity E CASE STUDY

1. Amenorrhea is a normal feature in prepubertal, pregnant, and postmenopausal women. The two categories of amenorrhea are primary and secondary amenorrhea. Primary amenorrhea is defined as either absence of menses by age 14, with absence of growth and development of secondary sexual characteristics, or absence of menses by age 16, with normal development of secondary sexual characteristics. Ninety-eight percent of American girls menstruate by age 16.
2. Causes of primary amenorrhea related to Alexa may include extreme weight gain or loss, stress from a major life event, excessive exercise, or eating disorders such as anorexia nervosa or bulimia. Primary amenorrhea is also caused by congenital abnormalities of the reproductive system, Cushing disease, polycystic ovarian syndrome, hypothyroidism, and Turner syndrome; other causes are imperforate hymen, chronic illness, pregnancy, cystic fibrosis, congenital heart disease, and ovarian or adrenal tumors.
3. The treatment of primary amenorrhea involves correcting any underlying disorders as well as

providing estrogen replacement therapy to stimulate the development of secondary sexual characteristics. If a pituitary tumor is the cause, it might be treated with drug therapy, surgical resection, or radiation therapy. Surgery might be needed to correct any structural abnormalities of the genital tract.

4. The nurse should address the diverse causes of amenorrhea, the relationship to sexual identity, and the possibility of infertility and more serious problems. In addition, the nurse should inform Alexa about the purpose of each diagnostic test, how it is performed, and when the results will be available. Sensitive listening, interviewing, and presenting treatment options are of paramount importance to gaining the client's cooperation and understanding. Nutritional counseling is also vital in managing this disorder, especially when the client has findings suggestive of an eating disorder. Although not all causes can be addressed by making lifestyle changes, the nurse can still emphasize maintaining a healthy lifestyle.

SECTION III: PRACTICING FOR NCLEX

Activity F NCLEX-STYLE QUESTIONS

1. **Answer: d**
   RATIONALE: When assessing a client for amenorrhea, the nurse should document facial hair and acne as possible evidence of androgen excess secondary to a tumor. The nurse may observe and should document hypothermia, bradycardia, hypotension, and reduced subcutaneous fat in women with anorexia nervosa; however, these are not symptoms of excess androgen.

2. **Answer: b**
   RATIONALE: The nurse should explain to the client that the fertility awareness method relies on the assumption that the "unsafe period" is approximately 6 days; 3 days before and 3 days after ovulation. The method also assumes that sperm can live up to 5 days, not just 24 hours after intercourse. An ovum lives up to 24 hours after being released from the ovary. The exact time of ovulation cannot be determined, so 2 to 3 days are added to the beginning and end to avoid pregnancy.

3. **Answer: b, d, & e**
   RATIONALE: When instructing a client with dysmenorrhea on how to manage her symptoms, the nurse should ask her to increase water consumption, use heating pads or take warm baths, and increase exercise and physical activity. Water consumption serves as a natural diuretic, heating pads or warm baths help increase comfort, and exercise increases endorphins and suppresses prostaglandin release. The nurse should also tell the client to limit salty foods to prevent fluid retention during menstruation and to keep legs elevated while lying down, because this helps increase comfort.

4. **Answer: d**
   RATIONALE: The nurse should prepare the client for a laparoscopy to obtain a definitive diagnosis; laparoscopy allows for direct visualization of the internal organs and helps confirm the diagnosis. A hysterosalpingogram assesses tubal patency, and a clomiphene citrate challenge test determines ovarian function; these tests are not used to determine the extent of endometriosis.

5. **Answer: d**
   RATIONALE: The nurse should instruct the client to deliver the semen sample to the laboratory for analysis within 1 to 2 hours after ejaculation. The client should also be instructed to collect the sample in a specimen container, not a condom or plastic bag. The client needs to abstain from sexual activity for at least 24 hours before giving the sample, but he need not avoid strenuous activity.

6. **Answer: c**
   RATIONALE: The nurse should explain that during ovulation, the cervix is high or deep in the vagina. The os is slightly open during ovulation. Under the influence of estrogen during ovulation, the cervical mucus is copious and slippery and can be stretched between two fingers without breaking. It becomes thick and dry after ovulation, under the influence of progesterone.

7. **Answer: c**
   RATIONALE: Recent studies have shown that the extended use of active OC pills carries the same safety profile as the conventional 28-day regimen. This option helps reduce the number of periods and is as effective as the conventional regimen. There is no evidence to suggest that discontinuation of active OCs will not ensure restoration of fertility. Depo-Provera, not active OC pills, prevents pregnancy for 3 months at a time.

8. **Answer: d**
   RATIONALE: The client should be instructed to take her temperature before rising and record it on a chart. If using this method by itself, the client should avoid unprotected intercourse until the BBT has been elevated for 3 days. The client should be informed that other fertility awareness methods should be used along with BBT for better results. The oral method is better suited than the axillary method for taking the temperature in this case.

9. **Answer: d**
   RATIONALE: The best option for a client who is not well educated would be the Standard Days Method with CycleBeads, as the 32 color-coded CycleBeads are easy to use and understand. An injection of Depo-Provera would also suit this client, as it works by suppressing ovulation and the production of FSH and LH by the pituitary gland and prevents pregnancy for 3 months at a time. BBT requires the client to take and chart her body temperature; this may be difficult for the client to

follow. Coitus interruptus is a method in which the man controls his ejaculation and ejaculates outside the vagina; this suggests that the client rely solely on the cooperation and judgment of her spouse. The lactational amenorrhea method works as a temporary method of contraception only for breastfeeding mothers.

10. **Answer: a, c, & e**
    RATIONALE: The nurse should tell the client to inspect the cervical cap before insertion for cracks, holes, or tears and to wait approximately 30 minutes after insertion before engaging in sexual intercourse to be sure that a seal has formed between the rim and the cervix. In addition, the cap should not be used during menses because of the potential for toxic shock syndrome; an alternative method such as condoms should be used during this time. The client should be told not to apply spermicide to the rim because it may interfere with the seal. It should be left in place for a minimum of 6 hours after sexual intercourse.

11. **Answer: b**
    RATIONALE: Considering the client's smoking habit, combination OCs may be contraindicated. OCs are highly effective when taken properly, but can aggravate many medical conditions, especially in women who smoke. The Lunelle injection, Depo-Provera, or copper intrauterine devices (IUDs) are not contraindicated in this client and can be used with certain precautions. Implantable contraceptives are subdermal time-release implants that deliver synthetic progestin; these are highly effective and are not contraindicated in this client.

12. **Answer: b**
    RATIONALE: The client is seeking a medical abortion. The nurse should inform the client that such medications are effectively used to terminate a pregnancy only during the first trimester, not the second. The medications are available as a vaginal suppository or in oral form and do not present a high risk of respiratory failure. Sterilization, not abortion, is considered a permanent end to fertility.

13. **Answer: b**
    RATIONALE: Since the client has multiple sex partners, condoms will help offer protection against STIs and are best suited for her needs. The client cannot use an IUD because of her history of various pelvic infections. Although OCs will help the client as a means of contraception, this method is not the best choice for her because it does not offer protection against STIs. Tubal ligation is a sterilization procedure and does not suit the client's purpose.

14. **Answer: b, c, & e**
    RATIONALE: The nurse needs to clear up misconceptions by explaining to clients that taking birth control pills does not protect against STIs and that irregular menstruation or douching after sex does not prevent pregnancy. The nurse also needs to confirm that breastfeeding does not protect against pregnancy and that pregnancy can occur during menses.

15. **Answer: a**
    RATIONALE: Since the client has a history of cardiac problems, long-term hormone replacement therapy is contraindicated. This is because there is an increased risk of heart attacks and strokes. The client should instead be asked to consider options with minimized risk, such as lipid-lowering agents, or nonhormonal therapies, such as bisphosphonates and selective estrogen receptor modulators.

16. **Answer: c**
    RATIONALE: The client is likely to be experiencing vaginal atrophy, which occurs during menopause because of declining estrogen levels. The condition can be managed with the use of over-the-counter moisturizers and lubricants. A positive outlook on sexuality and a supportive partner may make the sexual experience enjoyable and fulfilling, whereas a support group may reduce the client's anxiety. However, these will not alleviate the client's discomfort. Menopause can be a physically and emotionally challenging time for women because of the stigma of an "aging" body; the nurse should be sensitive to the client's feelings when discussing these changes.

17. **Answer: a**
    RATIONALE: The nurse should inform the client that IUSs cause monthly periods to become lighter, shorter, and less painful. Monthly periods reduce in number with use of OCs, but not with use of IUSs.

18. **Answer: b, c, & d**
    RATIONALE: The nurse should instruct the client to wet the sponge before inserting it, to insert it 24 hours before intercourse, and to leave it in place for at least 6 hours following intercourse, to be effective. The sponge should not be replaced every 2 hours because this will reduce its efficacy. A contraceptive sponge covers the cervix and releases spermicide. It does not protect against STIs. Therefore, keeping the sponge for more than 30 hours will not prevent STIs, but will increase risk of toxic shock syndrome.

CHAPTER 5

SECTION I: ASSESSING YOUR UNDERSTANDING

Activity A FILL IN THE BLANKS

1. Trichomoniasis
2. tertiary
3. Ectoparasites
4. Scabies
5. thrush
6. Syphilis
7. liver
8. chlamydia
9. CD4
10. chlamydia

Activity B LABELING

1. a. The disease in the photograph is genital herpes simplex.
   b. The clinical manifestations of genital herpes include blister-like lesions. Additional symptoms may include dysuria, headache, fever, and muscle aches.
   c. The disease is not curable. Pharmacologic management may include antiviral therapies such as acyclovir (Zovirax), famciclovir (Famvir), or valacyclovir (Valtrex).
2. a. The disease in the photograph is a STI known as genital warts.
   b. Risk factors associated with genital warts include multiple sex partners, age (15 to 25), sex with a male who has had multiple sexual partners, and first intercourse at 16 or younger.
   c. Treatments used in for genital warts include:
   - Topical trichloroacetic acid 80% to 90%
   - Liquid nitrogen Cryotherapy
   - Topical imiquimod 5% cream (Aldara)
   - Topical podophyllin 10% to 25%
   - Laser carbon dioxide vaporization
   - Client-applied Podofilox 0.5% solution or gel
   - Simple surgical excision
   - Loop electrosurgical excisional procedure
   - Intralesional interferon therapy

Activity C MATCHING

1. c **2.** a **3.** b **4.** f **5.** d **6.** e

Activity D SEQUENCING

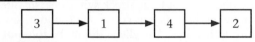

3 → 1 → 4 → 2

Activity E SHORT ANSWER

1. Predisposing factors that may increase the chances of vulvovaginal candidiasis include pregnancy; use of oral contraceptives with a high estrogen content; use of broad-spectrum antibiotics; diabetes mellitus; use of steroids and immunosuppressive drugs; HIV infection; wearing tight, restrictive clothes and nylon underpants; and trauma to vaginal mucosa from chemical irritants or douching.
2. Hepatitis A produces flulike symptoms with malaise, fatigue, anorexia, nausea, pruritus, fever, and upper-right-quadrant pain.
3. HIV is transmitted by intimate sexual contact; by sharing needles for intravenous drug use; from mother to fetus during pregnancy; or by transfusion of blood or blood products.
4. AIDS is a breakdown in the immune function caused by HIV, a retrovirus. The infected person develops opportunistic infections or malignancies that become fatal. Progression from HIV infection to AIDS occurs at a median of 11 years after infection.
5. There can be hundreds of causes of vaginitis, but more often than not the cause is infection by one of three organisms: Candida, a fungus; Trichomonas, a protozoan; or Gardnerella, a bacterium.
6. The clinical manifestations of Chlamydia are mucopurulent vaginal discharge, urethritis, bartholinitis, endometritis, salpingitis, and dysfunctional uterine bleeding.

SECTION II: APPLYING YOUR KNOWLEDGE

Activity F CASE STUDY

1. In pregnant women, gonorrhea is associated with chorioamnionitis, premature labor, premature rupture of membranes, and postpartum endometritis. It can also be transmitted to the newborn in the form of ophthalmia neonatorum during birth by direct contact with gonococcal organisms in the cervix. Ophthalmia neonatorum is highly contagious and, if untreated, leads to blindness of the newborn.

2. The nurse should be aware of the following factors:
   - Sensitivity and confidentiality: There is a social stigma attached to STIs, so women need to be reassured about confidentiality.
   - Education and counseling skills: The nurse should possess the necessary education and counseling skills to help the client deal with the infection.
   - Level of knowledge: The nurse's level of knowledge about chlamydia and gonorrhea should include treatment strategies, referral sources, and preventive measures.
   - Assessment: Assessment involves taking a health history that includes a comprehensive sexual history. Questions about the number of sex partners and the use of safer sex practices are appropriate. Previous and current symptoms should be reviewed. Seeking treatment and informing sex partners should be emphasized.
3. High-risk groups who may develop gonorrhea include individuals who
   - Have low socioeconomic status
   - Live in an urban area
   - Are single
   - Practice inconsistent use of barrier contraceptives
   - Have multiple sex partners

SECTION III: PRACTICING FOR NCLEX

Activity G NCLEX-STYLE QUESTIONS

1. **Answer: c**
   RATIONALE: As a preventive measure for the client with frequent vulvovaginal candidiasis, the nurse should instruct the client to wear white, 100% cotton underpants. The nurse should instruct the client to use pads instead of superabsorbent tampons, to avoid douching the affected area (as it washes away protective vaginal mucus), and to reduce her dietary intake of simple sugars and soda.

2. **Answer: a**
   RATIONALE: The nurse should instruct the client to use high-protein supplements such as Boost to provide quick and easy protein and calories. The nurse should also instruct the client to eat dry crackers upon arising, not after every meal, and to eat six small meals a day, not three. Drinking fluids constantly while eating is not recommended. The nurse should instruct the client to separate the intake of food and fluids.

3. **Answer: b**
   RATIONALE: The nurse should inform the client that even after warts are removed, HPV still remains and viral shedding will continue. The nurse should instruct the client to avoid applying steroid creams, sprays, or gels to vaginal area. All women above the age of 30 should undergo an HPV test, and women between 9 and 26 years of age should consider HPV vaccination with Gardasil. The use of latex condoms has been associated with a decreased risk, not an increased risk, of cervical cancer.

4. **Answer: d**
   RATIONALE: The nurse should counsel the client taking metronidazole to avoid alcohol during the treatment because mixing the two causes severe nausea and vomiting. Avoiding extremes of temperature to the genital area is a requirement for clients with genital ulcers, not trichomoniasis. The nurse should instruct the client to avoid sex, regardless of using condoms, until she and her sex partners are cured, that is, when therapy has been completed and both partners are symptom-free. It is not required to increase fluid intake during treatment.

5. **Answer: a**
   RATIONALE: Symptoms of bacterial vaginosis include a characteristic "stale fish" odor and thin, white homogeneous vaginal discharge, not heavy yellow discharge. Dysfunctional uterine bleeding is a sign of Chlamydia, not bacterial vaginosis. Erythema in the vulvovaginal area is a symptom of vulvovaginal candidiasis, not bacterial vaginosis.

6. **Answer: d**
   RATIONALE: Genital herpes simplex is characterized by lesions, frequently located on the vulva, vagina, and perineal areas. Rashes on the face are not symptoms of HSV. Alopecia is one of the symptoms of syphilis, not of primary HSV. Vaginal discharge during the primary stage of herpes is mucopurulent, not yellow-green.

7. **Answer: c**
   RATIONALE: As a nursing strategy to prevent the spread of STIs, the nurse should discuss reducing the number of sex partners to diminish the risk of acquiring STIs. Oral contraceptives are not effective in preventing STIs, and barrier methods (condoms, diaphragms) should be promoted. The nurse should counsel and encourage sex partners of persons with STIs to seek treatment. Maintaining good body hygiene or not sharing personal items with others does not reduce the risk of spreading STIs.

8. **Answer: b**
   RATIONALE: The nurse should instruct all community members to get vaccinated for prevention of hepatitis B. Ensuring that drinking water is disease free and educating people about the risks involved with injecting drugs may help prevent hepatitis A, not hepatitis B. Delaying the start of sexual activity by teenagers may not protect them from hepatitis B in the long run.

9. **Answer: a**
   RATIONALE: Although the reasons for bacterial vaginosis are not yet fully understood, sex with multiple partners increases the risk, and therefore it should be avoided. Using oral contraceptives and smoking have not been associated with bacterial vaginosis. A colposcopy test is recommended for clients with high-risk HPV, not for diagnosing bacterial vaginosis.

10. **Answer: c**
    RATIONALE: The nurse should inform the client that there is no evidence to suggest that antiviral therapy is completely safe during pregnancy. HSV cannot be cured completely, even with timely antiviral drug therapy, and there may be recurrences. The viral shedding process continues for 2 weeks during the primary episode, and kissing during this period may transmit the disease. Recurrent HSV-infection episodes are shorter and milder.

11. **Answer: b, c, & e**
    RATIONALE: The nurse should instruct the client with pelvic inflammatory disease to avoid douching, limit the number of sex partners, and complete the antibiotic therapy. Use of an intrauterine device is one of the risk factors associated with PID and should be avoided. Increasing fluid intake does not help alleviate the client's condition.

12. **Answer: a, c, & d**
    RATIONALE: The nurse should instruct the client to wear nonconstricting clothes and to wash her hands with soap and water after touching lesions to avoid autoinoculation. If urination is painful because of the ulcers, instruct the client to urinate in water but to avoid extremes of temperature such as ice packs or hot pads to the genital area. The client should abstain from intercourse during the prodromal period and when lesions are present. The ulcer disappears during the latency period.

13. **Answer: a, b, & c**
    RATIONALE: The nurse should give opportunities to practice negotiation techniques and encourage women to develop refusal skills so that they can respond positively in situations where they might be at risk for HIV infection. To reduce risk of HIV infection, the nurse should encourage the use of female condoms. Supporting youth-development activities to reduce sexual risk-taking and identifying or encouraging women to lead a healthy lifestyle may not be effective enough in empowering women to develop control over their lives.

14. **Answer: c, d, & e**
    RATIONALE: The nurse should ensure that the client understands the dosing regimen and schedule. The client should be informed that unpleasant side effects such as nausea and diarrhea are common. The nurse should provide written material describing diet, exercise, and

medications to promote compliance and ensure a healthy lifestyle. There is no evidence to suggest that exposure of the fetus to antiretroviral agents during pregnancy is completely safe in the long run. HIV is a lifelong condition, and antiretroviral therapy may delay the onset of AIDS but not prevent it.

15. **Answer: b, d, & e**
    RATIONALE: When educating the client about cervical cancer, the nurse should inform the client that recurrence of genital warts increases the risk of cervical cancer and that she should obtain regular Pap smears to detect cervical cancer. Use of latex condoms reduces the risk of cervical cancer. Abnormal vaginal discharge does not necessarily indicate cervical cancer. There is no significant link between use of broad-spectrum antibiotics and increased risk of cervical cancer.

16. **Answer: b**
    RATIONALE: The hepatitis B vaccine consists of a series of three injections given within 6 months. The vaccine is safe and well tolerated by most babies, including those who are underweight or premature. Vaccines are given after birth in most hospitals, not 6 months later. All babies are vaccinated, not just those whose mothers are identified as at high risk for hepatitis.

17. **Answer: b**
    RATIONALE: To prevent gonococcal ophthalmia neonatorum in the baby, the nurse should instill a prophylactic agent in the eyes of the newborn. Cephalosporins are administered to the mother during pregnancy to treat gonorrhea but not to prevent infection in the newborn. Performing a cesarean operation will not prevent gonococcal ophthalmia neonatorum in the newborn. An antiretroviral syrup is administered to the newborn only if the mother is HIV-positive and will not help prevent gonococcal ophthalmia neonatorum in the baby.

18. **Answer: d**
    RATIONALE: Antiretroviral syrup is administered to the infant within 12 hours after birth to reduce the risk of transmission of HIV to the baby. Delivering the baby via cesarean does not significantly lower the risk of transmitting AIDS to the baby. A triple-combination HAART is used to treat HIV in adults, not babies. The nurse should counsel the client to avoid breastfeeding and use formula instead, because HIV can be spread to the infant through breastfeeding.

Answers

CHAPTER 6

SECTION I: ASSESSING YOUR UNDERSTANDING

Activity A FILL IN THE BLANKS

1. Ultrasound
2. Brachytherapy
3. estrogen
4. Lumpectomy
5. Mammography
6. Chemotherapy
7. mastectomy
8. Hemoccult
9. Immunotherapy
10. Fibroadenomas

Activity B MATCHING

1. e   **2.** d   **3.** c   **4.** b   **5.** a

Activity C SEQUENCING

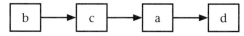

Activity D SHORT ANSWERS

1. A benign breast disorder is any noncancerous breast abnormality. Though not life threatening, benign disorders can cause pain and discomfort and account for a large number of visits to primary care providers. The most commonly encountered benign breast disorders in women include fibrocystic breasts, fibroadenomas, intraductal papilloma, mammary duct ectasia, and mastitis.
2. The three aspects on which breast cancers are classified are tumor size, extent of lymph node involvement, and evidence of metastasis.
3. Breast-conserving surgery, the least invasive procedure, is the wide local excision (or lumpectomy) of the tumor along with a 1-cm margin of normal tissue. A lumpectomy is often used for early-stage localized tumors. The goal of breast-conserving surgery is to remove the suspicious mass along with tissue free of malignant cells to prevent recurrence. The results are less drastic and emotionally less scarring to the woman. Women undergoing breast-conserving therapy receive radiation after lumpectomy with the goal of eradicating residual microscopic cancer cells to limit locoregional recurrence. In women who do not require adjuvant chemotherapy, radiation therapy typically begins 2 to 4 weeks after surgery to allow healing of the lumpectomy incision site. Radiation is administered to the entire breast at daily doses over a period of several weeks.
4. Adjunct therapy is supportive or additional therapy that is recommended after surgery. Adjunct therapies include local therapy such as radiation therapy and systemic therapies such as chemotherapy, hormonal therapy, and immunotherapy.
5. The typical side effects of chemotherapy include nausea and vomiting, diarrhea, or constipation.
6. The status of the axillary lymph nodes is an important prognostic indicator in early-stage breast cancer. The presence or absence of malignant cells in lymph nodes is highly significant. The more lymph nodes involved and the more aggressive the cancer, the more powerful chemotherapy will have to be, in terms of both the toxicity of drugs and the duration of treatment.

SECTION III: APPLYING YOUR KNOWLEDGE

Activity E CASE STUDY

1. The nurse should ask the following questions:
   - Where is the lump located, and is it freely moveable or fixed?
   - Does the client have any nipple discharge? If yes, describe its color and consistency.
   - Does the client have a feeling of fullness in the breast?
   - Is the pain dull, burning, or itchy?
   - Is there any skin dimpling or nipple retraction?
2. Mrs. Taylor needs the following education regarding breast health:
   - Monthly breast self-examination
   - Yearly clinical breast examination
   - Yearly mammography
3. The treatment modalities available to Mrs. Taylor in case of a malignancy are:
   - Local treatments such as surgery, and radiation
   - Systemic treatments such as chemotherapy, hormonal therapy, and immunotherapy

4. Mrs. Taylor will need the following community referrals:
   - Telephone counseling by the nurse
   - American Cancer Society's (ACS) Reach for Recovery
   - Organizations or charities that support cancer research
   - Participation in breast cancer walks to raise awareness
   - Emotional support groups

SECTION IV: PRACTICING FOR NCLEX

Activity F NCLEX-STYLE QUESTIONS

1. **Answer: c**
   RATIONALE: During menstrual cycles, hormonal stimulation of the breast tissue causes the glands and ducts to enlarge and swell. The breasts feel swollen, tender, and lumpy during this time, but after menses the swelling and lumpiness decline. Thus it is best to examine the breasts a week after the menses, when they are not swollen. For determining fibrocystic breast changes, it is not best to schedule the breast examination in the second phase of menstrual cycle or immediately after the client has completed her menses.

2. **Answer: b**
   RATIONALE: As the physician suspects fibroadenomas, it is important for the nurse to know whether the client is pregnant or lactating since the incidence of fibroadenomas is more frequent among pregnant and lactating women. Taking oral contraceptives assists a client with fibrocystic breast changes, but is not necessary for a client with fibroadenomas. Fibroadenomas usually occur in women between 20 and 30 years of age. Smoking and a high-fat diet will make the client more susceptible to cancer, not fibroadenomas.

3. **Answer: a**
   RATIONALE: The nurse should instruct the client with mastitis to increase her fluid intake. A client with mastitis is instructed to continue breastfeeding as tolerated and to frequently change positions while nursing. The nurse should also instruct the client to apply warm, not cold, compresses to the affected breast area or to take a warm shower before breastfeeding.

4. **Answer: b**
   RATIONALE: When preparing a client for mammography, the nurse should ensure the client has not applied deodorant or powder on the day of testing because they can appear on the x-ray film as calcium spots. It is not necessary for the client to avoid fluid intake an hour prior to testing. Mammography has to be scheduled just after the client's menses to reduce chances of breast tenderness, not when the client is going to start her menses. The client can take aspirin or Tylenol after the completion of the procedure to ease any discomfort, but these medications are not taken before mammography.

5. **Answer: d**
   RATIONALE: The side effects of chemotherapy are constipation, hair loss, weight loss, vomiting, diarrhea, immunosuppression, and, in extreme cases, bone marrow suppression. The nurse should monitor for these side effects when caring for the client undergoing chemotherapy. Vaginal discharge, headache, and chills are not side effects of chemotherapy. Vaginal discharge is one of the side effects of SERMs as a part of hormonal therapy, which is used to prevent cancer from spreading further into the body. Headache is a side effect of aromatase inhibitors under hormonal therapy to counter cancer. Chills are a side effect of immunotherapy.

6. **Answer: d**
   RATIONALE: The nurse should inform the client that intraductal papillomas and fibrocystic breasts, although considered benign, carry a cancer risk with prolific masses and hyperplastic changes within the breasts. Other benign breast disorders such as mastitis, mammary duct ectasia, and fibroadenomas carry little risk.

7. **Answer: a**
   RATIONALE: The nurse should inform the client that removing only the sentinel lymph node prevents side effects such as lymphedema, which is otherwise associated with a traditional axillary lymph node dissection. It does not help reveal the hormonal status of the cancer. Hormone-receptor status can be revealed through normal breast epithelium, which has hormone receptors and responds specifically to the stimulatory effects of estrogen and progesterone. A sentinel lymph node biopsy will determine how powerful a chemotherapy regimen the client will have to undergo, but undergoing a sentinel lymph node biopsy will not lessen the aggressiveness of the chemotherapy. Degree of HER-2/neu oncoprotein will be revealed through the HER-2/neu genetic marker, not through a sentinel lymph node biopsy.

8. **Answer: b**
   RATIONALE: When providing care to the client, the nurse should instruct the client to elevate the affected arm on a pillow. As part of the respiratory care, the nurse should instruct the client to turn, cough, and breathe deeply every 2 hours; rapid breathing is not encouraged. Active range-of-motion and arm exercises are necessary. To counter any pain experienced by the client, analgesics are administered as needed; intake of medication is not restricted.

9. **Answer: c**
   RATIONALE: Skin edema, redness, and warmth of the breast are symptoms of inflammatory breast cancer. Induced discharge is an indication of benign breast conditions, which are noncancerous. Cancer involves spontaneous nipple discharge. Papillomas and palpable mobile cysts are characteristics of fibroadenomas, intraductal papilloma, and mammary duct ectasia, which are benign breast conditions and are noncancerous.

10. **Answer: d**
    RATIONALE: The symptom of mammary duct ectasia that the nurse should assess for is the presence of green, brown, straw-colored, reddish, gray, or cream-colored nipple discharge with a consistency of toothpaste. Increased warmth of the breasts along with redness is a manifestation of mastitis but not mammary duct ectasia. Skin retractions on pulling are a sign of cancer, not mammary duct ectasia. The nurse has to observe nipple retraction. Tortuous tubular swellings are found only beneath the areola, not in the upper half of the breast, in mammary duct ectasia.

11. **Answer: c**
    RATIONALE: When caring for a client who is being administered selective estrogen receptor modulator, the nurse should monitor for side effects such as hot flashes, vaginal discharge, bleeding, and cataract formation. Weight loss is one of the side effects of chemotherapy, and fever and chills are the side effects of immunotherapy, not of SERM.

12. **Answer: a, c, & d**
    RATIONALE: The modifiable risk factors for breast cancer are postmenopausal use of estrogen and progestins, not having children until after the age of 30, and failing to breastfeed for up to a year after pregnancy. Early menarche or late menopause and previous abnormal breast biopsy are the nonmodifiable risk factors for breast cancer.

13. **Answer: d**
    RATIONALE: When performing the breast self-examination, the nurse should instruct the client to apply hard pressure down to the ribs. Light, not medium, pressure should be applied when moving the skin without moving the tissue underneath. Medium, not light, pressure should be applied midway into the tissue. Client need not specifically palpate the areolar area during breast self-examination.

14. **Answer: b**
    RATIONALE: Adverse effects of trastuzumab include cardiac toxicity, vascular thrombosis, hepatic failure, fever, chills, nausea, vomiting, and pain with first infusion. The nurse should monitor for these adverse effects with the first infusion of trastuzumab. Dyspnea, stroke, and myelosuppression are not side effects caused with the first infusion of trastuzumab. Dyspnea is a side effect of aromatase inhibitors as part of hormonal therapy. Stroke is an adverse effect of SERM, again as part of hormonal therapy. Myelosuppression is an extreme side effect of chemotherapy.

15. **Answer: a**
    RATIONALE: A nurse should closely monitor for signs of anorexia as it is a likely side effect of radiation therapy, along with swelling and heaviness of the breast, local edema, inflammation, and sunburn-like skin changes. Infection, fever, and nausea are not the side effects of radiation therapy. Infection and fever are the side effects of brachytherapy. Nausea is one of the side effects of chemotherapy.

16. **Answer: b**
    RATIONALE: When caring for a client who has just undergone surgery for intraductal papilloma, the nurse should instruct the client to continue monthly breast self-examinations along with yearly clinical breast examinations. Applying warm compresses to the affected breast and wearing a supportive bra 24 hours a day are instructions given in cases of mastitis but not for intraductal papilloma. The nurse should instruct clients to refrain from consuming salt in the diet in cases of fibrocystic breast changes but not in cases of intraductal papilloma.

17. **Answer: b, d, & e**
    RATIONALE: Lumpectomy is contraindicated for women who have previously undergone radiation to their affected breast, those whose connective tissue is reported to be sensitive to radiation, and those whose surgery will not result in a clean margin of tissue. Clients who have had an early menarche or late onset of menopause and clients who have failed to breastfeed for up to a year after pregnancy are at risk for developing breast cancer. Lumpectomy is a treatment option for clients with breast cancer.

18. **Answer: a, b, & d**
    RATIONALE: The client is more susceptible to lymphedema if the affected arm is used for drawing blood or measuring blood pressure, if she engages in activities like gardening without using gloves, or if she's not wearing a well-fitted compression sleeve to promote drainage return. Consuming foods rich in phytochemicals is essential to prevent the incidence of cancer, not lymphedema. Not consuming a diet high in fiber and protein will not make the client susceptible to lymphedema.

19. **Answer: b, d, & e**
    RATIONALE: The nurse should instruct the client with fibrocystic breast changes to avoid caffeine. Caffeine acts as a stimulant that can lead to discomfort. It is important to maintain a low-fat diet rich in fruits, vegetables, and grains to maintain a healthy body weight. Taking diuretics is important to counteract fluid retention and swelling of the breasts. Practicing good hand-washing techniques and increasing fluid intake are important for clients with mastitis but may not help clients with fibrocystic breast changes.

20. **Answer: a, b, & c**
    RATIONALE: The nurse should instruct the client to restrict intake of salted foods, limit intake of processed foods, and consume seven or more daily portions of complex carbohydrates, not proteins. Increasing liquid intake to 3 L daily will not reduce her risk of developing breast cancer.

Answers

CHAPTER 7

SECTION I: ASSESSING YOUR UNDERSTANDING

Activity A FILL IN THE BLANKS

1. Cystocele
2. prolapse
3. pessary
4. Polyps
5. leiomyomas
6. Kegel
7. rectum
8. urethra
9. Metrorrhagia
10. Transvaginal

Activity B MATCHING

1. a **2.** e **3.** b **4.** c **5.** d

Activity C SHORT ANSWERS

1. Pelvic organ prolapse could be caused by the following:
   - Constant downward gravity because of erect human posture
   - Atrophy of supporting tissues with aging and decline of estrogen levels
   - Weakening of pelvic support related to childbirth trauma
   - Reproductive surgery
   - Family history of pelvic organ prolapse
   - Young age at first birth
   - Connective tissue disorders
   - Infant birth weight of greater than 4,500 g
   - Pelvic radiation
   - Increased abdominal pressure secondary to lifting of children or heavy objects, straining due to chronic constipation, respiratory problems or chronic coughing, or obesity
2. Kegel exercises strengthen the pelvic-floor muscles to support the inner organs and prevent further prolapse. They help increase the muscle volume, which will result in a stronger muscular contraction. These exercises might limit the progression of mild prolapse and alleviate mild prolapse symptoms, including low back pain and pelvic pres-

sure. Clients with severe uterine prolapse may not benefit from Kegel exercises.
3. Several factors contribute to urinary incontinence:
   - Intake of fluids, especially alcohol, carbonated drinks, and caffeinated beverages
   - Constipation, which alters the position of pelvic organs and puts pressure on the bladder
   - Habitual preventive emptying, which may result in training the bladder to hold small amounts of urine
   - Anatomic changes due to advanced age, which decrease pelvic support
   - Pregnancy and childbirth, which cause damage to the pelvis structure during birthing process
   - Obesity, which increases abdominal pressure
4. The Colpexin sphere is a polycarbonate sphere with a locator string that is fitted above the hymenal ring to support the pelvis floor muscle. The sphere is used in conjunction with pelvic floor muscle exercises, which should be performed daily. The sphere supports the pelvic floor muscle and facilitates rehabilitation of the pelvic floor muscles.
5. Uterine fibroids may be medically managed by UAE. UAE is an option in which polyvinyl alcohol pellets are injected into selected blood vessels via a catheter to block circulation to the fibroid, causing shrinkage of the fibroid and resolution of the symptoms. After treatment, most fibroids are reduced by 50% within 3 months, but they might recur. The failure rate is approximately 10% to 15%, and this therapy should not be performed on women desiring to retain their fertility.
6. Bartholin glands are two mucus-secreting glandular structures with duct openings bilaterally at the base of the labia minora, near the opening of the vagina, that provide lubrication during sexual arousal. A Bartholin cyst is a fluid-filled, swollen, saclike structure that results from a blockage of one of the ducts of the Bartholin gland. The cyst may become infected and an abscess may develop in the gland. Bartholin cysts are the most common cystic growths in the vulva, affecting approximately 2% of women at some time in their lives.

SECTION II: APPLYING YOUR KNOWLEDGE

Activity D CASE STUDY

1. Pelvic support disorders increase with age and are a result of weakness of the connective tissue and muscular support of the pelvic organs. Vaginal childbirth, obesity, lifting, chronic cough, straining at defecation secondary to constipation, and estrogen deficiency all contribute to pelvic support disorders.

2. Symptoms of uterine prolapse include low back pain, pelvic pressure, urinary frequency, retention, and/or incontinence. These symptoms are likely to affect Mrs. Scott's daily activities.

3. Nonsurgical interventions include regular Kegel exercises, estrogen replacement therapy, dietary and lifestyle modifications, and pessaries. Kegel exercises might limit the progression of mild prolapse and alleviate mild prolapse symptoms, including low back pain and pelvic pressure. Estrogen replacement therapy may help to improve the tone and vascularity of the supporting tissue in perimenopausal and menopausal women by increasing blood perfusion and elasticity to the vaginal wall. Dietary and lifestyle modifications may help prevent pelvic relaxation and chronic problems later in life. Pessaries may be indicated for uterine prolapse or cystocele, especially among elderly clients for whom surgery is contraindicated. Surgical interventions include anterior and posterior colporrhaphy and vaginal hysterectomy. Anterior and posterior colporrhaphy may be effective for a first-degree prolapse. A vaginal hysterectomy is the treatment of choice for uterine prolapse because it removes the prolapsed organ that is bringing down the bladder and rectum with it.

SECTION III: PRACTICING FOR NCLEX

Activity E NCLEX-STYLE QUESTIONS

1. **Answer: c**
   RATIONALE: Weakening of the pelvic-floor muscles causes a feeling of dragging and a "lump" in the vagina; these are symptoms of pelvic organ prolapse. These symptoms do not indicate urinary incontinence, endocervical polyps, or uterine fibroids. Urinary incontinence is the involuntary loss of urine. The symptoms of endocervical polyps are abnormal vaginal bleeding or discharge. In cases of uterine fibroids, the uterus is enlarged and irregularly shaped.

2. **Answer: b**
   RATIONALE: Before starting estrogen replacement therapy, each woman must be evaluated on the basis of a thorough medical history to validate her risk for complications such as endometrial cancer, myocardial infarction, stroke, breast cancer, pulmonary emboli, or deep vein thrombosis. The effective dose of estrogen required, the dietary modifications, and the cost of estrogen replacement therapy can be discussed at a later stage when the client understands the risks associated with estrogen replacement therapy and decides to use hormone therapy.

3. **Answer: a**
   RATIONALE: The nurse should instruct the client to increase dietary fiber and fluids to prevent constipation. A high-fiber diet with an increase in fluid intake alleviates constipation by increasing stool bulk and stimulating peristalsis. Straining to pass a hard stool increases intra-abdominal pressure, which, over time, causes the pelvic organs to prolapse. Avoiding caffeine products would not help in the management of this condition. In addition to recommending increasing the amount of fiber in her diet, the nurse should also encourage the woman to drink eight 8-oz glasses of fluid daily. The nurse should instruct the client to avoid high-impact aerobics to minimize the risk of increasing intra-abdominal pressure.

4. **Answer: d**
   RATIONALE: The disadvantage of myomectomy is that the fibroids may grow back in the future. Fertility is not jeopardized because this procedure leaves the uterine wall intact. Weakening of the uterine walls, scarring, and adhesions are caused by laser treatment, not myomectomy.

5. **Answer: b**
   RATIONALE: Kegel exercises might limit the progression of mild prolapse and alleviate mild prolapse symptoms, including low back pain and pelvic pressure. Intake of food is not required before performing Kegel exercises. Surgical interventions do not interfere with Kegel exercises. Kegel exercises do not cause an increase in blood pressure.

6. **Answer: a, b, & d**
   RATIONALE: The predisposing factors for uterine fibroids are age (late reproductive years), nulliparity, obesity, genetic predisposition, and African American ethnicity. Smoking and hyperinsulinemia are not predisposing factors for uterine fibroids.

7. **Answer: b**
   RATIONALE: Vaginal dryness is one of the side effects of GnRH medications. The other side effects of GnRH medications are hot flashes, headaches, mood changes, musculoskeletal malaise, bone loss, and depression. Increased vaginal discharge, urinary tract infections, and vaginitis are side effects of a pessary, not GnRH medications.

8. **Answer: c**
   RATIONALE: The nurse should instruct the client using a pessary to report any discomfort or difficulty with urination or defecation. Avoiding high-impact aerobics, jogging, jumping, and lifting heavy objects, as well as wearing a girdle or abdominal support, are recommended for a client with prolapse as part of lifestyle modifications and may not be necessary for a client using a pessary.

9. **Answer: b**
   RATIONALE: The most common recommendation for pessary care is removing the pessary twice weekly and cleaning it with soap and water. In addition, douching with diluted vinegar or hydrogen peroxide helps to reduce urinary tract infections and odor, which are side effects of using a pessary. Estrogen cream is applied to make the vaginal mucosa more resistant to erosion and strengthen the vaginal walls. Removing the pessary before sleeping or intercourse is not part of the instructions for pessary care.

10. **Answer: d**
    RATIONALE: The nurse should monitor the client with ultrasound scans every 3 to 6 months. Monitoring gonadotropin level and blood sugar level and scheduling periodic Pap smears are not important assessments for the client with small ovarian cysts.

11. **Answer: a**
    RATIONALE: The nurse should teach the client turning, deep breathing, and coughing prior to the surgery to prevent atelectasis and respiratory complications such as pneumonia. Reducing activity level and the need for pelvic rest are instructions related to discharge planning after the client has undergone a hysterectomy. A high-fat diet need not be avoided before undergoing hysterectomy; avoiding a high-fat diet is required for clients with pelvic organ prolapse to reduce constipation.

12. **Answer: b, c, & e**
    RATIONALE: If the client is at high risk of recurrent prolapse after a surgical repair, is morbidly obese, or has chronic obstructive pulmonary disease, then the client is not a good candidate for surgical repair. Low back pain and pelvic pressure are common to almost all pelvic organ prolapses and do not help to decide whether the client should opt for surgical repair. A client with severe pelvic organ prolapse may be a candidate for surgical repair.

13. **Answer: a, b, & d**
    RATIONALE: The teaching guidelines include continuing pelvic floor (Kegel) exercises, increasing fiber in the diet to reduce constipation, and controlling blood glucose levels to prevent polyuria. The nurse should instruct the client to reduce the intake of fluids and foods that are bladder irritants, such as orange juice, soda, and caffeine, and the client should wipe from front to back to prevent urinary tract infections.

14. **Answer: a, d, & e**
    RATIONALE: The postoperative care plan for a client who has undergone a hysterectomy includes administering analgesics promptly and using a PCA pump, frequent ambulation, and administering antiemetics to control nausea and vomiting. The nurse should change the position of the client frequently and use pillows for support to promote comfort and pain management. Ambulation is key in the prevention of postoperative complications. An excess of carbonated beverages in the diet does not affect the postoperative healing process.

15. **Answer: a**
    RATIONALE: The nurse should stress follow-up care to the client with polycystic ovarian syndrome so that the client does not overlook this benign disorder. Increasing intake of fiber-rich foods, increasing fluid intake, and performing Kegel exercises help to control pelvic organ prolapse, not polycystic ovarian syndrome.

Answers

CHAPTER 8

SECTION I: ASSESSING YOUR UNDERSTANDING

Activity A FILL IN THE BLANKS

1. dysplasia
2. Colposcopy
3. Cryotherapy
4. Endometrial
5. Bethesda
6. Hysterectomy
7. CA-125
8. simplex
9. epithelium
10. Squamous

Activity B MATCHING

1. b   **2.** a   **3.** d   **4.** c

Activity C SEQUENCING

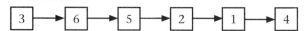

Activity D SHORT ANSWERS

1. Risk factors for developing cervical cancer are as follows:
   - Early age of first intercourse (within 1 year of menarche)
   - Lower socioeconomic status
   - Promiscuous male partners
   - Unprotected sexual intercourse
   - Family history of cervical cancer (mother or sisters)
   - Sexual intercourse with uncircumcised men
   - Female offspring of mothers who took diethylstilbestrol (DES)
   - Infections with genital herpes or chronic chlamydia
   - History of multiple sex partners
   - Cigarette smoking
   - Immunocompromised state
   - HIV infection
   - Oral contraceptive use
   - Moderate dysplasia on Pap smear within past 5 years
   - HPV infection

2. Treatment options for endometrial cancer are as follows:
   - Treatment of endometrial cancer depends on the stage of the disease and usually involves surgery, with adjunct therapy based on pathologic findings.
   - Surgery most often involves removal of the uterus (hysterectomy) and the fallopian tubes and ovaries (salpingo-oophorectomy).
   - In more advanced cancers, radiation and chemotherapy are used as adjunct therapies to surgery.
   - Routine surveillance intervals for follow-up care are typically every 3 to 4 months for the first 2 years, since 85% of recurrences occur in the first 2 years after diagnosis.

3. The following are possible risk factors for ovarian cancer:
   - Nulliparity
   - Early menarche (<12 years old)
   - Late menopause (>55 years old)
   - Increasing age (>50 years of age)
   - High-fat diet
   - Obesity
   - Persistent ovulation over time
   - First-degree relative with ovarian cancer
   - Use of perineal talcum powder or hygiene sprays
   - Older than 30 years at first pregnancy
   - Positive BRCA-1 and BRCA-2 mutations
   - Personal history of breast, bladder, or colon cancer
   - Hormone replacement therapy for more than 10 years
   - Infertility

4. Transvaginal ultrasound can be used to evaluate the endometrial cavity and measure the thickness of the endometrial lining. It can be used to detect endometrial hyperplasia.

5. The following are the nursing interventions in caring for clients with cancers of the female reproductive tract:
   - Validate the client's feelings and provide realistic hope.
   - Use basic communication skills in a sincere way during all interactions.
   - Provide useful, nonjudgmental information to all women.

- Individualize care to address the client's cultural traditions.
- Carry out postoperative care and instructions as prescribed.
- Discuss postoperative issues, including incision care, pain, and activity level.
- Instruct the client on health-maintenance activities after treatment.
- Inform the client and family about available support resources.

6. The following are the diagnostic options for endometrial cancer:
   - Endometrial biopsy: An endometrial biopsy is the procedure of choice to make the diagnosis. It can be done in the health care provider's office without anesthesia. A slender suction catheter is used to obtain a small sample of tissue for pathology. It can detect up to 90% of cases of endometrial cancer in the woman with postmenopausal bleeding, depending on the technique and experience of the health care provider. The woman may experience mild cramping and bleeding after the procedure for about 24 hours, but typically mild pain medication will reduce this discomfort.
   - Transvaginal ultrasound: A transvaginal ultrasound can be used to evaluate the endometrial cavity and measure the thickness of the endometrial lining. It can be used to detect endometrial hyperplasia. If the endometrium measures less than 4 mm, then the client is at low risk for malignancy.

SECTION II: APPLYING YOUR KNOWLEDGE

Activity E CASE STUDY

1. • Back pain
   - Abdominal bloating
   - Fatigue
   - Urinary frequency
   - Constipation
   - Abdominal pressure
2. The most common early symptoms include abdominal bloating, early satiety, fatigue, vague abdominal pain, urinary frequency, diarrhea or constipation, and unexplained weight loss or gain. The later symptoms include anorexia, dyspepsia, ascites, palpable abdominal mass, pelvic pain, and back pain. Early detection of ovarian cancer is possible if the clients are informed about yearly bimanual pelvic examination and transvaginal ultrasound to identify ovarian masses.
3. Disturbed body image related to:
   - Loss of body part
   - Loss of good health
   - Altered sexuality patterns
   Anxiety related to:
   - Threat of malignancy
   - Potential diagnosis

- Anticipated pain/discomfort
- Effect of condition treatment on future
Deficient knowledge related to:
- Disease process and prognosis
- Specific treatment options
- Diagnostic procedures needed

4. In Stage I, the ovarian cancer is limited to the ovaries. In Stage II, the growth involves one or both ovaries, with pelvic extension. In Stage III, the cancer spreads to the lymph nodes and other organs or structures inside the abdominal cavity. In Stage IV, the cancer has metastasized to distant sites. Treatment options for ovarian cancer vary, depending on the stage and severity of the disease. Usually a laparoscopy (abdominal exploration with an endoscope) is performed for diagnosis and staging, as well as evaluation for further therapy.

SECTION III: PRACTICING FOR NCLEX

Activity F NCLEX-STYLE QUESTIONS

1. **Answer: a**
   RATIONALE: The client should have Papanicolaou tests regularly to detect cervical cancer during the early stages. Blood tests for mutations in the BRCA genes indicate the lifetime risk of the client of developing breast or ovarian cancer. CA-125 is a biologic tumor marker associated with ovarian cancer, but it is not currently sensitive enough to serve as a screening tool. The transvaginal ultrasound can be used to detect endometrial abnormalities.

2. **Answer: a**
   RATIONALE: Early onset of sexual activity, within the first year of menarche, increases the risk of acquiring cervical cancer later on. Obesity, infertility, and hypertension are risk factors that are associated with endometrial cancer.

3. **Answer: c**
   RATIONALE: The nurse should inform the client that surgery most often involves removal of the uterus (hysterectomy) and the fallopian tubes and ovaries (salpingo-oophorectomy). Removal of the tubes and ovaries, not just the uterus, is recommended because tumor cells spread early to the ovaries, and any dormant cancer cells could be stimulated to grow by ovarian estrogen. In advanced cancers, radiation and chemotherapy are used as adjuvant therapies to surgery. Routine surveillance intervals for follow-up care are typically every 3 to 4 months for the first 2 years.

4. **Answer: b**
   RATIONALE: The client's present age increases her risk of developing ovarian cancer, as women who are older than 50 are at a greater risk. The client's age at menarche (older than 12) and menopause (younger than 55) are both normal. The client is underweight and not obese, so her weight is not a risk factor for ovarian cancer.

5. **Answer: c**
RATIONALE: To identify ovarian masses in their early stages, the client needs to have yearly bimanual pelvic examinations. Pap smears are not effective enough to detect ovarian masses. The U.S. Preventive Services Task Force recommends against routine screening for ovarian cancer with serum CA-125 because the potential harm could outweigh the potential benefits. X-rays of the pelvic area do not detect ovarian masses.

6. **Answer: a**
RATIONALE: Only 5% of ovarian cancers are genetic in origin. However, the nurse needs to tell the client to seek genetic counseling and thorough assessment to reduce her risk of ovarian cancer. Oral contraceptives reduce the risk of ovarian cancer and should be encouraged. Breastfeeding should be encouraged as a risk-reducing strategy. The nurse should instruct the client to avoid using perineal talc or hygiene sprays.

7. **Answer: c**
RATIONALE: The nurse should teach the client genital self-examination to assess for any unusual growths in the vulvar area. The nurse should instruct the client to seek care for any suspicious lesions and to avoid self-medication. Wearing restrictive undergarments is not associated with vulvar cancer.

8. **Answer: b, c, & e**
RATIONALE: To reduce the risk of cervical cancer, the nurse should encourage clients to avoid smoking and drinking. In addition, because STIs such as HPV increase the risk of cervical cancers, care should be taken to prevent STIs. Teenagers also should be counseled to avoid early sexual activity because it increases the risk of cervical cancer. The use of barrier methods of contraception, not IUDs, should be encouraged. Avoiding stress and high blood pressure will not have a significant impact on the risk of cervical cancer.

9. **Answer: a, c, & d**
RATIONALE: The responsibilities of a nurse while caring for a client with endometrial cancer include ensuring that the client understands all the treatment options available, suggesting the advantages of a support group and providing referrals, and offering the family explanations and emotional support throughout the treatment. The nurse should also discuss changes in sexuality with the client as well as stress the importance of regular follow-up care after the treatment and not just in cases where something unusual occurs.

10. **Answer: b, d, & e**
RATIONALE: Irregular vaginal bleeding, persistent low backache not related to standing, and elevated or discolored vulvar lesions are some of the symptoms that should be immediately brought to the notice of the primary health care provider. Increase in urinary frequency and irregular bowel movements are not symptoms related to cancers of the reproductive tract.

11. **Answer: b**
RATIONALE: The nurse should explain to the client that the colposcopy is done because the physician has observed abnormalities in Pap smears. The nurse should also explain to the client that the procedure is painless and there are no adverse effects, such as pain during urination. There is no need to avoid intercourse for a week after the colposcopy.

12. **Answer: b**
RATIONALE: According to the 2001 Bethesda system for classifying Pap smear results, a result of ASC-H means that the client is to be referred for colposcopy without HPV testing. Atypical squamous cells of undetermined significance (ASC-US) means that the test has to be repeated in 4 to 6 months or the client has to be referred for colposcopy. Atypical glandular cells (AGC) or adenocarcinoma in situ (AIS) results indicate immediate colposcopy, with the follow-up based on the results of findings.

13. **Answer: a**
RATIONALE: Abnormal and painless vaginal bleeding is a major initial symptom of endometrial cancer. Diabetes mellitus and liver disease are the risk factors, not symptoms, for endometrial cancer. Back pain is associated with ovarian cancer.

14. **Answer: a, b, & d**
RATIONALE: Although direct risk factors for the initial development of vaginal cancer have not been identified, associated risk factors include advancing age (>60 years old), HIV infection, smoking, previous pelvic radiation, exposure to DES in utero, vaginal trauma, history of genital warts (HPV infection), cervical cancer, chronic vaginal discharge, and low socioeconomic level. Persistent ovulation over time and hormone replacement therapy for more than 10 years are risk factors associated with ovarian cancer.

15. **Answer: a**
RATIONALE: The skin condition Lichen sclerosus has been linked with risk of vulvar cancer. Previous pelvic radiation and exposure to DES in utero are risk factors associated with vaginal rather than vulvar cancer, and tamoxifen use is a risk factor for endometrial cancer.

CHAPTER 9

SECTION I: ASSESSING YOUR UNDERSTANDING

Activity A FILL IN THE BLANKS

1. battered
2. Incest
3. Statutory
4. Rohypnol
5. circumcision
6. Acquaintance
7. sexual
8. hyperarousal
9. avoidance
10. honeymoon

Activity B MATCHING

1. d   **2.** b   **3.** a   **4.** c

Activity C SEQUENCING

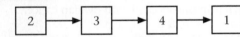

Activity D SHORT ANSWERS

1. The cycle of violence occurs in an abusive relationship. It includes three distinct phases: the tension-building phase, the acute battering phase, and the honeymoon phase. The cyclic behavior begins with a time of tension-building arguments, progresses to violence, and settles into a making-up or calm period. With time, this cycle of violence increases in frequency and severity as it is repeated over and over again. The cycle can cover a long or short period of time. The honeymoon phase gradually shortens and eventually disappears altogether.

2. An abuser may financially abuse the partner in the following ways:
   - Preventing the woman from getting a job
   - Sabotaging the current job
   - Controlling how all money is spent
   - Refusing to contribute financially

3. The potential nursing diagnoses related to violence against women include the following:

- Deficient knowledge related to understanding of the cycle of violence and availability of resources
- Fear related to possibility of severe injury to self or children during cycle of violence
- Low self-esteem related to feelings of worthlessness
- Hopelessness related to prolonged exposure to violence
- Compromised individual and family coping related to persistence of victim–abuser relationship

4. PTSD develops when an event outside the range of normal human experience occurs that produces marked distress in the person. Symptoms of PTSD are divided into three groups:
   - Intrusion (reexperiencing the trauma, including nightmares, flashbacks, recurrent thoughts)
   - Avoidance (avoiding trauma-related stimuli, social withdrawal, emotional numbing)
   - Hyperarousal (increased emotional arousal, exaggerated startle response, irritability)

5. The nurse should screen the client for the following signs to determine whether she is a victim of abuse:
   - Injuries: bruises, scars from blunt trauma, or weapon wounds on the face, head, and neck
   - Injury sequelae: headaches, hearing loss, joint pain, sinus infections, teeth marks, clumps of hair missing, dental trauma, pelvic pain, breast or genital injuries
   - The reported history of the injury doesn't seem to add up to the actual presenting problem
   - Mental health problems: depression, anxiety, substance abuse, eating disorders, suicidal ideation, or suicide attempts
   - Frequent health care visits for chronic, stress-related disorders such as chest pain, headaches, back or pelvic pain, insomnia, and gastrointestinal disturbances
   - Partner's behavior at the health care visit: appears overly solicitous or overprotective, unwilling to leave client alone with the health care provider, answers questions for her, and attempts to control the situation in the health care setting

6. Abuse during pregnancy threatens the well-being of the mother and fetus. Physical violence to the pregnant woman brings injuries to the head, face, neck, thorax, breasts, and abdomen. Mental health consequences are also significant. Women assaulted during pregnancy are at a risk for depression, chronic anxiety, insomnia, poor nutrition, excessive weight gain or loss, late entry into prenatal care, preterm labor, miscarriage, stillbirth, premature and low-birth-weight infants, placental abruption, uterine rupture, chorioamnionitis, vaginitis, STIs, urinary tract infections, or smoking and substance abuse.

SECTION II: APPLYING YOUR KNOWLEDGE

Activity E CASE STUDY

1. Some of the common symptoms of physical abuse include depression, sexual dysfunction, backaches, STIs, fear or guilt, or phobias.
2. Suzanne may not seek help in the abusive relationship for the following reasons:
   - She may feel responsible for the abuse.
   - She may feel she deserved the abuse.
   - She may have been abused as a child and has low self-esteem.
3. The following strategies may help Suzanne to manage the situation:
   - Teaching coping strategies to manage stress
   - Encouraging the establishment of realistic goals
   - Teaching problem-solving skills
   - Encouraging social activities to connect with other people
   - Explaining that abuse is never okay

SECTION III: PRACTICING FOR NCLEX

Activity F NCLEX-STYLE QUESTIONS

1. **Answer: c**
   RATIONALE: The nurse should inform the client that alcohol, drugs, money problems, depression, or jealousy do not cause violence and are excuses given by the abuser for losing control. Even though violence against women was common in the past, the police, justice system, and society are beginning to make domestic violence socially unacceptable. The nurse also needs to emphasize that physical abuse is not the result of provocation from the female but an expression of inadequacy of the perpetrator. Violence against women is widespread, and whatever the cause of the assault, there is no justification for physical or sexual assault.
2. **Answer: a**
   RATIONALE: The nurse should clearly explain to the client that whatever the cause of the incident, no one deserves to be a victim of physi-

cal abuse. Even though the partner appears to be genuinely contrite, most people who attack their spouses are serial abusers and there is no certainty that they will not repeat their actions. The client should realize that even if she tries her best not to upset her partner, her partner may abuse her again. The client should never accept battering as a normal part of any relationship.

3. **Answer: c**
   RATIONALE: Attacking pets and destroying valued possessions are examples of emotional abuse. Observing the client's movements closely may be a sign of suspicion. Throwing objects at the client is physical abuse. Forcing the client to have intercourse against her will is an act of sexual abuse.
4. **Answer: b**
   RATIONALE: Abusers are most likely to exhibit antisocial behavior or childlike aggression. They use aggression to control their victims. Abusers come from all walks of life; they are not just restricted to low-income groups, nor are they necessarily products of divorced parents. The physical characteristics of the abusers vary, and they are not necessarily physically imposing.
5. **Answer: d**
   RATIONALE: For every rape victim who turns up, the nurse should ensure that the appropriate law enforcement agencies are apprised of the incident. Victims should not be made to wait long hours in the waiting room, as they may leave if no one attends to them. Victims of rape should be treated with more sensitivity than other clients. Although the primary job of a nurse is to medically care for the rape victim, a nurse should also pay due attention to collecting evidence to substantiate the victim's claim in a court of law.
6. **Answer: c**
   RATIONALE: The nurse should tell the client that she is a victim of sexual abuse because her partner forces her to have intercourse against her will. The nurse should also explain to the client that she is in no way responsible for such incidents and that she has a right to refuse sexual intimacy. There is no justification for sexual abuse, and the client should not regard it as "normal" behavior.
7. **Answer: c**
   RATIONALE: The nurse should use pictures and diagrams to ensure that the client understands what is being explained. Instead of using medical terms, the nurse should use simple, accurate terms as much as possible. The nurse should look directly at the client while speaking to her and not at the interpreter. The nurse should not place any judgment on the cultural practice.

8. **Answer: b**
   RATIONALE: If the nurse suspects physical abuse, the nurse should attempt to interview the woman in private. Many abusers will not leave their partners for fear of being discovered. The nurse should use subtle ways of doing this, such as telling the woman a urine specimen is required and showing her the way to the restroom, providing the nurse and client some private time. Asking the partner directly if he was responsible will not help because the partner may not admit his culpability. Telling the partner to leave the room immediately may rouse the suspicions of the partner. Questioning the client about the injury in front of the partner may trigger another abusive episode and should be avoided. Precaution should be taken to prevent the abuser from punishing the woman when she returns home.

9. **Answer: a**
   RATIONALE: The nurse should use direct quotes and specific language as much as possible when documenting. The nurse should not obtain photos of the client without informed consent. The nurse should, however, document the refusal of the client to be photographed. Documentation must include details as to the frequency and severity of abuse and the location, extent, and outcome of injuries, not just a description of the interventions taken. The nurse is required by law to inform the police of any injuries that involve knives, firearms, or other deadly weapons or that present life-threatening emergencies. Hence, the nurse should explain to the client why the case has to be reported to the police.

10. **Answer: a**
    RATIONALE: The nurse should offer referrals to the client, such as support groups or specialists, so that the client gets professional help in recovering from the incident. The nurse should help the client cope with the incident rather than telling the client to forget about it. The nurse should also educate the client about the connection between the violence and some of the symptoms that she has developed recently, like palpitations. Confirming with the partner whether the client's story is true will create further problems for the client, and the nurse may lose the client's trust.

11. **Answer: a**
    RATIONALE: To minimize risk of pregnancy, the nurse should ensure that the client takes a double dose of emergency contraceptive pills: the first

dose within 72 hours of the rape and the second dose 12 hours after the first dose, if not sooner. It is better to use contraceptive measures immediately than to wait for signs of pregnancy. Using spermicidal creams or gels or regular oral contraceptive pills will not prove effective in preventing unwanted pregnancies.

12. **Answer: b, c, & d**
    RATIONALE: Some of the factors that may lead to abuse during pregnancy are resentment toward the interference of the growing fetus and change in the woman's shape, perception of the baby as a competitor once he or she is born, and insecurity and jealousy of the pregnancy and the responsibilities it brings. Concern for the child will never result in physical abuse, as the unborn child is also at risk through assault during pregnancy. Serial abusers may exhibit violent tendencies during pregnancy, and such behavior is unacceptable.

13. **Answer: a, b, & e**
    RATIONALE: Victims of human trafficking have restrictions on their daily movements, so the nurse should ask questions to learn whether the client can move around freely. The nurse should also find out if the client could leave her present job or situation if she wants to. Asking clients what their parents do or what their educational background is does not help determine whether they are victims of human trafficking.

14. **Answer: b, c, & e**
    RATIONALE: To screen for abuse, the nurse should assess for mental health problems or injuries. The nurse should also be alert for inconsistencies regarding the reporting of the injury and the actual problem. Having STIs frequently is not a sign of physical or sexual abuse. Usually, partners of suspected victims seem overprotective and they do not leave the client alone.

15. **Answer: a, b, & c**
    RATIONALE: To learn whether the client is having physical symptoms of PTSD, the nurse should ask the client if she is having trouble sleeping and whether she is emotionally stable or given to bursts of irritability. The nurse should also find out if the client experiences heart palpitations or sweating. Asking the client if she is feeling numb emotionally assesses the presence of avoidance reactions, not physical manifestation of PTSD. The nurse should ask the client whether she has upsetting thoughts and nightmares to assess for the presence of intrusive thoughts.

Answers

CHAPTER 10

SECTION I: ASSESSING YOUR UNDERSTANDING

Activity A FILL IN THE BLANKS

1. Allele
2. mutation
3. autosomes
4. amnion
5. Chromosomes
6. morula
7. karyotype
8. Polyploidy
9. genome
10. phenotype

Activity B LABELING

The image shows the foot of an infant with trisomy 13. The infant has supernumerary digits (polydactyly).

Activity C MATCHING

1. d   **2.** e   **3.** c   **4.** b   **5.** a

Activity D SEQUENCING

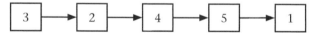

Activity E SHORT ANSWERS

1. For conception or fertilization to occur, a healthy ovum from the woman has to be released from the ovary. It passes into an open fallopian tube and starts its journey downward. Sperm from the male must be deposited into the vagina and be able to swim approximately 7 in to meet the ovum where one spermatozoa penetrates the ovum's thick outer membrane. Fertilization takes place in the outer third of the ampulla of the fallopian tube.

2. The three different stages of fetal development during pregnancy are:
   - Preembryonic stage: begins with fertilization through the 2nd week
   - Embryonic stage: begins 15 days after conception and continues through week 8
   - Fetal stage: begins from the end of the 8th week and lasts until birth

3. The sex of the zygote is determined at fertilization. It depends on whether the ovum is fertilized by a Y-bearing sperm or an X-bearing sperm. An XX zygote will become a female, and an XY zygote will become a male.

4. Concurrent with the development of the trophoblast and implantation, further differentiation of the inner cell mass of the zygote occurs. Some of the cells become the embryo itself, and others give rise to the membranes that surround and protect it. The three embryonic layers of cells formed are:
   - Ectoderm—forms the central nervous system, special senses, skin, and glands
   - Mesoderm—forms the skeletal, urinary, circulatory, and reproductive organs
   - Endoderm—forms the respiratory system, liver, pancreas, and digestive system

5. Amniotic fluid is derived from fluid transported from the maternal blood across the amnion and fetal urine. Its volume changes constantly as the fetus swallows and voids. Amniotic fluid is composed of 98% water and 2% organic matter. It is slightly alkaline and contains albumin, urea, uric acid, creatinine, bilirubin, lecithin, sphingomyelin, epithelial cells, vernix, and fine hair called lanugo.

6. The placenta produces hormones that control the basic physiology of the mother in such a way that the fetus is supplied with the necessary nutrients and oxygen needed for successful growth. The placenta produces the following hormones necessary for normal pregnancy:
   - Human chorionic gonadotropin
   - Human placental lactogen
   - Estrogen (estriol)
   - Progesterone (progestin)
   - Relaxin

SECTION II: APPLYING YOUR KNOWLEDGE

Activity F CASE STUDY

1. Shana should be reassured that she will continue to feel fetal movement throughout her pregnancy and that it is not common for a fetus to get "tangled in its umbilical cord."

2. The nurse should explain the following functions of the amniotic fluid:
- Helps maintain a constant body temperature for the fetus
- Permits symmetric growth and development of the fetus
- Cushions the fetus from trauma
- Allows the umbilical cord to be free of compression
- Promotes fetal movement to enhance musculoskeletal development
- Amniotic fluid volume can be important in determining fetal well-being

The nurse should explain the following functions of the placenta:
- Makes hormones to ensure implantation of the embryo and to control the mother's physiology to provide adequate nutrients and water to the growing fetus
- Transports oxygen and nutrients from the mother's bloodstream to the developing fetus
- Protects the fetus from immune attack by the mother
- Removes fetal waste products
- Near term, produces hormones to mature fetal organs in preparation for extrauterine life

The nurse should also explain the following about the umbilical cord:
- The lifeline from the mother to the fetus
- Formed from the amnion and contains one large vein and two small arteries
- Wharton jelly surrounds the vessels to prevent compression
- At term, the average length is 22 in and the average width is 1 in

SECTION III: PRACTICING FOR NCLEX

Activity G NCLEX-STYLE QUESTIONS

1. Answer: b
RATIONALE: This disorder is not X-linked. Either the father or the mother can pass the gene along regardless of whether their mate has the gene or not. The only way that an autosomal-dominant gene is not expressed is if it does not exist. If only one of the parents has the gene, then there is a 50% chance it will be passed on to the child.

2. Answer: c
RATIONALE: The nurse should instruct the client to stop using drugs, alcohol, and tobacco, as these harmful substances may be passed on to the fetus from the mother. There is no need to avoid exercise during pregnancy as long as the client follows the prescribed regimen. Wearing comfortable clothes is not as important as the client's health. The client need not stay indoors during pregnancy.

3. Answer: c
RATIONALE: The nurse should find out the age and cause of death for deceased family members, as it will help establish a genetic pattern. Although inquiry of a history of premature birth or depression

during pregnancy are important and should be included in the data collection, they do not relate to genetically inherited disorders. A family history of drinking or drug abuse does not increase the risk of genetic disorders.

4. Answer: a
RATIONALE: The risk of trisomies such as Klinefelter syndrome increases with the age of the mother at the time of pregnancy. Klinefelter syndrome occurs only in males. Having twins does not increase the risk of Klinefelter syndrome for the babies, nor does the client's previous smoking habit have any bearing on the risk for Klinefelter syndrome.

5. Answer: b
RATIONALE: Down syndrome occurs because of the presence of an extra chromosome in the body. Down syndrome is not genetically inherited. Both males and females are equally at risk for Down syndrome. Most children with Down syndrome have mild to moderate intellectual disability.

6. Answer: d
RATIONALE: While obtaining the genetic history of the client, the nurse should find out if the members of the couple are related to each other or have blood ties, as this increases the risk of many genetic disorders. The socioeconomic status or the physical characteristics of family members do not have any significant bearing on the risk of genetic disorders. The nurse should ask questions about race or ethnic background because some races are more susceptible to certain disorders than others.

7. Answer: c
RATIONALE: After the client has seen the specialist, the nurse should review what the specialist has discussed with the family and clarify any doubts the couple may have. The nurse should never make the decision for the client but rather should present all the relevant information and aid the couple in making an informed decision. There is no need for the nurse to refer the client to another specialist or for further diagnostic and screening tests unless instructed to do so by the specialist.

8. Answer: a
RATIONALE: Tay–Sachs disease affects both male and female babies. The age of the client does not significantly increase the risk of Tay–Sachs disease. Even though the client and her husband are not related by blood, because of their background their baby is at a greater risk. There is a chance that the offspring may have Tay–Sachs disease even if both parents don't have it because they could be carriers.

9. Answer: b, d, & e
RATIONALE: The nurse should explain to the client that individuals with hemophilia are usually males. Female carriers have a 50% chance of transmitting the disorder to their sons, and females are affected by the condition if it is a dominant X-linked disorder. Offspring of nonhemophiliac parents may be hemophilic. Daughters of an affected male are usually carriers.

10. **Answer: a, b, & d**

 RATIONALE: The responsibilities of the nurse while counseling the client include knowing basic genetic terminology and inheritance patterns and explaining basic concepts of probability and disorder susceptibility. The nurse should ensure complete informed consent to facilitate decisions about genetic testing. The nurse should explain ethical and legal issues related to genetics as well. The nurse should never instruct the client on which decision to make and should let the client make the decision.

11. **Answer: d**

 RATIONALE: The embryonic stage of development begins at day 15 after conception and continues through week 8. Basic structures of all major body organs and the main external features are completed during this time period, including internal organs. Lung development sufficient so sustain life is not completed until the third trimester of gestation.

12. **Answer: a, c, & d**

 RATIONALE: Identical twins (also called monozygotic twins) occur when one fertilized egg splits and develops into two (or occasionally more) fetuses. The fetuses usually share one placenta. Identical twins have the same genes, so they generally look alike and are the same sex. Fraternal twins (also called dizygotic twins) develop when two separate eggs are fertilized by two different sperm. Each twin usually has its own placenta. Fraternal twins (like other siblings) share about 50% of their genes, so they can be different sexes. They generally do not look any more alike than brothers or sisters born from different pregnancies.

14. **Answer: d**

 RATIONALE: Prepregnancy screening with a genetic counselor would be helpful to the client who has a history of fetal loss as a result of a genetic disorder. The screening would allow the family to closely be evaluated for risk factors and have access to potential screening options.

15. **Answer: d**

 RATIONALE: The pictorial analysis of the number, form, and size of an individual's chromosomes is referred to as a karyotype. This analysis commonly uses white blood cells and fetal cells in amniotic fluid. The chromosomes are numbered from the largest to the smallest, 1 to 22, and the sex chromosomes are designated by the letter X or the letter Y. The severity and related complications of a disorder are not determined by the karyotype. Condition management is not determined by the karyotype.

CHAPTER 11

SECTION I: ASSESSING YOUR UNDERSTANDING

Activity A FILL IN THE BLANKS

1. cortisol
2. Ambivalence
3. Oxytocin
4. placenta
5. estrogen
6. sacroiliac
7. hemorrhoids
8. progesterone
9. Colostrum
10. leukorrhea

Activity B LABELING

1. The condition illustrated is supine hypotensive syndrome.
2. When the inferior vena cava is in the supine position, vena cava compression results from pressure of the gravid uterus. This causes a reduction in venous return and decreases cardiac output and blood pressure, with increasing orthostatic stress.
3. Symptoms associated with supine hypotensive include weakness, lightheadedness, nausea, dizziness, or syncope.

Activity C MATCHING

1. e   2. a   3. c   4. d   5. b

Activity D SEQUENCING

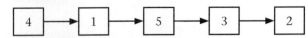

Activity E SHORT ANSWERS

1. Striae gravidarum, or stretch marks, are irregular reddish streaks that may appear on the abdomen, breasts, and buttocks in about half of pregnant women. Striae are most prominent by 6 to 7 months and occur in up to 90% of pregnant women. They are caused by reduced connective tissue strength resulting from elevated adrenal steroid levels and stretching of the structures secondary to growth. They are more common in younger women, women with larger infants, and women with higher body mass indices. Nonwhites and women with a history of breast or thigh striae or a family history of striae gravidarum are also at higher risk.

2. There is slight hypertrophy, or enlargement of the heart, during pregnancy to accommodate the increase in blood volume and cardiac output. The heart works harder and pumps more blood to supply the oxygen needs of the fetus as well as those of the mother. Both heart rate and venous return are increased in pregnancy, contributing to the increase in cardiac output seen throughout gestation.

3. Iron requirements during pregnancy increase because of the oxygen and nutrient demands of the growing fetus and the resulting increase in maternal blood volume. The fetal tissues take predominance over the mother's tissues with respect to use of iron stores. With the accelerated production of RBCs, iron is necessary for hemoglobin formation, the oxygen-carrying component of RBCs.

4. Pica is the compulsive ingestion of nonfood substances. The three main substances consumed by women with pica are soil or clay (geophagia), ice (pagophagia), and laundry starch (amylophagia). Nutritional implications of pica include iron-deficiency anemia, parasitic infection, and constipation.

5. Oxytocin is responsible for stimulating uterine contractions. After delivery, oxytocin secretion causes the myometrium to contract and helps constrict the uterine blood vessels, decreasing the amount of vaginal bleeding after delivery. Oxytocin is also responsible for milk ejection during breastfeeding. Stimulation of the breasts through sucking or touching stimulates the secretion of oxytocin from the posterior pituitary gland.

6. Varicose veins during pregnancy are the result of venous distention and instability, from poor circulation secondary to prolonged standing or sitting. Venous compression from the heavy gravid uterus places pressure on the pelvic veins, also preventing efficient venous return.

SECTION II: APPLYING YOUR KNOWLEDGE

Activity F CASE STUDY

1. The realization of a pregnancy can lead to fluctuating responses, possibly at opposite ends of the spectrum. For example, regardless of whether the pregnancy was planned, it is normal to be fearful and anxious of the implications. The woman's reaction may be influenced by several factors, including the way she was raised by her family, her current family situation, the quality of the relationship with the expectant father, and her hopes for the future. It is common for some women to express concern over the timing of the pregnancy, wishing that goals and life objectives had been met before becoming pregnant. Other women may question how a newborn or infant will affect their careers or their relationships with friends and family. These feelings can cause conflict and confusion about the impending pregnancy.
   Ambivalence, or having conflicting feelings at the same time, is a universal feeling and is considered normal when preparing for a lifestyle change and new role. Pregnant women commonly experience ambivalence during the first trimester. Usually ambivalence evolves into acceptance by the second trimester, when fetal movement is felt.

2. A pregnant woman may withdraw and become increasingly preoccupied with herself and her fetus. As a result, participation with the outside world may be less, and she may appear passive to her family and friends. This introspective behavior is a normal psychological adaptation to motherhood for most women. Introversion seems to heighten during the first and third trimesters, when the woman's focus is on behaviors that will ensure a safe and healthy pregnancy outcome. Women may also feel disinterested in certain activities because of nausea and fatigue experienced in the first trimester. Couples need to be aware of this behavior and be informed about measures to maintain and support the focus on the family.

3. During the second trimester, as the pregnancy progresses, the physical changes of the growing fetus, along with an enlarging abdomen and fetal movement, bring reality and validity to the pregnancy. The pregnant woman feels fetal movement and may hear the heartbeat. She may see the fetal image on an ultrasound screen and feel distinct parts, which allow her to identify the fetus as a separate individual. Many women will verbalize positive feelings of the pregnancy and will conceptualize the fetus. In addition, a reduction in physical discomfort will bring about an improvement in mood and physical well-being in the second trimester.

4. Frequently, pregnant women will start to cry without any apparent cause. Some feel as though they are riding an "emotional roller coaster."

These extremes in emotion can make it difficult for partners and family members to communicate with the pregnant woman without placing blame on themselves for the woman's mood changes. Emotional liability is characteristic throughout most pregnancies. One moment a woman can feel great joy, and within a short time span feel shock and disbelief.

SECTION III: PRACTICING FOR NCLEX

Activity G NCLEX-STYLE QUESTIONS

1. **Answer: b**
   RATIONALE: Absence of menstruation, or skipping a period, along with consistent nausea, fatigue, breast tenderness, and urinary frequency, are the presumptive signs of pregnancy. A positive home pregnancy test, abdominal enlargement, and softening of the cervix are the probable signs of pregnancy.

2. **Answer: c**
   RATIONALE: During pregnancy, the vaginal secretions become more acidic, white, and thick. Most women experience an increase in a whitish vaginal discharge, called leukorrhea, during pregnancy. The nurse should inform the client that the vaginal discharge is normal except when it is accompanied by itching and irritation, possibly suggesting Candida albicans infection, a monilial vaginitis, which is a very common occurrence in this glycogen-rich environment. Monilial vaginitis is a benign fungal condition and is treated with local antifungal agents. The client need not refrain from sexual activity when there is an increase in a thick, whitish vaginal discharge.

3. **Answer: a**
   RATIONALE: Estrogen aids in developing the ductal system of the breasts in preparation for lactation during pregnancy. Prolactin stimulates the glandular production of colostrum. During pregnancy, the ability of prolactin to produce milk is opposed by progesterone. Progesterone supports the endometrium of the uterus to provide an environment conducive to fetal survival. Oxytocin is responsible for uterine contractions, both before and after delivery. Oxytocin is also responsible for milk ejection during breastfeeding.

4. **Answer: d**
   RATIONALE: The maternal emotional response experienced by the client is ambivalence. Ambivalence, or having conflicting feelings at the same time, is universal and is considered normal when preparing for a lifestyle change and new role. Pregnant women commonly experience ambivalence during the first trimester. The client is not experiencing introversion, acceptance, or mood swings. Introversion, or focusing on oneself, is common during the early part of pregnancy. The woman may withdraw and become increasingly preoccupied with herself and her fetus. Acceptance

is the common maternal emotional response during the second trimester. As the pregnancy progresses, the physical changes of the growing fetus, along with an enlarging abdomen and fetal movement, bring reality and validity to the pregnancy. Although mood swings are common during pregnancy, this client is not experiencing mood swings.

5. **Answer: a, c, & e**
   RATIONALE: Constipation during pregnancy is due to changes in the gastrointestinal system. Constipation can result from decreased activity level, use of iron supplements, intestinal displacement secondary to a growing uterus, slow transition time of food throughout the GI tract, a low-fiber diet, and reduced fluid intake. Increase in progesterone, not estrogen levels, causes constipation during pregnancy. Reduced stomach acidity does not cause constipation. Morning sickness has been linked to stomach acidity.

6. **Answer: a, b, & d**
   RATIONALE: hCG levels in a normal pregnancy usually double every 48 to 72 hours, until they reach a peak at approximately 60 to 70 days after fertilization. This elevation of hCG corresponds to the morning sickness period of approximately 6 to 12 weeks during early pregnancy. Reduced stomach acidity and high levels of circulating estrogens are also believed to cause morning sickness. Elevation of hPL and RBC production do not cause morning sickness. hPL increases during the second half of pregnancy, and it helps in the preparation of mammary glands for lactation and is involved in the process of making glucose available for fetal growth by altering maternal carbohydrate, fat, and protein metabolism. The increase in RBCs is necessary to transport the additional oxygen required during pregnancy.

7. **Answer: c**
   RATIONALE: Spontaneous, irregular, painless contractions, called Braxton Hicks contractions, begin during the first trimester. These contractions are not the signs of preterm labor, infection of the GI tract, or acid indigestion. Acid indigestion causes heartburn. Acid indigestion or heartburn (pyrosis) is caused by regurgitation of the stomach contents into the upper esophagus and may be associated with the generalized relaxation of the entire digestive system.

8. **Answer: d**
   RATIONALE: The symptoms experienced by the client indicate supine hypotension syndrome. When the pregnant woman assumes a supine position, the expanding uterus exerts pressure on the inferior vena cava, causing a reduction in blood flow to the heart, most commonly during the third trimester. The nurse should place the client in the left lateral position to correct this syndrome and optimize cardiac output and uterine perfusion. Elevating the client's legs, placing the client in an orthopneic position, or keeping the head of the bed elevated will not help alleviate the client's condition.

9. **Answer: a**
   RATIONALE: The nurse should instruct the parents to provide constant reinforcement of love and care to reduce the sibling's fear of change and possible replacement by the new family member. The parents should neither avoid talking to the child about the new arrival nor pay less attention to the child. The nurse should urge parents to include siblings in this event and make them feel a part of the preparations for the new infant. The nurse should instruct the parents to continue to focus on the older sibling after the birth to reduce regressive or aggressive behavior that might manifest toward the newborn. The child is exhibiting sibling rivalry, which results from the child's fear of change in the security of his relationships with his parents. This behavior is common and does not require the intervention of a child psychologist.

10. **Answer: b**
    RATIONALE: Monilial vaginitis is a benign fungal condition that is uncomfortable for women; it can be transmitted from an infected mother to her newborn at birth. Neonates develop an oral infection known as thrush, which presents as white patches on the mucus membranes of the mouth. Although rubella, toxoplasmosis, and cytomegalovirus are infections transmitted to the newborn by the mother, this newborn is not experiencing any of these infections. Rubella causes fetal defects, known as congenital rubella syndrome; common defects of rubella are cataracts, deafness, congenital heart defects, cardiac disease, and intellectual disability. Possible fetal effects due to toxoplasmosis include stillbirth, premature delivery, microcephaly, hydrocephaly, seizures, and intellectual disability, whereas possible effects of cytomegalovirus infection include small for gestational age (SGA), microcephaly, hydrocephaly, and intellectual disability.

11. **Answer: a**
    RATIONALE: Between 38 and 40 weeks of gestation, the fundal height drops as the fetus begins to descend and engage into the pelvis. Because it pushes against the diaphragm, many women experience shortness of breath. By 40 weeks, the fetal head begins to descend and engage into the pelvis. Although breathing becomes easier because of this descent, the pressure on the urinary bladder now increases, and women experience urinary frequency. The fundus reaches its highest level at the xiphoid process at approximately 36, not 39, weeks. By 20 weeks' gestation, the fundus is at the level of the umbilicus and measures 20 cm. At between 6 and 8 weeks of gestation, the cervix begins to soften (Goodell sign) and the lower uterine segment softens (Hegar sign).

12. **Answer: c**
RATIONALE: The skin and complexion of pregnant women undergo hyperpigmentation, primarily as a result of estrogen, progesterone, and melanocyte-stimulating hormone levels. The increased pigmentation that occurs on the breasts and genitalia also develops on the face to form the "mask of pregnancy," or facial melisma (chloasma). This is a blotchy, brownish pigment that covers the forehead and cheeks in dark-haired women. The symptoms experienced by the client do not indicate linea nigra, striae gravidarum, or vascular spiders. The skin in the middle of the abdomen may develop a pigmented line called the linea nigra, which extends from the umbilicus to the pubic area. Striae gravidarum, or stretch marks, are irregular reddish streaks that appear on the abdomen, breasts, and buttocks in about 50% of pregnant women after month 5 of gestation. Vascular spiders appear as small, spider-like blood vessels in the skin and are usually found above the waist and on the neck, thorax, face, and arms.

13. **Answer: c**
RATIONALE: During pregnancy, there is an increase in the client's blood components. These changes, coupled with venous stasis secondary to venous pooling, which occurs during late pregnancy after standing long periods of time (with the pressure exerted by the uterus on the large pelvic veins), contribute to slowed venous return, pooling, and dependent edema. These factors also increase the woman's risk for venous thrombosis. The symptoms experienced by the client do not indicate that she is at risk for hemorrhoids, embolism, or supine hypotension syndrome. Supine hypotension syndrome occurs when the uterus expands and exerts pressure on the inferior vena cava, which causes a reduction in blood flow to the heart. A client with supine hypotension syndrome experiences dizziness, clamminess, and a marked decrease in blood pressure.

14. **Answer: a, c, & e**
RATIONALE: Changes in the structures of the respiratory system take place to prepare the body for the enlarging uterus and increased lung volume. Increased vascularity of the respiratory tract is influenced by increased estrogen levels, leading to congestion. This congestion gives rise to nasal and sinus stuffiness and to epistaxis (nosebleed). As muscles and cartilage in the thoracic region relax, the chest broadens with a conversion

from abdominal breathing to thoracic breathing. Persistent cough, Kussmaul respirations, and dyspnea are not associated with the changes in the respiratory tract during pregnancy.

15. **Answer: d**
RATIONALE: During the second trimester, many women will verbalize positive feelings about the pregnancy and will conceptualize the fetus. The woman may accept her new body image and talk about the new life within her. Generating a discussion about the woman's feelings and offering support and validation at prenatal visits are important nursing interventions. The nurse should encourage the client in her first trimester to focus on herself, not on the fetus; this is not required when the client is in her second trimester. The client's feelings are normal for the second trimester of pregnancy; hence, it is not necessary either to inform the primary health care provider about the client's feelings or to tell the client that it is too early to conceptualize the fetus.

16. **Answer: b**
RATIONALE: The nurse should instruct the client to change sexual positions to increase comfort as the pregnancy progresses. Although the nurse should also encourage her to engage in alternative, noncoital modes of sexual expression, such as cuddling, caressing, and holding, the client need not restrict herself to such alternatives. It is not advisable to perform frequent douching, because this is believed to irritate the vaginal mucosa and predispose the client to infection. Using lubricants or performing stress-relieving and relaxation exercises will not alleviate discomfort during sexual activity.

17. **Answer: b**
RATIONALE: During the second trimester of pregnancy, partners go through acceptance of their role of breadwinner, caretaker, and support person. They come to accept the reality of the fetus when movement is felt, and they experience confusion when dealing with the woman's mood swings and introspection. During the first trimester, the expectant partner may experience couvade syndrome—a sympathetic response to the partner's pregnancy—and may also experience ambivalence with extremes of emotions. During the third trimester, the expectant partner prepares for the reality of the new role and negotiates what his or her role will be during the labor and birthing process.

Answers

CHAPTER 12

SECTION I: ASSESSING YOUR UNDERSTANDING

Activity A FILL IN THE BLANKS

1. doula
2. primipara
3. Fundal
4. Montgomery
5. Chadwick
6. Pica
7. Amniocentesis
8. liver
9. nonstress
10. Hemorrhoids

Activity B MATCHING

1. d   2. e   3. a   4. b   5. c

Activity C SEQUENCING

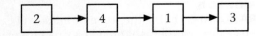

Activity D SHORT ANSWERS

1. The nurse should include the following key areas when providing preconception care:
   - Immunization status
   - Underlying medical conditions, such as cardiovascular or respiratory problems or genetic disorders
   - Reproductive health data such as pelvic examinations, use of contraceptives, and STIs
   - Sexuality and sexual practices, such as safe sex practices and body image issues
   - Nutrition
   - Lifestyle practices, including occupation and recreational activities
   - Psychosocial issues such as levels of stress and exposure to abuse and violence
   - Medication and drug use, including use of tobacco, alcohol, over-the-counter and prescription medications, and illicit drugs
   - Support system, including family, friends, and community
2. Nurses can enter into a collaborative partnership with a woman and her partner, enabling them to examine their own health and its influence on the health of their future baby. The nurse performs the following interventions as part of preconception care to ensure a positive impact on the pregnancy:
   - Stress the importance of taking folic acid to prevent neural tube defects.
   - Urge the woman to achieve optimal weight before pregnancy.
   - Ensure that the woman's immunizations are up to date.
   - Address substance use issues, including smoking and taking drugs.
   - Identify victims of violence and assist them in getting help.
   - Manage chronic conditions such as diabetes and asthma.
   - Educate the woman about environmental hazards, including metals and herbs.
   - Offer genetic counseling to identify carriers.
   - Suggest the availability of support systems, if needed.
3. The assessments to be made by a nurse on a client's initial prenatal visit are as follows:
   - Screen for factors that place the client and her fetus at risk.
   - Educate the client about changes that will affect her life.
4. Counseling and educating the pregnant client and her partner are important to healthy outcomes for the mother and her infant. The role of a nurse in providing counseling and education to the client during a prenatal visit is as follows:
   - Provide anticipatory guidance.
   - Make appropriate community referrals.
   - Answer questions that the client and her partner may have regarding the pregnancy. It is important for the nurse to clarify all the misinformation or misconceptions in the minds of the client and her partner.
5. The nurse should perform the following assessments when conducting a chest examination of the client:
   - Auscultate heart sounds, noting any abnormalities.
   - A soft systolic murmur caused by the increase in blood volume may be noted.

- Anticipate an increase in heart rate by 10 to 15 beats per minute secondary to increases in cardiac output and blood volume.
- Note adaptation of the body with peripheral dilatation.
- Auscultate the chest for breath sounds, which should be clear.
- Note symmetry of chest movement and thoracic breathing patterns.
- Expect a slight increase in respiratory rate to accommodate the increase in tidal volume and oxygen consumption.
- Inspect and palpate the breasts: Increases in estrogen and progesterone and blood supply make the breasts feel full and more nodular, with increased sensitivity to touch.
- Blood vessels become more visible, and there is an increase in breast size.
- Striae gravidarum may be visible in women with large breasts.
- Darker pigmentation of the nipple and areola is present, along with enlargement of Montgomery glands.
- Teach and reinforce breast self-examination.

6. The nurse should perform the following assessments during a follow-up visit:
   - Weight and blood pressure, which are compared to baseline values
   - Urine testing for protein, glucose, ketones, and nitrites
   - Fundal height measurement to assess fetal growth
   - Assessment for quickening/fetal movement to determine well-being
   - Assessment of fetal heart rate (should be 120 to 160 bpm)
   - Answer questions
   - Provide anticipatory guidance and education
   - Review nutritional guidelines
   - Evaluate the client for compliance with prenatal vitamin therapy
   - Encourage the woman's partner to participate if possible

SECTION II: APPLYING YOUR KNOWLEDGE

Activity E CASE STUDY

1. The items in the checklist used by the nurse to ensure that the client is well prepared for the newborn's birth and homecoming are as follows:
   - Attend childbirth preparation classes and practice breathing techniques.
   - Purchase an infant safety seat.
   - Select a feeding method.
   - Decide whether a boy will be circumcised.
   - Select and arrange for a birth setting.
   - Tour the birthing facility.
   - Choose a family planning method to be used after the birth.

- Communicate needs and desires concerning pain management.
- Understand signs and symptoms of labor.
- Provide for care of other siblings during labor (when applicable).
- Discuss the possibility of a cesarean birth.
- Prepare for the birthing facility when labor starts.
- Discuss possible names for the newborn.
- Know how to reach a health care professional when labor starts.
- Decide on a pediatrician.

2. The nurse should perform the following interventions in preparing a client for breastfeeding:
   - Encourage the client to attend a La Leche League or breastfeeding class.
   - Provide the client with sources of information about infant feeding.
   - Suggest that the client read a good reference book about lactation.

3. The nurse should educate the pregnant client about the following advantages of breastfeeding:
   - Human milk is digestible, is economical, and requires no preparation
   - Promotes bonding between mother and child
   - Costs less than purchasing formula
   - Suppresses ovulation
   - Reduces the risk of ovarian cancer and premenopausal breast cancer
   - Uses extra calories, which promotes weight loss gradually without dieting
   - Releases oxytocin, which promotes rapid uterine involution with less bleeding
   - Suckling helps in developing the muscles in the infant's jaw
   - Improves absorption of lactose and minerals in the newborn
   - Helps prevent infections in the baby
   - Composition of breast milk adapts to meet the infant's changing needs
   - Prevents constipation in the baby, with adequate intake
   - Helps lessen chance that the baby will develop food allergies
   - Reduces the incidence of otitis media and upper respiratory infections in the infant and the risk of adult obesity
   - Makes the baby less prone to vomiting

SECTION III: PRACTICING FOR NCLEX

Activity F NCLEX-STYLE QUESTIONS

1. **Answer: c**
   RATIONALE: When preparing the client for a physical examination, the nurse should instruct the client to empty her bladder; the nurse should then collect the urine sample so that it can be sent for laboratory tests to detect possibilities of a urinary tract infection. The client need not

lie down, take deep breaths, or have the family present; however, it is important for the nurse to ensure that the client feels comfortable.

2. **Answer: a**
   RATIONALE: To reduce the client's urinary frequency, the nurse should instruct the client to avoid consuming caffeinated drinks, since caffeine stimulates voiding patterns. The nurse instructs the client to drink fluids between meals rather than with meals if the client complains of nausea and vomiting. The nurse instructs the client to avoid an empty stomach at all times, to prevent fatigue. The nurse also instructs the client to munch on dry crackers or toast early in the morning before arising if the client experiences nausea and vomiting; this would not help the client experiencing urinary frequency.

3. **Answer: a, b, & c**
   RATIONALE: When documenting a comprehensive health history while caring for a client, it is important for the nurse to prepare a care plan that suits the client's lifestyle, to develop a trusting relationship with the client, and to prepare a plan of care for the pregnancy. The nurse does not need to assess the client's partner's sexual health during the history-taking process or urge the client to achieve an optimal body weight. Achieving optimal body weight before conception helps the client to achieve a positive impact on the pregnancy.

4. **Answer: a, d, & e**
   RATIONALE: While conducting a physical examination of the head and neck, the nurse assesses for any previous injuries and sequelae, evaluates for limitations in range of motion, and palpates the thyroid gland for enlargement. The nurse should also assess for any edema of the nasal mucosa or hypertrophy of gingival tissue, as well as palpate for enlarged lymph nodes or swelling. The nurse need not check the client's eye movements; pregnancy does not affect the eye muscles. The nurse should check for levels of estrogen when examining the extremities of the client.

5. **Answer: d**
   RATIONALE: In the 12th week of gestation, the nurse should palpate the fundus at the symphysis pubis. The nurse should palpate for the fundus below the ensiform cartilage when the client is in the 36th week of gestation; midway between symphysis and umbilicus in the 16th week of gestation; and at the umbilicus in the 20th week of gestation.

6. **Answer: c**
   RATIONALE: While examining external genitalia, the nurse should assess for any infection due to hematomas, varicosities, inflammation, lesions, and discharge. The nurse assesses for a long, smooth, thick, and closed cervix when examining the internal genitalia. Other assessments when examining the internal genitalia include assessing for bluish coloration of cervix and vaginal mucosa and conducting a rectal examination to assess for lesions, masses, prolapse, or hemorrhoids.

7. **Answer: b**
   RATIONALE: When assessing fetal well-being through abdominal ultrasonography, the nurse should instruct the client to refrain from emptying her bladder. The nurse must ensure that abdominal ultrasonography is conducted on a full bladder and should inform the client that she is likely to feel cold, not hot, initially in the test. The nurse should obtain the client's vital records and instruct the client to report the occurrence of fever when the client has to undergo amniocentesis, not ultrasonography.

8. **Answer: a**
   RATIONALE: The nurse should inform the client that sexual activity is permissible during pregnancy unless there is a history of incompetent cervix, vaginal bleeding, placenta previa, risk of preterm labor, multiple gestation, premature rupture of membranes, or presence of any infection. Anemia and facial and hand edema would be contraindications to exercising but not intercourse. Freedom from anxieties and worries contributes to adequate sleep promotion.

9. **Answer: a**
   RATIONALE: To help alleviate constipation, the nurse should instruct the client to ensure adequate hydration and bulk in the diet. The nurse should instruct the client to avoid spicy or greasy foods when a client complains of heartburn or indigestion. The nurse also should instruct the client to avoid lying down for 2 hours after meals if the client experiences heartburn or indigestion. The nurse should instruct the client to practice Kegel exercises when the client experiences urinary frequency.

10. **Answer: d**
    RATIONALE: To promote easy and safe travel for the client, the nurse should instruct the client to always wear a three-point seat belt to prevent ejection or serious injury from collision. The nurse should instruct the client to deactivate the air bag if possible. The nurse should instruct the client to apply a nonpadded shoulder strap properly, ensuring that it crosses between the breasts and over the upper abdomen, above the uterus. The nurse should instruct the client to use a lap belt that crosses over the pelvis below—not over—the uterus.

11. **Answer: b**
    RATIONALE: Naegele's rule can be used to establish the estimated date of birth (EDB). Using this rule, the nurse should subtract 3 months and then add 7 days to the first day of the last normal menstrual period. On the basis of Naegele's rule, the EDB will be December 17, because the client started her last menstrual period on March 10. January 7, February 21, and January 30 are not the EDB according to Naegele's rule.

12. **Answer: a**
RATIONALE: Pica is characterized by a craving for substances that have no nutritional value. Consumption of these substances can be dangerous to the client and her developing fetus. The nurse should monitor the client for iron-deficiency anemia as a manifestation of the client's compulsion to consume soil. Consumption of ice due to pica is likely to lead to tooth fractures. The nurse should monitor for inefficient protein metabolism if the client has been consuming laundry starch as a result of pica. The nurse should monitor for constipation in the client if she has been consuming clay.

13. **Answer: b, c, & e**
RATIONALE: When caring for a pregnant client who follows a vegetarian diet, the nurse should monitor her for iron-deficiency anemia, decreased mineral absorption, and low gestational weight gain. Risk of epistaxis and increased risk of constipation are not reported to be associated with a vegetarian diet.

14. **Answer: a**
RATIONALE: In a client's second trimester of pregnancy, the nurse should educate the client to look for vaginal bleeding as a danger sign of pregnancy needing immediate attention from the physician. Generally, painful urination, severe/persistent vomiting, and lower abdominal and shoulder pain are the danger signs that the client has to monitor for during the first trimester of pregnancy.

15. **Answer: c**
RATIONALE: The nurse should instruct the client to serve the formula to her infant at room temperature. The nurse should instruct the client to follow the directions on the package when mixing the powder because different formulas may have different instructions. The infant should be fed every 3 to 4 hours, not every 8 hours. The nurse should specifically instruct the client to avoid

refrigerating the formula for subsequent feedings. Any leftover formula should be discarded.

16. **Answer: d**
RATIONALE: According to the Lamaze method of preparing for labor and childbirth, the nurse must remain quiet during the client's period of imagery and focal point visualization to avoid breaking her concentration. The nurse should ensure deep abdominopelvic breathing by the client according to the Bradley method, along with ensuring the client's concentration on pleasurable sensations. The Bradley method emphasizes the pleasurable sensations of childbirth and involves teaching women to concentrate on these sensations when "turning on" to their own bodies. The nurse should ensure abdominal breathing during contractions when using the Dick-Read method.

17. **Answer: b**
RATIONALE: To help the client alleviate varicosities of the legs, the nurse should instruct the client to refrain from crossing her legs when sitting for long periods. The nurse should instruct the client to avoid standing, not sitting, in one position for long periods of time. The nurse should instruct the client to wear support stockings to promote better circulation, though the client should stay away from constrictive stockings and socks. Applying heating pads on the extremities is not reported to alleviate varicosities of the legs.

18. **Answer: b, e, c, a, & d**
RATIONALE: The client who is to undergo a non-stress test should have a meal before the procedure. The client is then placed in a lateral recumbent position to avoid supine hypotension syndrome. An external electronic fetal monitoring device is applied to her abdomen. The client is handed an "event marker" with a button that she pushes every time she perceives fetal movement. When the button is pushed, the fetal monitor strip is marked to identify that fetal movement has occurred.

Answers

CHAPTER 13

SECTION I: ASSESSING YOUR UNDERSTANDING

Activity A FILL IN THE BLANKS

1. gynecoid
2. effacement
3. sagittal
4. Zero
5. Lightening
6. contractions
7. decidua
8. passageway
9. nesting
10. molding

Activity B LABELING

1. The pelvic shapes in images A to D are as follows. The gynecoid shape (Figure A) is the most favorable shape for a vaginal delivery.
    A. **Gynecoid:** This is considered the true female pelvis, occurring in about 50% of all women. Vaginal birth is most favorable with this type of pelvis because the inlet is round and the outlet is roomy.
    B. **Android:** This type of pelvic is characterized by its funnel shape. Descent of the fetal head into the pelvis is slow, and failure of the fetus to rotate is common. Prognosis for labor is poor, subsequently leading to cesarean birth.
    C. **Anthropoid:** Vaginal birth is more favorable with this pelvic shape (deep pelvis, wider front-to-back than side-to-side) compared to the android or platypelloid shape.
    D. **Platypelloid** (or flat pelvis): This is the least common type of pelvic structure. The pelvic cavity is shallow but widens at the pelvic outlet, making it difficult for the fetus to descend through the midpelvis. It is not favorable for a vaginal birth unless the fetal head can pass through the inlet. Women with this type of pelvis usually require cesarean birth.
2. The figure[K2] shows four breech presentations which are identified below. Breech presentations are associated with prematurity, placenta previa,

multiparity, uterine abnormalities (fibroids), and some congenital anomalies such as hydrocephaly.
    A. Frank breech
    B. Complete breech
    C. Single footling breech
    D. Double footling breech

Activity C MATCHING

1. a **2.** b **3.** e **4.** d **5.** c

Activity D SEQUENCING

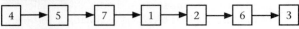

Activity E SHORT ANSWERS

1. Well-controlled research validates that nonmoving, back-lying positions during labor are not healthy. Despite this, most women lie flat on their backs. This position is preferred during labor mostly for the following reasons:
    • Laboring women need to conserve their energy and not tire themselves.
    • Nurses can keep track of clients more easily if they are not ambulating.
    • The supine position facilitates vaginal examinations and external belt adjustment.
    • A bed is simply where one is usually supposed to be in a hospital setting.
    • It is believed that this practice is convenient for the delivering health professional.
    • Laboring women are "connected to things" that impede movement.
2. The nurse should encourage the pregnant client to adopt the upright or lateral position because such a position
    • Reduces the duration of the second stage of labor
    • Reduces the number of assisted deliveries (vacuum and forceps)
    • Reduces episiotomies and perineal tears
    • Contributes to fewer abnormal fetal heart-rate patterns
    • Increases comfort and reduces requests for pain medication
    • Enhances a sense of control reported by mothers
    • Alters the shape and size of the pelvis, which assists descent

- Assists gravity to move the fetus downward
- Reduces the length of labor

3. Maternal physiologic responses that occur as a woman progresses through childbirth include:
   - Increase in heart rate, by 10 to 20 bpm
   - Increase in cardiac output, by 12% to 31% during the first stage of labor and by 50% during the second stage of labor
   - Increase in blood pressure, up to 35 mm Hg during uterine contractions in all labor stages
   - Increase in white blood cell count, to 25,000 to 30,000 cells per mm^3, perhaps as a result of tissue trauma
   - Increase in respiratory rate, along with greater oxygen consumption, related to the increase in metabolism
   - Decrease in gastric motility and food absorption, which may increase the risk of nausea and vomiting during the transition stage of labor
   - Decrease in gastric emptying and gastric pH, which increases the risk of vomiting with aspiration
   - Slight elevation in temperature, possibly as a result of an increase in muscle activity
   - Muscular aches/cramps, as a result of a stressed musculoskeletal system involved in the labor process
   - Increase in basal metabolic rate (BMR) and decrease in blood glucose levels because of the stress of labor

4. The factors that influence the ability of a woman to cope with labor stress include:
   - Previous birth experiences and their outcomes
   - Current pregnancy experience
   - Cultural considerations
   - Involvement of support system
   - Childbirth preparation
   - Expectations of the birthing experience
   - Anxiety level and fear of labor experience
   - Feelings of loss of control
   - Fatigue and weariness
   - Anxiety levels

5. The signs of separation that indicate the placenta is ready to deliver are the following:
   - Uterus rises upward.
   - Umbilical cord lengthens.
   - Blood trickles suddenly from the vaginal opening.
   - Uterus changes its shape to globular.

6. The following factors ensure a positive birth experience for the pregnant client:
   - Clear information on procedures
   - Positive support; not being alone
   - Sense of mastery, self-confidence
   - Trust in staff caring for her
   - Positive reaction to the pregnancy
   - Personal control over breathing
   - Preparation for the childbirth experience

SECTION II: APPLYING YOUR KNOWLEDGE

Activity F CASE STUDY

1. Many women fear being sent home from the hospital with "false labor." All women feel anxious when they feel contractions, but they should be informed that labor can be a long process, especially if it is their first pregnancy. With first pregnancies, the cervix can take up to 20 hours to dilate completely. False labor is a condition occurring during the latter weeks of some pregnancies, in which irregular uterine contractions are felt but the cervix is not affected. In contrast, true labor is characterized by contractions occurring at regular intervals that increase in frequency, duration, and intensity with the contraction starting in the back and radiating around toward the front of the abdomen. True labor contractions bring about progressive cervical dilation and effacement.

2. The client should follow the instructions of her health care provider, but generally the client is instructed to stay home until contractions are 5 minutes apart, lasting 45 to 60 seconds and strong enough so that a conversation during one is not possible. Variables, such as rural versus urban setting, time to the hospital/distance from hospital, traffic at certain times of day, are taken into consideration when giving instructions on when to leave to travel to the hospital. She should be instructed to drink fluids and walk to assess if there is any change in her contractions. In true labor, contractions are regular, become closer together, and become stronger with time. The contraction starts in the back and radiates around toward the front of the abdomen.

3. Changing positions and moving around during labor and birth do offer several benefits. Maternal position can influence pelvic size and contours. Changing position and walking affect the pelvis joints, which facilitates fetal descent and rotation. Squatting enlarges the pelvic diameter, whereas a kneeling position removes pressure on the maternal vena cava and assists to rotate the fetus in the posterior position.
   The client should be encouraged to ask the nurse caring for her during labor if she can walk and have the nurse suggest positions to try.

4. Pushing occurs during the second stage of labor, which begins with complete cervical dilation (10 cm) and effacement and ends with the birth of the newborn. Although the previous stage of labor primarily involved the thinning and opening of the cervix, this stage involves moving the fetus through the birth canal and out of the body. The cardinal movements of labor occur during the early phase of passive descent in the second stage of labor.
   Additional second-stage characteristics that help indicate that pushing can occur includes

contractions that occur every 2 to 3 minutes, last 60 to 90 seconds, and are described as strong by palpation. During this expulsive stage, the client may feel more in control and less irritable and agitated and be focused on the work of pushing. During the second stage of labor, pushing can either follow a spontaneous urge or be directed by the nurse and/or health provider.

SECTION III: PRACTICING FOR NCLEX

Activity G NCLEX-STYLE QUESTIONS

1. **Answer: b**
   RATIONALE: The nurse knows that the client is experiencing lightening. Lightening occurs when the fetal presenting part begins to descend into the maternal pelvis, and may occur 2 weeks or more before labor. The uterus lowers and moves into a more anterior position. The client may report increased respiratory capacity, decreased dyspnea, increased pelvic pressure, cramping, and low back pain. She may also note edema of the lower extremities as a result of the increased stasis of blood pooling, an increase in vaginal discharge, and more frequent urination. Some women report a sudden increase in energy before labor. This is sometimes referred to as nesting. Bloody show is a pink-tinged secretion that occurs when a small amount of blood released by cervical capillaries mixes with mucus. Braxton Hicks contractions are typically felt as a tightening or pulling sensation of the top of the uterus.

2. **Answer: a, b, & d**
   RATIONALE: Upon seeing the increased prostaglandin levels, the nurse should assess for myometrial contractions, leading to a reduction in cervical resistance and subsequent softening and thinning of the cervix. The uterus of the client will appear boggy during the fourth stage of delivery, after the completion of pregnancy and birth. Hypotonic character of the bladder is also marked during the fourth stage of pregnancy, not when the prostaglandin levels rise, marking the onset of labor.

3. **Answer: a**
   RATIONALE: Braxton Hicks contractions assist in labor by ripening and softening the cervix and moving the cervix from a posterior position to an anterior position. Prostaglandin levels increase late in pregnancy secondary to elevated estrogen levels; this is not due to the occurrence of Braxton Hicks contractions. Braxton Hicks contractions do not help in bringing about oxytocin sensitivity. Occurrence of lightening, not Braxton Hicks contractions, makes maternal breathing easier.

4. **Answer: c**
   RATIONALE: The labor of a first-time-pregnant woman lasts longer because during the first pregnancy the cervix takes between 12 and 16 hours to dilate completely. The intensity of the Braxton Hicks contractions stays the same during the first and second pregnancies. Spontaneous rupture of membranes may occur before the onset of labor during each delivery, not only during the first delivery.

5. **Answer: d**
   RATIONALE: The advantage of adopting a kneeling position during labor is that it helps to rotate the fetus in a posterior position. Facilitating vaginal examinations, facilitating external belt adjustment, and helping the woman in labor to save energy are advantages of the back-lying maternal position.

6. **Answer: a, b, & c**
   RATIONALE: When caring for a client in labor, the nurse should monitor for an increase in the heart rate by 10 to 20 bpm, an increase in blood pressure by as much as 35 mm Hg, and an increase in respiratory rate. During labor, the nurse should monitor for a slight elevation in body temperature as a result of an increase in muscle activity. The nurse should also monitor for decreased gastric emptying and gastric pH, which increases the risk of vomiting with aspiration.

7. **Answer: d**
   RATIONALE: When monitoring fetal responses in a client experiencing labor, the nurse should monitor for a decrease in circulation and perfusion to the fetus secondary to uterine contractions. The nurse should monitor for an increase, not a decrease, in arterial carbon dioxide pressure. The nurse should also monitor for a decrease, not an increase, in fetal breathing movements throughout labor. The nurse should monitor for a decrease in fetal oxygen pressure with a decrease in the partial pressure of oxygen.

8. **Answer: c**
   RATIONALE: The nurse must massage the client's uterus briefly after placental expulsion to constrict the uterine blood vessels and minimize the possibility of hemorrhage. Massaging the client's uterus will not lessen the chances of conducting an episiotomy. In addition, an episiotomy, if required, is conducted in the second stage of labor, not the third. The client's uterus may appear boggy only in the fourth stage of labor, not in the third stage. Ensuring that all sections of the placenta are present and that no piece is left attached to the uterine wall is confirmed through a placental examination after expulsion.

9. **Answer: d**
   RATIONALE: The first stage of labor terminates with the dilation of the cervix diameter to 10 cm. Diffused abdominal cramping and rupturing of the fetal membrane occurs during the first stage of labor. Regular contractions occur at the beginning of the latent phase of the first stage; they do not mark the end of the first stage of labor.

10. **Answer: a, c, & e**

    RATIONALE: The nurse knows that lower uterine segment distention, stretching and tearing of the structures, and dilation of the cervix cause pain in the first stage. The fetus moves along the birth canal during the second stage of labor, when the client is more in control and less agitated. Spontaneous expulsion of the placenta occurs in the third stage of labor, not the first.

11. **Answer: b**

    RATIONALE: The nurse, along with the physician, has to assess for fetal anomalies, which are usually associated with a shoulder presentation during a vaginal birth. The other conditions include placenta previa and multiple gestations. Uterine abnormalities, congenital anomalies, and prematurity are conditions associated with a breech presentation of the fetus during a vaginal birth.

12. **Answer: a, b, & c**

    RATIONALE: To ensure a positive childbirth experience for the client, the nurse should provide the client clear information on procedures involved, encourage the client to have a sense of mastery and self-control, and encourage the client to have a positive reaction to pregnancy. Instructing the client to spend some time alone is not an appropriate intervention; instead, the nurse should instruct the client to obtain positive support and avoid being alone. The client does not need to change the home environment; this does not ensure a positive childbirth experience.

13. **Answer: c**

    RATIONALE: If the long axis of the fetus is perpendicular to that of the mother, then the client's fetus is in the transverse lie position. If the long axis of the fetus is parallel to that of the mother, the client's fetus is in the longitudinal lie position. The long axis of the fetus being at 45° or 60° to that of the client does not indicate any specific position of the fetus.

14. **Answer: d**

    RATIONALE: The pauses between contractions during labor are important because they allow the restoration of blood flow to the uterus and the placenta. Shortening of the upper uterine segment, reduction in length of the cervical canal, and effacement and dilation of the cervix are other processes that occur during uterine contractions.

15. **Answer: a, c, & d**

    RATIONALE: To provide comfort to the pregnant client, the nurse should make use of massage, hand holding, and acupressure to bring comfort to the pregnant client during labor. It is not advisable to provide chewing gum to a client in labor; it may cause accidental asphyxiation. Pain killers are not prescribed for a client experiencing labor.

Answers

CHAPTER 14

SECTION I: ASSESSING YOUR UNDERSTANDING

Activity A FILL IN THE BLANKS

1. Nonpharmacologic
2. hypoglycemia
3. fern
4. uteroplacental
5. ischial
6. uterine
7. tocotransducer
8. Artifact
9. parasympathetic
10. accelerations

Activity B MATCHING

1. c   2. b   3. a   4. d

Activity C SEQUENCING

1. b → a → c → e → d

Activity D SHORT ANSWERS

1. The nurse should include biographical data such as the woman's name and age and the name of the delivering health care provider, prenatal record data, past health and family history, prenatal education, medications, risk factors, reason for admission, history of previous preterm births, allergies, the last time the client ate, method for infant feeding, name of birth attendant and pediatrician, and pain management plan.
2. The Apgar score assesses five parameters—heart rate (absent, slow, or fast), respiratory effort (absent, weak cry, or good strong yell), muscle tone (limp, or lively and active), response to irritation stimulus, and color—that evaluate a newborn's cardiorespiratory adaptation after birth.
3. The purpose of vaginal examination is to assess the amount of cervical dilation, the percentage of cervical effacement, and the fetal membrane status, and to gather information about presentation, position, and station. If the presentation is cephalic, the degree of fetal head flexion and presence of

fetal skull swelling or molding can be determined during the vaginal examination.
4. Advantage: Electronic fetal monitoring produces a continuous record of the FHR, unlike intermittent auscultation, when gaps are likely.
   Disadvantage: Continuous monitoring can limit maternal movement and encourages her to lie in the supine position, which reduces placental perfusion.
5. The typical signs of the second stage of labor are as follows:
   - Increase in apprehension or irritability
   - Spontaneous rupture of membranes
   - Sudden appearance of sweat on upper lip
   - Increase in blood-tinged show
   - Low grunting sounds from the woman
   - Complaints of rectal and perineal pressure
   - Beginning of involuntary bearing-down efforts
6. Positions used for the second stage of labor are as follows:
   - Lithotomy with feet up in stirrups: most convenient position for caregivers
   - Semisitting with pillows underneath knees, arms, and back
   - Lateral/side-lying with curved back and upper leg supported by partner
   - Sitting on birthing stool: opens pelvis, enhances the pull of gravity, and helps with pushing
   - Squatting/supported squatting: gives the woman a sense of control
   - Kneeling with hands on bed and knees comfortably apart

SECTION II: APPLYING YOUR KNOWLEDGE

Activity E CASE STUDY

1. If there was no vaginal bleeding on admission, the nurse should perform a vaginal examination to assess cervical dilation, after which it is monitored periodically as necessary to identify progress.
2. The purpose of vaginal examination is to assess the amount of cervical dilation, the percentage of cervical effacement, and the fetal membrane status and to gather information about presentation, position, and station. If the presentation is cephalic, the degree of fetal head flexion and presence of

fetal skull swelling or molding can be assessed. The vaginal examination will also reveal the presence of a breech presentation.

3. Procedure for conducting vaginal examination:
   - Instruct the client on the purpose of the vaginal examination.
   - Place the client in a lithotomy position.
   - Put on sterile gloves.
   - Use water as lubricant to check membrane status, if needed.
   - Use antiseptic solution to prevent infection if the membrane has ruptured.
   - Insert index and middle fingers into the vaginal introitus.
   - Palpate cervix to assess dilation, effacement, and position.

SECTION III: PRACTICING FOR NCLEX

Activity F NCLEX-STYLE QUESTIONS

1. **Answer: a**
   RATIONALE: When a nurse first comes in contact with a pregnant client during the admission assessment, it is important to first ascertain whether the woman is in true or false labor. Information regarding the number of pregnancies, addiction to drugs, or history of drug allergy is not important criteria for admitting the client.

2. **Answer: a, c, & d**
   RATIONALE: When conducting an admission assessment on the phone for a pregnant client, the nurse needs to obtain information regarding the estimated due date, characteristics of contractions, and appearance of vaginal blood to evaluate the need to admit her. History of drug abuse or a drug allergy is usually recorded as part of the client's medical history.

3. **Answer: b**
   RATIONALE: When a pregnant client is in the active phase of labor, the nurse should monitor the vital signs every 30 minutes. The nurse should monitor the vital signs every 30 to 60 minutes if the client is in the latent phase of labor and every 15 to 30 minutes during the transition phase of labor. Temperature is usually monitored every 4 hours in the active phase of labor.

4. **Answer: a**
   RATIONALE: In a cephalic presentation, the FHR is best heard in the lower quadrant of the maternal abdomen. In a breech presentation, it is heard at or above the level of the maternal umbilicus.

5. **Answer: a**
   RATIONALE: Analysis of the FHR using external electronic fetal monitoring is one of the primary evaluation tools used to determine fetal oxygen status indirectly. Fetal pulse oximetry measures fetal oxygen saturation directly and in real time. It is used with electronic fetal monitoring as an adjunct method of assessment when the FHR pattern is nonreassuring or inconclusive. Fetal scalp

blood is obtained to measure the pH. The fetal position can be determined through ultrasonography or abdominal palpation but is not indicative of fetal oxygenation.

6. **Answer: a**
   RATIONALE: Increased sedation is an adverse effect of lorazepam. Diazepam and midazolam cause central nervous system depression for both the woman and the newborn. Opioids are associated with newborn respiratory depression and decreased alertness.

7. **Answer: d**
   RATIONALE: General anesthesia is administered in emergency cesarean births. Local anesthetic is injected into the superficial perineal nerves to numb the perineal area generally before an episiotomy. Although an epidural block is used in cesarean births, it is contraindicated in clients with spinal injury. Regional anesthesia is contraindicated in cesarean births.

8. **Answer: b**
   RATIONALE: During the latent phase of labor, the nurse should monitor the FHR every 30 to 60 minutes. FHR should be monitored every 30 minutes in the active phase and every 15 to 30 minutes in the transition phase of labor. Continuous monitoring is done when an electronic fetal monitor is used.

9. **Answer: b**
   RATIONALE: If vaginal bleeding is absent during admission assessment, the nurse should perform vaginal examination to assess the amount of cervical dilation. Hydration status is monitored as part of the physical examination. A urine specimen is obtained for urinalysis to obtain a baseline. Vital signs are monitored frequently throughout the maternal assessment.

10. **Answer: c**
    RATIONALE: The Nitrazine tape shows a pH between 5 and 6, which indicates an acidic environment with the presence of vaginal fluid and less blood. If the membranes had ruptured, amniotic fluid was present, or there was excess blood, the Nitrazine test tape would have indicated an alkaline environment.

11. **Answer: a, b, & e**
    RATIONALE: The nurse should assess the frequency of contractions, intensity of contractions, and uterine resting tone to monitor uterine contractions. Monitoring changes in temperature and blood pressure is part of the general physical examination and does not help to monitor uterine contraction.

12. **Answer: a, b, & c**
    RATIONALE: Leopold maneuvers help the nurse to determine the presentation, position, and lie of the fetus. The approximate weight and size of the fetus can be determined with ultrasound sonography or abdominal palpation.

13. **Answer: a, c, & d**
    RATIONALE: The nurse should turn the client on her left side to increase placental perfusion, administer oxygen by mask to increase fetal oxygenation, and assess the client for any underlying contributing causes. The client's questions should not be ignored; instead, the client should be reassured that interventions are to effect FHR pattern change. A reduced IV rate would decrease intravascular volume, affecting the FHR further.

14. **Answer: c**
    RATIONALE: The client should be administered oxygen by mask because the nonreassuring FHR pattern could be due to inadequate oxygen reserves in the fetus. Because the client is in preterm labor, it is not advisable to apply vibroacoustic stimulation, tactile stimulation, or fetal scalp stimulation.

15. **Answer: a**
    RATIONALE: The nurse must monitor for respiratory depression. Accidental intrathecal blockade, inadequate or failed block, and postdural puncture headache are possible complications associated with combined spinal–epidural analgesia.

16. **Answer: b**
    RATIONALE: The nurse should provide supplemental oxygen if a client who has been administered combined spinal–epidural analgesia exhibits signs of hypotension and associated FHR changes. The client should be assisted to a semi-Fowler position; the client should not be kept in a supine position or be turned on her left side. Discontinuing IV fluid will cause dehydration.

17. **Answer: b**
    RATIONALE: The nurse should monitor the client for uterine relaxation. Pruritus, inadequate or failed block, and maternal hypotension are associated with combined spinal–epidural analgesia.

18. **Answer: a**
    RATIONALE: The recommendation for initiating hydrotherapy is that women be in active labor (>5 cm dilated) to prevent the slowing of labor contractions secondary to muscular relaxation. Women are encouraged to stay in the bath or shower as long as they feel they are comfortable. The water temperature should not exceed body temperature. The woman's membranes can be intact or ruptured.

19. **Answer: b**
    RATIONALE: For slow-paced breathing, the nurse should instruct the woman to inhale slowly through her nose and exhale through pursed lips. In shallow or modified-pace breathing, the woman should inhale and exhale through her mouth at a rate of 4 breaths every 5 seconds. In pattern-paced breathing, the breathing is punctuated every few breaths by a forceful exhalation through pursed lips. Holding the breath for 5 seconds after every three breaths is not recommended in any of the three levels of patterned breathing.

20. **Answer: a, b, & d**
    RATIONALE: The nurse should check for any abnormality of the spine, hypovolemia, or coagulation defects in the client. An epidural is contraindicated in women with these conditions. Varicose veins and skin rashes or bruises are not contraindications for an epidural block. They are contraindications for massage used for pain relief during labor.

Answers

CHAPTER 15

SECTION I: ASSESSING YOUR UNDERSTANDING

Activity A FILL IN THE BLANKS

1. pelvis
2. subinvolution
3. Afterpains
4. engorgement
5. uterus
6. Oxytocin
7. nonlactating
8. Lactation
9. Prolactin
10. diaphoresis

Activity B MATCHING

1. d   **2.** e   **3.** a   **4.** b   **5.** c

Activity C SEQUENCING

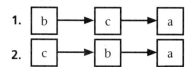

1. b → c → a
2. c → b → a

Activity D SHORT ANSWERS

1. The timing of the first menses and ovulation after birth differs considerably in lactating and nonlactating women. In nonlactating women, menstruation resumes 7 to 9 weeks after giving birth; the first cycle is anovulatory. In lactating women, the return of menses depends on the frequency and duration of breastfeeding. It usually resumes anytime from 2 to 18 months after childbirth, and the first postpartum menses is usually heavier and frequently anovulatory. However, ovulation may occur before menstruation, so breastfeeding is not a reliable method of contraception.

2. Afterpains are more acute in multiparous women secondary to repeated stretching of the uterine muscles, which reduces muscle tone, allowing for alternate uterine contraction and relaxation.

3. Factors that facilitate uterine involution are
   - Complete expulsion of amniotic membranes and placenta at birth
   - Complication-free labor and birth process
   - Breastfeeding
   - Ambulation

4. Factors that inhibit involution include
   - Prolonged labor and difficult birth
   - Incomplete expulsion of amniotic membranes and placenta
   - Uterine infection
   - Overdistention of uterine muscles due to
   a. Multiple gestation, hydramnios, or large singleton fetus
   b. Full bladder, which displaces uterus and interferes with contractions
   c. Anesthesia, which relaxes uterine muscles
   d. Close childbirth spacing, leading to frequent and repeated distention and thus decreasing uterine tone and causing muscular relaxation

5. Women who have had cesarean births tend to have less flow because the uterine debris is removed manually with delivery of the placenta.

6. Afterpains are usually stronger during breastfeeding because oxytocin released by the sucking reflex strengthens uterine contractions. Mild analgesics can be used to reduce this discomfort.

SECTION II: APPLYING YOUR KNOWLEDGE

Activity E CASE STUDY

1. The nurse should suggest the following measures to resolve engorgement in the client who is breastfeeding:
   Empty the breasts frequently to minimize discomfort and resolve engorgement.
   Stand in a warm shower or apply warm compresses to the breasts to provide some relief.

2. The nurse should suggest the following relief measures for the client with nonbreastfeeding engorgement:
   - Wear a tight, supportive bra 24 hours daily.
   - Apply ice to the breasts for approximately 15 to 20 minutes every other hour.
   - Do not stimulate the breasts by squeezing or manually expressing milk from the nipples.
   - Avoid exposing the breasts to warmth.

SECTION III: PRACTICING FOR NCLEX

Activity F **NCLEX-STYLE QUESTIONS**

1. **Answer: a, c, & d**
   RATIONALE: Involution involves three retrogressive processes. The first of these is contraction of muscle fibers, which serves to reduce those previously stretched during pregnancy. Next, catabolism reduces enlarged, individual myometrial cells. Finally, there is regeneration of uterine epithelium from the lower layer of the decidua after the upper layers have been sloughed off and shed during lochia. The breasts do not return to their prepregnancy size as the uterus does. Urinary retention inhibits uterine involution.

2. **Answer: d**
   RATIONALE: Displacement of the uterus from the midline to the right and frequent voiding of small amounts suggests urinary retention with overflow. Catheterization may be necessary to empty the bladder to restore tone. A warm shower and warm compresses are recommended for clients with breastfeeding engorgement. Good body mechanics are recommended to prevent lower back and joint pains.

3. **Answer: b, c, & d**
   RATIONALE: The nurse should tell the client to use warm sitz baths, witch hazel pads, and anesthetic sprays to provide local comfort. Using good body mechanics and maintaining a correct position are important to prevent lower back pain and injury to the joints.

4. **Answer: a**
   RATIONALE: The nurse should recommend that the client practice Kegel exercises to improve pelvic floor tone, strengthen the perineal muscles, and promote healing. Sitz baths are useful in promoting local comfort in a client who had an episiotomy during the birth. Abdominal crunches would not be advised during the initial postpartum period and would not help tone the pelvic floor as much as Kegel exercises.

5. **Answer: a, b, & d**
   RATIONALE: Many women have difficulty with feeling the sensation to void after giving birth if they have received an anesthetic block during labor, which inhibits neural functioning of the bladder. This client will be at risk for incomplete emptying, bladder distention, difficulty voiding, and urinary retention. Ambulation difficulty and perineal lacerations are due to episiotomy.

6. **Answer: c**
   RATIONALE: Postpartum diuresis is due to the buildup and retention of extra fluids during pregnancy. Bruising and swelling of the perineum, swelling of tissues surrounding the urinary meatus, and decreased bladder tone due to anesthesia cause urinary retention.

7. **Answer: b**
   RATIONALE: The nurse should recommend that clients maintain correct position and good body mechanics to prevent pain in the lower back, hips, and joints. Avoiding carrying her baby and soaking several times per day is unrealistic. Application of ice is suggested to help relieve breast engorgement in nonbreastfeeding clients.

8. **Answer: a**
   RATIONALE: The nurse should suggest that the father care for the newborn by holding and talking to the child. Reading up on parental care and speaking to his friends or the physician will not help the father resolve his fears about caring for the child.

9. **Answer: c**
   RATIONALE: The nurse should encourage the client to change her pajamas to prevent chilling and reassure the client that it is normal to have postpartal diaphoresis. Drinking cold fluids at night will not prevent postpartum diaphoresis.

10. **Answer: c**
    RATIONALE: The nurse should tell the client that poor perineal muscular tone may cause urinary incontinence later in life. Kegel exercises are important to improve perineal muscular tone. Pain in the joints and lower back is due to improper body position. Postpartum diuresis is observed in the first week after birth.

11. **Answer: c**
    RATIONALE: The nurse should tell the client to frequently empty the breasts to improve milk supply. Encouraging cold baths and applying ice on the breasts are recommended to relieve engorgement in nonbreastfeeding clients. Kegel exercises are encouraged to promote pelvic floor tone.

12. **Answer: a**
    RATIONALE: The nurse should explain to the client that lochia rubra is a deep red mixture of mucus, tissue debris, and blood. Discharge consisting of leukocytes, decidual tissue, RBCs, and serous fluid is called lochia serosa. Discharge consisting of only RBCs and leukocytes is blood. Discharge consisting of leukocytes and decidual tissue is called lochia alba.

13. **Answer: d**
    RATIONALE: The nurse should explain to the client that the afterpains are due to oxytocin released by the sucking reflex, which strengthens uterine contractions. Prolactin, estrogen, and progesterone cause synthesis and secretion of colostrum.

14. **Answer: d**
    RATIONALE: The abdominal organs, including the diaphragm, typically return to prepregnancy state within 1 to 3 weeks after birth. Discomforts such as shortness of breath and rib aches lessen, and tidal volume and vital capacity return to normal values.

15. **Answer: a, c, & d**
RATIONALE: Many people of Latin American, African, and Asian descent believe that good health involves a balance of heat and cold. The blood loss during childbirth is considered loss of warmth, leaving the woman in a cold state. Therefore, cold foods are avoided during this time. Hot soup and mashed potatoes with gravy would provide the warm foods that are desired.

16. **Answer: c**
RATIONALE: The taking-in phase occurs during the first 24 to 48 hours following the delivery of the newborn and is characterized by the mother taking on a very passive role in caring for herself, as well as recounting her labor experience. The second maternal adjustment phase is the taking-hold phase and usually lasts several weeks after the delivery. This phase is characterized by both dependent and independent behavior, with increasing autonomy. During the letting-go phase the mother reestablishes relationships with others and accepts her new role as a parent. Acquaintance/attachment phase is a newer term that refers to the first 2 to 6 weeks following birth when the mother is learning to care for her baby and is physically recuperating from the pregnancy and delivery.

Answers

CHAPTER 16

SECTION I: ASSESSING YOUR UNDERSTANDING

Activity A FILL IN THE BLANKS

1. peribottle
2. mastitis
3. hypertension
4. Pain
5. Orthostatic
6. fundus
7. cesarean
8. Reciprocity
9. Commitment
10. colostrum

Activity B MATCHING

1. c   2. a   3. d   4. b   5. e

Activity C SHORT ANSWERS

1. Postpartum assessment of the mother typically includes vital signs, pain level, and a systematic head-to-toe review of the body systems: breasts, uterus, bladder, bowels, lochia, episiotomy/perineum, extremities, and emotional status.
2. The new mother might ignore her own needs for health and nutrition. She should be encouraged to take good care of herself and eat a healthy diet so that the nutrients lost during pregnancy can be replaced and she can return to a healthy weight. The nurse should provide nutritional recommendations, such as
   - Eating a wide variety of foods with high nutrient density
   - Using foods and recipes that require little or no preparation
   - Avoiding high-fat, fast foods and fad weight-reduction diets
   - Drinking plenty of fluids
   - Avoiding harmful substances such as alcohol, tobacco, and drugs
   - Avoiding excessive intake of fat, salt, sugar, and caffeine
   - Eating the recommended daily servings from each food group

3. The physical stress of pregnancy and birth, the required caregiving tasks associated with a newborn, meeting the needs of other family members, and fatigue can cause the postpartum period to be quite stressful for the mother.
4. Postpartum danger signs include
   - Fever more than 38° C (100.4° F) after the first 24 hours following birth
   - Foul-smelling lochia or an unexpected change in color or amount
   - Visual changes, such as blurred vision or spots, or headaches
   - Calf pain experienced with dorsiflexion of the foot
   - Swelling, redness, or discharge at the episiotomy site
   - Dysuria, burning, or incomplete emptying of the bladder
   - Shortness of breath or difficulty breathing
   - Depression or extreme mood swings
5. The nurse should model behavior to family members as follows:
   - Holding the newborn close and speaking positively
   - Referring to the newborn by name in front of the parents
   - Speaking directly to the newborn in a calm voice
   - Encouraging both parents to pick up and hold the newborn
   - Monitoring newborn's response to parental stimulation
   - Pointing out positive physical features of the newborn
6. The nurse should suggest the following to the family to avoid sibling rivalry:
   - Expect and tolerate some regression
   - Discuss the new infant during relaxed family times
   - Teach safe handling of the newborn with a doll
   - Encourage older children to verbalize emotions about the newborn
   - Move the sibling from the crib to a youth bed months in advance of the birth of the newborn

SECTION II: APPLYING YOUR KNOWLEDGE

Activity D CASE STUDY

1. The nurse should perform the following assessments in a client intending to breastfeed her baby:
   - Inspect the breasts for size, contour, asymmetry, engorgement, or areas of erythema.
   - Check the nipples for cracks, redness, fissures, or bleeding.
   - Palpate the breasts to ascertain if they are soft, filling, or engorged, and document findings.
   - Palpate the breasts for any nodules, masses, or areas of warmth, which may indicate a plugged duct that may progress to mastitis if not treated promptly.
   - Describe and document any discharge from the nipple that is not creamy yellow or bluish white.

2. The client is encouraged to offer frequent feedings, at least every 2 to 3 hours, using manual expression just before feeding to soften the breast so the newborn can latch on more effectively. The client should be told to allow the newborn to feed on the first breast until it softens before switching to the other side.

SECTION III: PRACTICING FOR NCLEX

Activity E NCLEX-STYLE QUESTIONS

1. **Answer: b**
   RATIONALE: Postpartum assessment is typically performed every 15 minutes for the first hour. After the second hour, assessment is performed every 30 minutes. The client has to be monitored closely during the first hour after delivery; assessment frequencies of 45 or 60 minutes are too long.

2. **Answer: c**
   RATIONALE: Tachycardia in the postpartum woman can suggest anxiety, excitement, fatigue, pain, excessive blood loss, infection, or underlying cardiac problems. Pulmonary edema, atelectasis, and pulmonary embolism are associated with out-of-normal-range changes in respiratory rate.

3. **Answer: d**
   RATIONALE: A boggy or relaxed uterus is a sign of uterine atony. This can be the result of bladder distention, which displaces the uterus upward and to the right, or retained placental fragments. Foul-smelling urine and purulent drainage are signs of infections but are not related to uterine atony. The firm fundus is normal and is not a sign of uterine atony.

4. **Answer: b**
   RATIONALE: "Scant" would describe a 1- to 2-in lochia stain on the perineal pad, or an approximate 10-mL loss. "Light" or "small" would describe an approximate 4-in stain, or a 10- to

25-mL loss. "Moderate" lochia would describe a 4- to 6-in stain, with an estimated loss of 25 to 50 mL. A large or heavy lochia loss would describe pad saturation within an hour after changing it.

5. **Answer: d**
   RATIONALE: The nurse should classify the laceration as fourth degree because it continues through the anterior rectal wall. First-degree laceration involves only skin and superficial structures above muscle; second-degree laceration extends through perineal muscles; and third-degree laceration extends through the anal sphincter muscle but not through the anterior rectal wall.

6. **Answer: c**
   RATIONALE: The nurse should ensure that the ice pack is changed frequently to promote good hygiene and to allow for periodic assessments. Ice packs are wrapped in a disposable covering or clean washcloth and then applied to the perineal area, not directly. The nurse should apply the ice pack for 20 minutes, not 40 minutes. Ice packs should be used for the first 24 hours, not for a week after delivery.

7. **Answer: d**
   RATIONALE: Routine exercise should be resumed gradually, beginning with Kegel exercises on the first postpartum day. The client should be allowed to perform abdominal, buttock, and thigh-toning exercises only during the second week after delivery and not earlier.

8. **Answer: a**
   RATIONALE: The nurse should reassure the mother that some newborns "latch on and catch on" right away, and some newborns take more time and patience; this information will help to reduce the feelings of frustration and uncertainty about their ability to breastfeed. The nurse should also explain that breastfeeding is a learned skill for both parties. It would not be correct to say that breastfeeding is a mechanical procedure. In fact, the nurse should encourage the mother to cuddle and caress the newborn while feeding. The nurse should allow sufficient time to the mother and child to enjoy each other in an unhurried atmosphere. The nurse should teach the mother to burp the newborn frequently. Different positions, such as cradle and football holds and side-lying positions, should be shown to the mother.

9. **Answer: c**
   RATIONALE: The nurse should observe positioning and latching-on technique while breastfeeding so that she may offer suggestions based on observation to correct positioning/latching. This will help minimize trauma to the breast. The client should use only water, not soap, to clean the nipples to prevent dryness. Breast pads with plastic liners should be avoided. Leaving the nursing bra flaps down after feeding allows nipples to air dry.

10. **Answer: b**
   RATIONALE: The nurse should inform the client that intercourse can be resumed if bright-red bleeding stops. Use of water-based gel lubricants can be helpful and should not be avoided. Pelvic floor exercises may enhance sensation and should not be avoided. Barrier methods such as a condom with spermicidal gel or foam should be used instead of oral contraceptives.

11. **Answer: c**
   RATIONALE: The nurse should ensure that the follow-up appointment is fixed for within 2 weeks after hospital discharge. One week after hospital discharge is too early for a follow-up visit, whereas 3 weeks after discharge is too long because the client can develop complications that would go undiagnosed. For clients with an uncomplicated vaginal birth, an office visit is usually scheduled for between 4 and 6 weeks after childbirth.

12. **Answer: a**
   RATIONALE: Mothers who are Rh-negative and have given birth to an infant who is Rh-positive should receive an injection of Rh immunoglobulin within 72 hours after birth; this prevents a sensitization reaction to Rh-positive blood cells received during the birthing process. It may be too late to administer Rh immunoglobulin after 72 hours.

13. **Answer: a & b**
   RATIONALE: Engorged breasts are hard and tender, and the nurse should assess for these signs. Improper positioning of the infant on the breast, not engorged breasts, results in cracked, blistered, fissured, bruised, or bleeding nipples in the breastfeeding woman.

14. **Answer: b, d, & e**
   RATIONALE: Finding active bowel sounds, verification of passing gas, and a nondistended abdomen are normal assessment results. The abdomen should be nontender and soft. Abdominal pain is not a normal assessment finding and should be immediately looked into.

15. **Answer: b, c, & e**
   RATIONALE: The nurse should show mothers how to initiate breastfeeding within 30 minutes of birth. To ensure bonding, place the baby in uninterrupted skin-to-skin contact with the mother. Breastfeeding on demand should be encouraged. Pacifiers do not help fulfill nutritional requirements and are not a part of breastfeeding instruction. The nurse should also ensure that no food or drink other than breast milk is given to newborns.

Answers

CHAPTER 17

SECTION I: ASSESSING YOUR UNDERSTANDING

Activity A FILL IN THE BLANKS

1. Habituation
2. reflex
3. acquired
4. Meconium
5. intestinal
6. amniotic
7. Jaundice
8. hemolysis
9. hemoglobin
10. hypothalamus

Activity B LABELING

A. Conduction
B. Convection
C. Evaporation
D. Radiation

Activity C MATCHING

1. d   2. a   3 c   4. b   5. e

Activity D SHORT ANSWERS

1. The newborn's response to auditory and visual stimuli is demonstrated by the following:
   - Moving the head and eyes to focus on stimulus
   - Staring at the object intently
   - Using sensory capacity to become familiar with people and objects
2. The expected neurobehavioral responses of the newborn include
   - Orientation
   - Habituation
   - Motor maturity
   - Self-quieting ability
   - Social behaviors
3. The following events must occur before the newborn's lungs can maintain respiratory function:
   - Initiation of respiratory movement
   - Expansion of the lungs
   - Establishment of functional residual capacity (ability to retain some air in the lungs on expiration)
   - Increased pulmonary blood flow
   - Redistribution of cardiac output
4. The amniotic fluid is removed from the lungs of a newborn by the following actions:
   - The passage through the birth canal squeezes the thorax, which helps eliminate the fluids in the lungs
   - The action of the pulmonary capillaries and lymphatics removes the remaining fluid
5. The nurse should look for the following signs of abnormality in the newborn's respiration:
   - Labored respiratory effort
   - Respiratory rate less than 30 breaths per minute or greater than 60 breaths per minute
   - Asymmetric chest movements
   - Periodic breathing
   - Apneic periods lasting more than 15 seconds with cyanosis and heart rate changes
6. The nursing interventions that may help minimize regurgitation are
   - Avoiding overfeeding
   - Stimulating frequent burping

SECTION II: APPLYING YOUR KNOWLEDGE

Activity E CASE STUDY

1. Normal factors that increase the heart rate and blood pressure in a newborn are
   - Wakefulness
   - Movement
   - Crying
2. Normal factors affecting the hematologic values of a newborn are
   - Site of the blood sampling
   - Placental transfusion
   - Gestational age
3. The benefits of delayed cord clamping after birth are
   - Improved cardiopulmonary adaptation and oxygen transport
   - Prevention of anemia
   - Increased blood pressures and RBC flow

SECTION III: PRACTICING FOR NCLEX

Activity F NCLEX-STYLE QUESTIONS

1. Answer: b
RATIONALE: The nurse should instruct the mother to keep the newborn wrapped in a blanket, with a cap on its head. This ensures that the newborn is kept warm and helps prevent cold stress. Allowing cool air to circulate over the newborn's body leads to heat loss and is not desirable. Holding the newborn close to the body after taking a shower is not recommended, as the mother's body temperature will be lower than normal after a shower. The nurse need not instruct the client to refrain from using clothing and blankets in the crib. Using clothing and blankets in the crib is actually an effective means of reducing the newborn's exposed surface area and providing external insulation.

2. Answer: a
RATIONALE: Breast milk is a major source of IgA, so breastfeeding is believed to have significant immunologic advantages over formula feeding. The newborn does not depend on IgD and IgE for defense mechanisms. IgM is found in blood and lymph fluid.

3. Answer: a, c, & d
RATIONALE: Limited sweating ability, a crib that is too warm or one that is placed too close to a sunny window, and limited insulation are factors that predispose a newborn to overheating. The immaturity of the newborn's central nervous system makes it difficult to create and maintain balance between heat production, heat gain, and heat loss. Underdeveloped lungs do not increase the risk of overheating. Lack of brown fat will make the infant feel cold, because the infant will not have enough fat stores to burn in response to cold; it does not, however, increase the risk of overheating.

4. Answer: c
RATIONALE: The nurse should look for signs of lethargy and hypotonia in the newborn in order to confirm the occurrence of cold stress. Cold stress does not lead to any color change in the newborn's skin or urine. Cold stress leads to a decrease, not increase, in the newborn's body temperature.

5. Answer: b
RATIONALE: Risk factors for the development of jaundice include drugs such as oxytocin, diazepam, and sulfisoxazole/erythromycin. Breastfeeding, not formula feeding, and male gender are other risk factors. Administering hepatitis A vaccine does not increase the risk of jaundice.

6. Answer: d
RATIONALE: The possibility of fluid overload is increased and must be considered by a nurse when administering IV therapy to a newborn. IV therapy does not significantly increase heart rate or change blood pressure unless fluid overload occurs.

7. Answer: b
RATIONALE: The nurse should tell the client not to worry because it is perfectly normal for the stools of a formula-fed newborn to be greenish, loose, pasty, or formed in consistency, with an unpleasant odor. There is no need to administer vitamin K supplements, increase the newborn's fluid intake, or switch from formula to breast milk.

8. Answer: b
RATIONALE: The ideal caloric intake for a term newborn to regain weight lost in the first week is 108 kcal/kg/day. Eighty-five kcal/kg/day is too little to meet the newborn's requirements, and 156 or 212 kcal/kg/day will be greater than the newborn's requirements.

9. Answer: a
RATIONALE: Preterm newborns are at a greater risk for cold stress than term or postterm newborns. Formula-fed newborns and larger-than-average newborns are not at a greater risk for cold stress than preterm newborns.

10. Answer: a
RATIONALE: The hand-to-mouth movement of the baby indicates the self-quieting ability of a newborn. Movement of the head and eyes, movements of the legs, and hyperactivity do not indicate the self-quieting ability of a newborn.

11. Answer: c
RATIONALE: Typically, a newborn's blood glucose levels are assessed with use of a heel stick sample of blood on admission to the nursery, not 5 or 24 hours after admission to the nursery. It is also not necessary or even reasonable to check the glucose level only after the newborn has been fed.

12. Answer: a
RATIONALE: The nurse should promote early breastfeeding to provide fuels for nonshivering thermogenesis. The nurse can bathe the newborn if he or she is medically stable. The nurse can also use a radiant heat source while bathing the newborn to maintain the temperature. Skin-to-skin contact with the mother should be encouraged, not discouraged, if the newborn is stable. The infant transporter should be kept fully charged and heated at all times.

13. Answer: c
RATIONALE: The nurse should place the temperature probe over the newborn's liver. Skin temperature probes should not be placed over a bony area like the forehead, or an area with brown fat such as the buttocks. The newborn should be in a supine or side-lying position.

14. **Answer: a**
RATIONALE: The nurse should monitor for yellow skin or mucous membranes in a newborn at risk for developing jaundice due to a high bilirubin level. Pinkish appearance of the tongue and bluish skin discoloration are not consequences of increased bilirubin levels. A heart rate of 130 bpm is normal for a newborn.

15. **Answer: d & e**
RATIONALE: The stools of a breastfed newborn are yellowish gold in color. They are not firm in shape or solid. The smell is usually sour. A formula-fed infant's stools are formed in consistency, whereas a breastfed infant's stools are stringy to pasty in consistency.

Answers

CHAPTER 18

SECTION I: ASSESSING YOUR UNDERSTANDING

Activity A FILL IN THE BLANKS

1. Apgar
2. Lanugo
3. Postmature
4. large
5. prothrombin
6. acrocyanosis
7. Milia
8. Harlequin
9. anterior
10. Cephalhematoma

Activity B LABELING

The figure depicts (A) caput succedaneum and (B) cephalhematoma, which are one of several variations in head sizes and appearance for the newborn after delivery. Caput succedaneum describes localized edema on the scalp that occurs from the pressure of the birth process. It is commonly observed after prolonged labor. Cephalhematoma is localized effusion of blood beneath the periosteum of the skull. This condition is due to disruption of the vessels during birth. It occurs after prolonged labor and use of obstetric interventions such as low forceps or vacuum extraction.

Activity C MATCHING

1. b   **2.** a   **3.** c   **4.** d

Activity D SEQUENCING

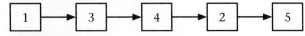

1 → 3 → 4 → 2 → 5

Activity E SHORT ANSWERS

1. The football hold is achieved by holding the infant's back and shoulders in the palm of the mother's hand and tucking the infant under the mother's arm. The infant's ear, shoulder, and hip should be in a straight line. The mother's hand should support the breast and bring it to the infant's lips to latch on until the infant begins to nurse. This position allows the mother to see the infant's mouth as she guides her infant to the nipple. Mothers who have had a cesarean birth can avoid pressure on the incision lines by adopting the football hold position for breastfeeding.

2. Colostrum is a thick, yellowish substance secreted during the first few days after birth. It is high in protein, minerals, and fat-soluble vitamins. It is rich in immunoglobulins (e.g., IgA), which help protect the newborn's GI tract against infections. It is a natural laxative to help rid the intestinal tract of meconium quickly.

3. Fiber optic pads (Biliblanket or Bilivest) are used for treatment of physiologic jaundice and can be wrapped around newborns or newborns can lie upon them. These pads consist of a light that is delivered from a tungsten–halogen bulb through a fiber optic cable and is emitted from the sides and ends of the fibers inside a plastic pad. They work on the premise that phototherapy can be improved by delivering higher-intensity therapeutic light to decrease bilirubin levels. The pads do not produce appreciable heat like banks of lights or spotlights do, so insensible water loss is not increased. Eye patches are also not needed; thus, parents can feed and hold their newborns continuously to promote bonding.

4. The Moro reflex, or the embrace reflex, occurs when the neonate is startled. To elicit this reflex, the newborn is placed on his back. The upper body weight of the supine newborn is supported by the arms with use of a lifting motion, without lifting the newborn off the surface. When the arms are released suddenly, the newborn will throw the arms outward and flex the knees; arms then return to the chest. The fingers also spread to form a C. The newborn initially appears startled and then relaxes to a normal resting position.

5. Caput succedaneum is a localized edema on the scalp that occurs from the pressure of the birth process. It is commonly observed after prolonged labor. Clinically, it appears as a poorly demarcated soft tissue swelling that crosses suture lines. Pitting

edema and overlying petechiae and ecchymosis are noted. The swelling will gradually dissipate in about 3 days without any treatment. Newborns who were delivered via vacuum extraction usually have a caput in the area where the cup was used.

6. Erythema toxicum is a benign, idiopathic, very common, generalized, transient rash occurring in as many as 70% of all newborns during the first week of life. It consists of small papules or pustules on the skin resembling flea bites. The rash is common on the face, chest, and back. One of the chief characteristics of this rash is its lack of pattern. It is caused by the newborn's eosinophils reacting to the environment as the immune system matures. It does not require any treatment, and it disappears in a few days.

SECTION II: APPLYING YOUR KNOWLEDGE

Activity F CASE STUDY

1. The nurse should inform the mother that newborns usually sleep for up to 20 hours daily, for periods of 2 to 4 hours at a time, but not through the night. This is because their stomach capacity is too small to go long periods of time without nourishment. All newborns develop their own sleep patterns and cycles.

2. The nurse should ask the mother to place the newborn on her back to sleep; remove all fluffy bedding, quilts, sheepskins, stuffed animals, and pillows from the crib to prevent potential suffocation. Parents should avoid unsafe conditions such as placing the newborn in the prone position, using a crib that does not meet federal safety guidelines, allowing window cords to hang loose and in close proximity to the crib, or having the room temperature too high, causing overheating.

3. The nurse should educate Karen about potential risks of bed-sharing. Bringing a newborn into bed to nurse or quiet her down and then falling asleep with the newborn is not a safe practice. Infants who sleep in adult beds are up to 40 times more likely to suffocate than those who sleep in cribs. Suffocation also can occur when the infant gets entangled in bedding or caught under pillows, or slips between the bed and the wall or the headboard and mattress. It can also happen when someone accidentally rolls against or on top of them. Therefore, the safest sleeping location for all newborns is in their crib, without any movable objects close.

SECTION III: PRACTICING FOR NCLEX

Activity G NCLEX-STYLE QUESTIONS

1. **Answer: b**
RATIONALE: The nurse should complete the second assessment for the newborn within the first 2 to 4 hours, when the newborn is in the nursery. The nurse should complete the initial newborn assessment in the birthing area and the third assessment before the newborn is discharged.

2. **Answer: d**
RATIONALE: The nurse should place the newborn skin-to-skin with mother. This would help to maintain baby's temperature as well as promote breastfeeding and bonding between the mother and baby. The nurse can weigh the infant as long as a warmed cover is placed on the scale. The stethoscope should be warmed before it makes contact with the infant's skin, rather than using the stethoscope over the garment because it may obscure the reading. The newborn's crib should not be placed close to the outer walls in the room to prevent heat loss through radiation.

3. **Answer: a**
RATIONALE: Skin turgor is checked by pinching the skin over chest or abdomen and noting the return to original position; if the skin remains "tented" after pinching, it denotes dehydration. Stork bites or salmon patches, unopened sebaceous glands, and blue or purple splotches on buttocks are common skin variations not related to skin turgor.

4. **Answer: c**
RATIONALE: As per the recommendations of AAP, all newborns should receive a daily supplement of vitamin D during the first 2 months of life to prevent rickets and vitamin D deficiency. There is no need to feed the newborn water, as breast milk contains enough water to meet the newborn's needs. Iron supplements need not be given, as the newborn is being breastfed. Infants over 6 months of age are given fluoride supplementation if they are not receiving fluoridated water.

5. **Answer: a**
RATIONALE: The nurse should instruct the woman to use the sealed and chilled milk within 24 hours. The nurse should not instruct the woman to use frozen milk within 6 months of obtaining it, to use microwave ovens to warm chilled milk, or to refreeze the used milk and reuse it. Instead, the nurse should instruct the woman to use frozen milk within 3 months of obtaining it, to avoid using microwave ovens to warm chilled milk, and to discard any used milk and never refreeze it.

6. **Answer: a**
RATIONALE: The nurse should ask the mother to hold the baby upright with the baby's head on her mother's shoulder. Alternatively, the nurse can also suggest the mother sit with the newborn on her lap with the newborn lying face down. Gently rubbing the baby's abdomen or giving frequent sips of warm water to the infant will not significantly induce burping; burping is induced by the newborn's position. Placing the baby on her back while trying to elicit burping after feeding may cause choking or aspiration.

7. **Answer: b**
   RATIONALE: A sign of adequate formula intake is when the newborn seems satisfied and is gaining weight regularly. The formula fed newborn should take 30 minutes or less to finish a bottle, not less than 15 minutes. The newborn does normally produce several stools per day, but should wet 6 to 10 diapers rather than 3 to 4 per day. The newborn should consume approximately 2 oz of formula per pound of body weight per day, not per feeding.

8. **Answer: d**
   RATIONALE: A concentration of immature blood vessels causes salmon patches. Mongolian spots are caused by a concentration of pigmented cells and usually disappear within the first 4 years of life. Erythema toxicum is caused by the newborn's eosinophils reacting to the environment as the immune system matures, and Harlequin sign is a result of immature autoregulation of blood flow and is commonly seen in low-birth-weight newborns.

9. **Answer: c**
   RATIONALE: The nurse should obtain a newborn's temperature by placing an electronic temperature probe in the midaxillary area. The nurse should not tape an electronic thermistor probe to the abdominal skin, as this method is applied only when the newborn is placed under a radiant heat source. Rectal temperatures are no longer taken because of the risk of perforation. Oral temperature readings are not taken for newborns.

10. **Answer: c**
    RATIONALE: The nurse should conclude that the newborn is facing moderate difficulty in adjusting to extrauterine life. The nurse need not conclude severe distress in adjusting to extrauterine life, better condition of the newborn, or abnormal central nervous system status. If the Apgar score is 8 points or higher, it indicates that the condition of the newborn is better. An Apgar score of 0 to 3 points represents severe distress in adjusting to extrauterine life.

11. **Answer: a**
    RATIONALE: The nurse should instruct the parent to expose the newborn's bottom to air several times per day to prevent diaper rashes. Use of plastic pants and products such as powder and items with fragrance should be avoided. The parent should be instructed to place the newborn's buttocks in warm water after having had a diaper on all night.

12. **Answer: b, d, & e**
    RATIONALE: The nurse should give the newborn oxygen, ensure the newborn's warmth, and observe the newborn's respiratory status frequently. The nurse need not give the newborn warm water to drink or massage the newborn's back.

13. **Answer: a, c, & e**
    RATIONALE: The nurse should monitor the newborn for lethargy, cyanosis, and jitteriness. Low-pitched crying or rashes on the infant's skin are not signs generally associated with hypoglycemia.

14. **Answer: a, c, & e**
    RATIONALE: To relieve breast engorgement in the client, the nurse should educate the client to take warm-to-hot showers to encourage milk release, express some milk manually before breastfeeding, and apply warm compresses to the breasts before nursing. The mother should be asked to feed the newborn in a variety of positions—sitting up and then lying down. The breasts should be massaged from under the axillary area, down toward the nipple.

15. **Answer: a, c, & e**
    RATIONALE: Mongolian spots, swollen genitals in the female baby, and a short, creased neck are normal findings in a newborn. Mongolian spots are blue or purple splotches that appear on the lower back and buttocks of newborns. Female babies may have swollen genitals as a result of maternal estrogen. The newborn's neck will appear almost nonexistent because it is so short. Creases are usually noted. Enlarged fontanelles are associated with malnutrition; hydrocephaly; congenital hypothyroidism; trisomies 13, 18, and 21; and various bone disorders such as osteogenesis imperfecta. Low-set ears are characteristic of many syndromes and genetic abnormalities such as trisomies 13 and 18 and internal organ abnormalities involving the renal system.

Answers

CHAPTER 19

SECTION I: ASSESSING YOUR UNDERSTANDING

Activity A FILL IN THE BLANKS

1. Oligohydramnios
2. Clonus
3. latent
4. hyperreflexia
5. incompatibility
6. Monozygotic
7. infection
8. spontaneous
9. first
10. Gestational

Activity B MATCHING

1. c   **2.** e   **3.** a   **4.** b   **5.** d

Activity C SEQUENCING

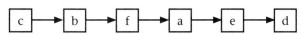

Activity D SHORT ANSWERS

1. Possible complications of hyperemesis gravidarum include persistent, uncontrollable nausea, dehydration, acid–base imbalances, electrolyte imbalances, and weight loss. If the condition is allowed to continue, it jeopardizes fetal well-being.
2. Conditions commonly associated with early bleeding (first half of pregnancy) include spontaneous abortion, ectopic pregnancy, and gestational trophoblastic disease.
3. Ectopic pregnancies usually result from conditions that obstruct or slow the passage of the fertilized ovum through the fallopian tube to the uterus. This may be a physical blockage in the tube or failure of the tubal epithelium to move the zygote (the cell formed after the egg is fertilized) down the tube into the uterus. In the general population, most cases are the result of tubal scarring secondary to PID. Organisms such as *Neisseria gonorrhoeae* and *Chlamydia trachomatis* preferentially attack the fallopian tubes, producing silent infections.

4. Risk factors for hyperemesis gravidarum include young age, nausea and vomiting with previous pregnancy, history of intolerance of oral contraceptives, nulliparity, trophoblastic disease, multiple gestation, emotional or psychological stress, gastroesophageal reflux disease, primigravida status, obesity, hyperthyroidism, and *Helicobacter pylori* seropositivity.
5. A nurse should include the following in prevention education for ectopic pregnancies:
   - Reducing risk factors such as sexual intercourse with multiple partners or intercourse without a condom
   - Avoiding contracting STIs that lead to PID
   - Obtaining early diagnosis and adequate treatment of STIs
   - Avoiding the use of an intrauterine contraception (IUC) as a contraceptive method to reduce the risk of repeat ascending infections responsible for tubal scarring
   - Using condoms to decrease the risk of infections that cause tubal scarring
   - Seeking prenatal care early if pregnant, to confirm location of pregnancy
6. The Kleihauer–Betke test detects fetal RBCs in the maternal circulation, determines the degree of fetal–maternal hemorrhage, and helps calculate the appropriate dosage of RhoGAM to give for Rh-negative clients.

SECTION II: APPLYING YOUR KNOWLEDGE

Activity E CASE STUDY

1. Recognizing preterm labor at an early stage requires that the expectant mother and her health care team identify the subtle symptoms of preterm labor. These may include
   - Change or increase in vaginal discharge
   - Pelvic pressure (pushing down sensation)
   - Low, dull backache
   - Menstrual-like cramps
   - Uterine contractions, with or without pain
   - Intestinal cramping, with or without diarrhea
2. The nurse must teach Jenna how to palpate and time uterine contractions. Provide written

materials to support this education at a level and in a language appropriate for her. Also, educate Jenna about the importance of prenatal care, risk reduction, and recognizing the signs and symptoms of preterm labor. The nurse may also include

- Stressing good hydration and consumption of a nutritious diet
- Advising against any activity, such as sexual activity or nipple stimulation, that might stimulate oxytocin release and initiate uterine contractions
- Assessing stress levels of client and family and making appropriate referrals
- Providing emotional support and client empowerment throughout
- Emphasizing the possible need for more frequent office visits and for notifying the health care provider if she has questions or concerns.

SECTION III: PRACTICING FOR NCLEX

Activity F NCLEX-STYLE QUESTIONS

1. **Answer: c**
   RATIONALE: The nurse should instruct the client with hyperemesis gravidarum to eat small, frequent meals throughout the day to minimize nausea and vomiting. The nurse should also instruct the client to avoid lying down or reclining for at least 2 hours after eating and to increase the intake of carbonated beverages. The nurse should instruct the client to try foods that settle the stomach such as dry crackers, toast, or soda.

2. **Answer: a**
   RATIONALE: A temperature elevation or an increase in the pulse of a client with PROM would indicate infection. Increase in the pulse does not indicate preterm labor or cord compression. The nurse should monitor FHR patterns continuously, reporting any variable decelerations suggesting cord compression. Respiratory distress syndrome is one of the perinatal risks associated with PROM.

3. **Answer: c**
   RATIONALE: The nurse should closely assess the woman for hemorrhage after giving birth by frequently assessing uterine involution. Assessing skin turgor and blood pressure and monitoring hCG titers will not help to determine hemorrhage.

4. **Answer: b**
   RATIONALE: When meconium is present in the amniotic fluid, it typically indicates fetal distress related to hypoxia. Meconium stains the fluid yellow to greenish brown, depending on the amount present. A decreased amount of amniotic fluid reduces the cushioning effect, thereby making cord compression a possibility. A foul odor of amniotic fluid indicates infection. Meconium in the amniotic fluid does not indicate CNS involvement.

5. **Answer: d**
   RATIONALE: The nurse should institute and maintain seizure precautions such as padding the side rails and having oxygen, suction equipment, and call light readily available to protect the client from injury. The nurse should provide a quiet, darkened room to stabilize the client. The nurse should maintain the client on complete bed rest in the left lateral lying position and not in a supine position. Keeping the head of the bed slightly elevated will not help maintain seizure precautions.

6. **Answer: a**
   RATIONALE: If the client is receiving magnesium sulfate to suppress or control seizures, assess deep tendon reflexes to determine the effectiveness of therapy. Common sites utilized to assess deep tendon reflexes are the biceps reflex, triceps reflex, patellar reflex, Achilles reflex, and plantar reflex. Assessing the mucous membranes for dryness and skin turgor for dehydration are the required interventions when caring for a client with hyperemesis gravidarum. Monitoring intake and output will not help to determine the effectiveness of therapy.

7. **Answer: d**
   RATIONALE: A previous myomectomy to remove fibroids can be associated with the cause of placenta previa. Risk factors also include advanced maternal age (greater than 30 years old). A structurally defective cervix cannot be associated with the cause of placenta previa. However, it can be associated with the cause of cervical insufficiency. Alcohol ingestion is not a risk factor for developing placenta previa but is associated with abruptio placenta.

8. **Answer: b**
   RATIONALE: The nurse should encourage a client with mild elevations in blood pressure to rest as much as possible in the lateral recumbent position to improve uteroplacental blood flow, reduce blood pressure, and promote diuresis. The nurse should maintain the client with severe preeclampsia on complete bed rest in the left lateral lying position. Keeping the head of the bed slightly elevated will not help to improve the condition of the client with mild elevations in blood pressure.

9. **Answer: d**
   RATIONALE: The first choice for fluid replacement is generally 5% dextrose in lactated Ringer solution with vitamins and electrolytes added. If the client does not improve after several days of bed rest, "gut rest," IV fluids, and antiemetics, then total parenteral nutrition or percutaneous endoscopic gastrostomy tube feeding is instituted to prevent malnutrition.

10. **Answer: c**
    RATIONALE: The classic manifestations of abruptio placenta are painful dark red vaginal bleeding,

"knife-like" abdominal pain, uterine tenderness, contractions, and decreased fetal movement. Painless bright red vaginal bleeding is the clinical manifestation of placenta previa. Generalized vasospasm is the clinical manifestation of preeclampsia and not of abruptio placenta.

11. **Answer: a**
    RATIONALE: The symptoms if rupture or hemorrhaging occurs before successfully treating the pregnancy are lower abdomen pain, feelings of faintness, phrenic nerve irritation, hypotension, marked abdominal tenderness with distension, and hypovolemic shock. Painless bright red vaginal bleeding occurring during the second or third trimester is the clinical manifestation of placenta previa. Fetal distress and tetanic contractions are not the symptoms observed in a client if rupture or hemorrhaging occurs before successfully treating an ectopic pregnancy.

12. **Answer: d**
    RATIONALE: When the woman arrives and is admitted, assessing her vital signs, the amount and color of the bleeding, and current pain rating on a scale of 1 to 10 are the priorities. Assessing the signs of shock, monitoring uterine contractility, and determining the amount of funneling are not priority assessments when a pregnant woman complaining of vaginal bleeding is admitted to the hospital.

13. **Answer: c**
    RATIONALE: A nurse should closely monitor the client's vital signs, bleeding (peritoneal or vaginal) to identify hypovolemic shock that may occur with tubal rupture. Beta-hCG level is monitored to diagnose an ectopic pregnancy or impending abortion. Monitoring the mass with transvaginal ultrasound and determining the size of the mass are done for diagnosing an ectopic pregnancy. Monitoring the FHR does not help to identify hypovolemic shock.

14. **Answer: a**
    RATIONALE: The current recommendation is that every Rh-negative nonimmunized woman receives RhoGAM at 28 weeks' gestation and again within 72 hours after giving birth. Consuming a well-balanced nutritional diet and avoiding sexual activity until after 28 weeks will not help to prevent complications of blood incompatibility. Transvaginal ultrasound helps to validate the position of the placenta and will not help to prevent complications of blood incompatibility.

15. **Answer: c**
    RATIONALE: The nurse should know that coma usually follows an eclamptic seizure. Muscle rigidity occurs after facial twitching. Respirations do not become rapid during the seizure; they cease. Coma usually follows the seizure activity, with respiration resuming.

16. **Answer: d**
    RATIONALE: The nurse should know that dependent edema may be seen in the sacral area if the client is on bed rest. Pitting edema leaves a small depression or pit after finger pressure is applied to a swollen area and can be measured. Dependent edema may occur in clients who are both ambulatory and on bed rest.

17. **Answer: a, c, & d**
    RATIONALE: Signs such as a change or increase in vaginal discharge, rupture of membranes, and uterine contractions should be further assessed as a possible sign of preterm labor. Phrenic nerve irritation and hypovolemic shock are the symptoms if rupture or hemorrhaging occurs before successfully treating the ectopic pregnancy.

18. **Answer: a, b, & e**
    RATIONALE: The associated conditions and complications of premature rupture of the membranes are infection, prolapsed cord, abruptio placenta, and preterm labor. Spontaneous abortion and placenta previa are not associated conditions or complications of premature rupture of the membranes.

19. **Answer: b, d, & e**
    RATIONALE: The signs and symptoms of HELLP syndrome are nausea, malaise, epigastric pain, upper right quadrant pain, demonstrable edema, and hyperbilirubinemia. Blood pressure higher than 160/110 and oliguria are the symptoms of severe preeclampsia rather than HELLP syndrome.

20. **Answer: b, d, & e**
    RATIONALE: Adverse effects commonly associated with misoprostol include dyspepsia, hypotension, tachycardia, diarrhea, abdominal pain, and vomiting. Constipation and headache are not adverse effects commonly associated with misoprostol.

Answers

CHAPTER 20

SECTION I: ASSESSING YOUR UNDERSTANDING

Activity A FILL IN THE BLANKS

1. somatotropin
2. Gestational
3. airway
4. lung
5. Anemia
6. Group B streptococcus
7. Toxoplasmosis
8. Adolescence
9. Nicotine
10. cocaine

Activity B MATCHING

1. f   **2.** e   **3.** d   **4.** c   **5.** b   **6.** a

Activity C SHORT ANSWERS

1. The most common complications in a pregnant client with hypertension are
   - Increased risk for developing preeclampsia
   - Decreased uteroplacental perfusion
2. The nurse should include the following elements during the physical examination of pregnant clients with asthma:
   - Rate, rhythm, and depth of respirations
   - Auscultation of lung sounds
   - Skin color
   - Blood pressure
   - Pulse rate
   - Evaluation for signs of fatigue
3. The nurse should include the following factors in the teaching plan for a client with asthma:
   - Signs and symptoms of asthma progression and exacerbation
   - Importance and safety of medication to fetus and to herself
   - Warning signs; potential harm to fetus and self by undertreatment or delay in seeking help
   - Prevention and avoidance of known triggers
   - Home use of metered-dose inhalers
   - Adverse effects of medications

4. Assessment of tuberculosis in pregnant clients includes the following:
   - At antepartum visits, the nurse should be alert for clinical manifestations of tuberculosis such as fatigue, fever or night sweats, nonproductive cough, slow weight loss, anemia, hemoptysis, and anorexia.
   - If tuberculosis is suspected or the woman is at risk for developing tuberculosis, the nurse should anticipate screening with purified protein derivative administered by intradermal injection; if the client has been exposed to tuberculosis, a reddened induration will appear within 72 hours.
   - A follow-up chest X-ray with a lead shield over the abdomen and sputum cultures will confirm the diagnosis.
5. The developmental tasks associated with adolescent behavior are
   - Seeking economic and social stability
   - Developing a personal value system
   - Building meaningful relationships with others
   - Becoming comfortable with their changing bodies
   - Working to become independent from their parents
   - Learning to verbalize conceptually
6. The effects of sedatives by the mother on her infant are as follows:
   - Sedatives easily cross the placenta and cause birth defects and behavioral problems
   - Infants born to mothers who abuse sedatives may be physically dependent on the drugs and prone to respiratory problems, feeding difficulties, disturbed sleep, sweating, irritability, and fever

SECTION II: APPLYING YOUR KNOWLEDGE

Activity D CASE STUDY

1. The greatest increase in asthma attacks in the pregnant client usually occurs between 24 and 36 weeks' gestation; flare-ups are rare during the last 4 weeks of pregnancy and during labor.
2. Successful management of asthma in pregnancy involves
   - Drug therapy

- Client education
- Elimination of environmental triggers

3. The following are the nursing interventions involved when caring for the pregnant client with asthma during labor:
   - Monitor client's oxygen saturation by pulse oximetry.
   - Provide pain management through epidural analgesia.
   - Continuously monitor the fetus for distress during labor and assess FHR patterns for indications of hypoxia.
   - Assess the newborn for signs and symptoms of hypoxia.

SECTION III: PRACTICING FOR NCLEX

Activity E NCLEX-STYLE QUESTIONS

1. **Answer: b**
   RATIONALE: The nurse should identify postprandial hyperglycemia as the effect of insulin resistance in the client. Hypertension, hypercholesterolemia, and myocardial infarction are not the effects of insulin resistance in a diabetic client.

2. **Answer: a**
   RATIONALE: The nurse should identify respiratory distress syndrome as a major risk that can be faced by the offspring of a client with cardiovascular disease. Congenital varicella syndrome can occur in an offspring of a mother infected with varicella during early pregnancy. SIDS can occur in an offspring of a mother who smokes during pregnancy. Prune belly syndrome is a fetal anomaly associated with cocaine use in early pregnancy.

3. **Answer: b**
   RATIONALE: The nurse should stress the positive benefits of a healthy lifestyle during the preconception counseling of a client with chronic hypertension. The client need not avoid dairy products or increase intake of vitamin D supplements. It may not be advisable for a client with chronic hypertension to exercise without consultation.

4. **Answer: a**
   RATIONALE: Swelling of the face is a symptom of cardiac decompensation, along with moist, frequent cough and rapid respirations. Dry, rasping cough; slow, labored respiration; and an elevated temperature are not symptoms of cardiac decompensation.

5. **Answer: d**
   RATIONALE: The nurse should assess the client with heart disease for cardiac decompensation, which is most common from 28 to 32 weeks of gestation and in the first 48 hours postpartum. Limiting sodium intake, inspecting the extremities for edema, and ensuring that the client consumes a high-fiber diet are interventions during pregnancy, not in the first 48 hours postpartum.

6. **Answer: b**
   RATIONALE: The nurse should evaluate for signs of fatigue during the physical examination of a client with asthma. The nurse need not monitor the client's temperature, frequency of headache, or feelings of nausea because these conditions are not related to asthma.

7. **Answer: a**
   RATIONALE: The nurse should instruct the pregnant client with tuberculosis to maintain adequate hydration as a health-promoting activity. The client need not avoid direct sunlight or red meat, or wear light clothes; these have no impact on the client's condition.

8. **Answer: c**
   RATIONALE: The nurse should identify preterm birth as a risk associated with anemia during pregnancy. Anemia during pregnancy does not increase the risk of a newborn with heart problems, an enlarged liver, or fetal asphyxia.

9. **Answer: a, b, c, & d**
   RATIONALE: The nurse should assess for possible fluid overload in a client with cardiovascular disease who has just delivered. Signs of fluid overload in the client who has just labored include cough, progressive dyspnea, edema, palpitations, and crackles in the lung bases. Hemoglobin and hematocrit levels are not affected by laboring of the client with cardiovascular disease.

10. **Answer: a**
    RATIONALE: The nurse should stress the importance of good hand-washing and use of sound hygiene practices to reduce transmission of the virus to a client who could pass the virus on to her fetus. Drinking plenty of fluids will not help minimize this risk. The client need not take antibiotics if she has not been infected. It is not practical for the client to avoid interaction with children.

11. **Answer: d**
    RATIONALE: The nurse should address the client's knowledge of child development during assessment of the pregnant adolescent client. The nurse need not address the sexual development of the client or whether sex was consensual. This would not be an opportune time to discuss birth control methods to be used after the pregnancy.

12. **Answer: d**
    RATIONALE: Class I recommendations (no physical activity limitations) are suggested for client's who are asymptomatic and exhibit no objective evidence of cardiac disease. The functional classifications system consists of Class I to IV, based on past and present disability and physical signs resulting from cardiac disease.

13. **Answer: d**
    RATIONALE: The nurse should stress the avoidance of breastfeeding when counseling a pregnant client who is HIV positive. The client's

relationship with the spouse, contact with the infant, and the plan for future pregnancies is not the highest priority at this time.

14. **Answer: b**
RATIONALE: RAFFT is the acronym for a screening tool used to help in determining the abuse of drugs during the assessment of a client. The "R" in raft refers to asking the client if she drinks or takes drugs to relax, improve her self-image, or help her fit in.

15. **Answer: b**
RATIONALE: The nurse should make the client aware of increased risk of anemia as a possible effect of maternal coffee consumption during pregnancy, as it decreases iron absorption. Maternal coffee consumption during pregnancy does not increase the risk of heart disease, rickets, or scurvy.

16. **Answer: a, b, & e**
RATIONALE: To minimize risk of toxoplasmosis, the nurse should instruct the client to eat meat that has been cooked to an internal temperature of 160° F throughout and to avoid cleaning the cat's litter box or performing activities such as gardening. Avoiding children with colds is unreasonable when working with children, and contact with children with colds is not a cause of toxoplasmosis. The cat should be kept indoors to prevent it from hunting and eating birds or rodents.

17. **Answer: c, d, & e**
RATIONALE: Obesity, hypertension, and a previous infant weighing more than 9 lb are risk factors for developing gestational diabetes. Maternal age less than 18 years and genitourinary tract abnormalities do not increase the risk of developing gestational diabetes.

18. **Answer: a, d, & e**
RATIONALE: The nurse caring for a pregnant client with sickle cell anemia should teach the client meticulous hand-washing to prevent the risk of infection, assess the hydration status of the client at each visit, and urge the client to drink 8 to 10 glasses of fluid daily. The nurse need not assess serum electrolyte levels of the client at each visit or instruct the client to consume protein-rich food.

19. **Answer: a**
RATIONALE: The nurse should assess for small head circumference in a newborn being assessed for fetal alcohol spectrum disorder. Fetal alcohol spectrum disorder does not cause decreased blood glucose level, a poor breathing pattern, or wide eyes.

20. **Answer: b**
RATIONALE: The nurse should stress the inclusion of complex carbohydrates in the diet in the dietary plan for a pregnant woman with pregestational diabetes. The pregnant client with pregestational diabetes need not include more dairy products in the diet, eat only two meals per day, or eat at least one egg per day; these have no impact on the client's condition.

Answers

CHAPTER 21

SECTION I: ASSESSING YOUR UNDERSTANDING

Activity A FILL IN THE BLANKS

1. dystocia
2. Breech
3. Leopold
4. Tocolytic
5. Steroids
6. fibronectin
7. Bishop
8. Hygroscopic
9. amniotomy
10. Oxytocin

Activity B LABELING

The figures depict prolapsed cord. **A.** Prolapse within the uterus. **B.** Prolapse with the cord visible at the vulva.

Activity C MATCHING

1. c **2.** a **3.** e **4.** b **5.** d

Activity D SEQUENCING

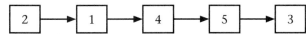

Activity E SHORT ANSWERS

1. The symptoms of preterm labor are
   - Change or increase in vaginal discharge
   - Pelvic pressure (pushing down sensation)
   - Low, dull backache
   - Menstrual-like cramps
   - Heaviness or aching in the thighs
   - Uterine contractions, with or without pain
   - Intestinal cramping, with or without diarrhea
2. Cervical ripeness is an assessment of the readiness of the cervix to efface and dilate in response to uterine contractions. It is an important variable when labor induction is being considered. A ripe cervix is shortened, centered (anterior), softened, and partially dilated. An unripe cervix is long, closed, posterior, and firm. Cervical ripening usually begins before the onset of labor

contractions and is necessary for cervical dilatation and the passage of the fetus.

3. Uterine rupture is a catastrophic tearing of the uterus at the site of a previous scar into the abdominal cavity. The onset is often marked only by sudden fetal bradycardia, and the obliteration of intrauterine pressure/cessation of contractions. Treatment requires rapid surgical attention. In uterine rupture, fetal morbidity occurs secondary to catastrophic hemorrhage, fetal anoxia, or both.
4. Indications of amnioinfusion are severe variable decelerations due to cord compression, oligohydramnios due to placental insufficiency, postmaturity or rupture of membranes, preterm labor with premature rupture of membranes, and thick meconium fluid. Vaginal bleeding of unknown origin, umbilical cord prolapse, amnionitis, uterine hypertonicity, and severe fetal distress are contraindications to amnioinfusion.
5. The nurse assesses each client to help predict her risk status. The nurse should be aware that cord prolapse is more common in pregnancies involving malpresentation, growth restriction, prematurity, ruptured membranes with a fetus at a high station, hydramnios, grand multiparity, and multifetal gestation. The client and fetus should be thoroughly assessed to detect changes and evaluate the effectiveness of any interventions performed.
6. Shoulder dystocia can cause postpartum hemorrhage, secondary to uterine atony or vaginal lacerations in the mother. In the fetus, shoulder dystocia can result in transient and/or permanent Erb or Duchenne brachial plexus palsies and clavicular or humeral fractures, as well as hypoxic encephalopathy.

SECTION II: APPLYING YOUR KNOWLEDGE

Activity F CASE STUDY

1. The nurse should perform the following interventions during amnioinfusion to prevent maternal and fetal complications:
   - Explain the need for the procedure, what it involves, and how it may solve the problem.

- Inform the mother that she will need to remain on bed rest during the procedure.
- Assess the mother's vital signs and associated discomfort level.
- Maintain adequate intake and output records.
- Assess the duration and intensity of uterine contractions frequently to identify overdistention or increased uterine tone.
- Monitor FHR pattern to determine whether the amnioinfusion is improving the fetal status.
- Prepare the mother for a possible cesarean birth if the FHR does not improve after the amnioinfusion.

SECTION III: PRACTICING FOR NCLEX

Activity G NCLEX-STYLE QUESTIONS

1. **Answer: a**
   RATIONALE: A forceps-and-vacuum-assisted birth is required for the client having a prolonged second stage of labor. In cases of uterine rupture, the baby has to be immediately delivered by cesarean section. Oligohydramnios due to placental insufficiency and preterm labor with premature rupture of membranes are treated with amnioinfusion.

2. **Answer: d**
   RATIONALE: The nurse should know that gestational hypertension leads to placental abruption. Other factors leading to placental abruption include preeclampsia, seizure activity, uterine rupture, trauma, smoking, cocaine use, coagulation defects, previous history of abruption, domestic violence, and placental pathology. These conditions may force blood into the under layer of the placenta and cause it to detach. Gestational diabetes, cardiovascular disease, and excess weight gain during pregnancy, though dangerous conditions, are not known to specifically cause placental abruption.

3. **Answer: a & e**
   RATIONALE: The nurse should monitor cyanosis and pulmonary edema when caring for a client with amniotic fluid embolism. Other signs and symptoms of this condition include hypotension, cyanosis, seizures, tachycardia, coagulation failure, disseminated intravascular coagulation, uterine atony with subsequent hemorrhage, adult respiratory distress syndrome, and cardiac arrest. Arrhythmia, hematuria, and hyperglycemia are not known to occur in cases of amniotic fluid embolism. Hematuria is seen in clients having uterine rupture.

4. **Answer: a**
   RATIONALE: Chorioamnionitis is an indication for labor induction. Complete placenta previa, abruptio placenta, and transverse fetal lie are contraindications for labor induction.

5. **Answer: a**
   RATIONALE: The nurse should ensure that the client does not have uterine hypertonicity to confirm that amnioinfusion is not contraindicated. Other factors that enforce contraindication of amnioinfusion include vaginal bleeding of unknown origin, umbilical cord prolapse, amnionitis, and severe fetal distress. Active genital herpes infection, abruptio placentae, and invasive cervical cancer are conditions that enforce contraindication of labor induction rather than amnioinfusion.

6. **Answer: d**
   RATIONALE: The nurse should identify nerve damage as a risk to the fetus in cases of shoulder dystocia. Other fetal risks include asphyxia, clavicle fracture, central nervous system injury or dysfunction, and death. Bladder injury, infection, and extensive lacerations are poor maternal outcomes due to the occurrence of shoulder dystocia.

7. **Answer: a**
   RATIONALE: A Bishop score of less than 6 indicates that a cervical ripening method should be used before inducing labor. A low Bishop score is not an indication for cesarean birth; there are several other factors that need to be considered for a cesarean birth. A Bishop score of less than 6 indicates that vaginal birth will be unsuccessful and prolonged because the duration of labor is inversely correlated with the Bishop score.

8. **Answer: a**
   RATIONALE: When caring for a client who has undergone a cesarean section, the nurse should assess the client's uterine tone to determine fundal firmness. The nurse should assist with breastfeeding initiation and offer continued support. The nurse can also suggest alternate positioning techniques to reduce incisional discomfort while breastfeeding. Delaying breastfeeding may not be required. The nurse should encourage the client to cough, perform deep-breathing exercises, and use the incentive spirometer every 2 hours. The nurse should assist the client with early ambulation to prevent respiratory and cardiovascular problems.

9. **Answer: d**
   RATIONALE: Overdistended uterus is a contraindication for oxytocin administration. Postterm status, dysfunctional labor pattern, and prolonged ruptured membranes are indications for administration of oxytocin.

10. **Answer: a**
    RATIONALE: The nurse caring for the client in labor with shoulder dystocia of the fetus should assist with positioning the client in squatting position. The client can also be helped into the

hands and knees position or lateral recumbent position for birth, to free the shoulders. Assessing for complaints of intense back pain in first stage of labor, anticipating possible use of forceps to rotate to anterior position at birth, and assessing for prolonged second stage of labor with arrest of descent are important interventions when caring for a client with persistent occiput posterior position of fetus.

11. **Answer: a**
    RATIONALE: The nurse should assess infertility treatment as a contributor to increased probability of multiple gestations. Multiple gestations do not occur with an adolescent delivery; instead, chances of multiple gestations are known to decrease due to the increasing number of women giving birth at older ages. Medications and advanced maternal age are not known to cause multiple gestations.

12. **Answer: d**
    RATIONALE: Cephalopelvic disproportion is associated with postterm pregnancy. Underdeveloped suck reflex, congenital heart defects, and intraventricular hemorrhage are associated with preterm pregnancy.

13. **Answer: c**
    RATIONALE: The nurse should assess for fetal complications such as head trauma associated with intracranial hemorrhage, nerve damage, and

hypoxia in cases of precipitous labor. Facial and scalp lacerations, facial nerve injury, and cephalhematoma are all newborn traumas associated with the use of the forceps of vacuum extractors during birth. These conditions are not neonatal complications associated with precipitous labor.

14. **Answer: c & e**
    RATIONALE: Prolonged pregnancy and hypertension are causes of intrauterine fetal demise in late pregnancy that the nurse should be aware of. Other factors resulting in intrauterine fetal demise include infection, advanced maternal age, Rh disease, uterine rupture, diabetes, congenital anomalies, cord accident, abruption, premature rupture of membranes, or hemorrhage. Hydramnios, multifetal gestation, and malpresentation are not the causes of intrauterine fetal demise in late pregnancy; they are causes of umbilical cord prolapse.

15. **Answer: a**
    RATIONALE: The nurse should monitor for fetal hypoxia in cases of umbilical cord prolapse. Because this is the fetus's only lifeline, fetal perfusion deteriorates rapidly. Complete occlusion renders the fetus helpless and oxygen deprived. Preeclampsia, coagulation defects, and placental pathology are not risks associated with umbilical cord prolapse.

Answers

CHAPTER 22

SECTION I: ASSESSING YOUR UNDERSTANDING

Activity A FILL IN THE BLANKS

1. atony
2. Subinvolution
3. decrease
4. thrombus
5. thromboembolism
6. Metritis
7. mastitis
8. early
9. accreta
10. inversion

Activity B MATCHING

1. b   2. a   3. d   4. c   5. e

Activity C SEQUENCING

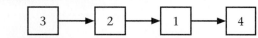

Activity D SHORT ANSWERS

1. Overdistention of the uterus can be caused by multifetal gestation, fetal macrosomia, polyhydramnios, fetal abnormality, or placental fragments. Other causes might include prolonged or rapid, forceful labor, especially if stimulated; bacterial toxins; use of anesthesia; and magnesium sulfate used in the treatment of preeclampsia. Overdistention of the uterus is a major risk factor for uterine atony, the most common cause of early postpartum hemorrhage, which can lead to hypovolemic shock.

2. Idiopathic thrombocytopenic purpura (ITP) is characterized by increased platelet destruction caused by the development of autoantibodies to platelet-membrane antigens. The incidence of ITP in adults is approximately 66 cases per 1 million per year. The characteristic features of the disorder are thrombocytopenia, capillary fragility, and increased bleeding time. Clients with ITP present with easy bruising, bleeding from mucous membranes, menorrhagia, epistaxis, bleeding gums, hematomas, and severe hemorrhage after a cesarean birth or lacerations.

3. Postpartum infections are usually polymicrobial and involve *Staphylococcus aureus*, *Escherichia coli*, *Klebsiella* species, *Gardnerella vaginalis*, gonococci, coliform bacteria, group A or B hemolytic streptococci, *Chlamydia trachomatis*, and the anaerobes that are common to bacterial vaginosis.

4. Most postpartum women experience baby blues. The woman exhibits mild depressive symptoms of anxiety, irritability, mood swings, tearfulness, and increased sensitivity, feelings of being overwhelmed, and fatigue after the birth of the baby. The condition typically peaks on postpartum days 4 and 5 and usually resolves by postpartum day 10. Baby blues are usually self-limiting and require no formal treatment other than reassurance and validation of the woman's experience, as well as assistance in caring for herself and the newborn.

5. Symptoms of postpartum psychosis surface within 3 weeks of giving birth. The main symptoms include sleep disturbances, fatigue, depression, and hypomania. The mother will be tearful, confused, and preoccupied with feelings of guilt and worthlessness. The symptoms may escalate to delirium, hallucinations, anger toward herself and her infant, bizarre behavior, manifestations of mania, and thoughts of hurting herself and the infant. The mother frequently loses touch with reality and experiences a severe regressive breakdown, associated with a high risk of suicide or infanticide.

6. A thrombosis refers to the development of a blood clot in the blood vessel. It can cause an inflammation of the blood vessel lining, which in turn can lead to a possible thromboembolism. Thrombi can involve the superficial or deep veins in the legs or pelvis:
   - Superficial venous thrombosis usually involves the saphenous venous system and is confined to the lower leg. The lithotomy position during birth can cause superficial thrombophlebitis in some women.
   - Deep venous thrombosis (DVT) can involve deep veins from the foot to the calf, to the thighs, or to the pelvis.

In both locations, thrombi can dislodge and migrate to the lungs, causing a pulmonary embolism.

SECTION II: APPLYING YOUR KNOWLEDGE

Activity E CASE STUDY

1. The major causes of thrombus formation are venous stasis, injury to the innermost layer of the blood vessel, and hypercoagulation. Venous stasis and hypercoagulation are common in the postpartum period. The risk factors for thrombosis are as follows:
   - Prolonged bed rest
   - Diabetes
   - Obesity
   - Cesarean birth
   - Smoking
   - Severe anemia
   - History of previous thrombosis
   - Varicose veins
   - Advanced maternal age (greater than 35 years)
   - Multiparity
   - Use of oral contraceptives before pregnancy
2. The nurse should perform the following nursing interventions to prevent thromboembolic complications in a client:
   - Educate the client on the need for early and frequent ambulation.
   - Encourage activities that cause leg muscles to contract (leg exercises and walking) to promote venous return in order to prevent venous stasis.
   - Use intermittent sequential compression devices, which cause passive leg contractions until the client is ambulatory.
   - Elevate the client's legs above heart level to promote venous return.
   - Ensure antiembolism stockings are applied and removed every day for inspections of the legs.
   - Encourage the client to perform passive exercises on the bed.
   - Ensure that the client is involved in postoperative deep-breathing exercises; this improves venous return.
   - In order to prevent venous pooling, avoid placing pillows under the knees or keeping the legs in stirrups for a long time or using the knee gatch on the bed.
   - Ensure the use of bed cradles; this helps in keeping linens and blankets off the extremity.
3. For clients with superficial venous thrombosis, the nurse should perform the following interventions:
   - Administer NSAIDs for analgesic effect as prescribed.
   - Provide rest and elevation of the affected leg.
   - Apply warm compresses over the affected area to promote healing.
   - Use antiembolism stockings, which promote circulation to the extremities.

SECTION III: PRACTICING FOR NCLEX

Activity F NCLEX-STYLE QUESTIONS

1. **Answer: c**
   RATIONALE: The nurse should monitor the client for swelling in the calf. Swelling in the calf, erythema, and pedal edema are early manifestations of DVT, which may lead to pulmonary embolism if not prevented at an early stage. Sudden change in the mental status, difficulty in breathing, and sudden chest pain are manifestations of pulmonary embolism, beyond the stage of prevention.

2. **Answer: d**
   RATIONALE: When caring for a client with DVT, the nurse should instruct the client to avoid using oral contraceptives. Cigarette smoking, use of oral contraceptives, sedentary lifestyle, and obesity increase the risk for developing DVT. The nurse should encourage the client with DVT to wear compression stockings. The nurse should instruct the client to avoid using products containing aspirin when caring for clients with bleeding, but not for clients with DVT. Prolonged rest periods should be avoided. Prolonged rest involves staying motionless; this could lead to venous stasis, which needs to be avoided in cases of DVT.

3. **Answer: b**
   RATIONALE: When caring for a client with ITP, the nurse should administer platelet transfusions as ordered to control bleeding. Glucocorticoids, intravenous immunoglobulins, and intravenous anti-Rho D are also administered to the client. The nurse should not administer NSAIDs when caring for this client since nonsteroidal anti-inflammatory drugs cause platelet dysfunction. ITP is a disorder of increased platelet destruction due to the presence of autoantibodies to platelet-membrane antigens. As the client is bleeding, the nurse should continue with the administration of oxytocics, which helps to control the bleeding. Continuous firm uterine massage results in uterine exhaustion, leading to augmentation of bleeding.

4. **Answer: a**
   RATIONALE: The nurse should monitor for foul-smelling vaginal discharge to verify the presence of an episiotomy infection. Sudden onset of shortness of breath, and apprehension and diaphoresis are signs of pulmonary embolism and do not indicate episiotomy infection. Pain in the lower leg is indicative of a thrombosis.

5. **Answer: a**
   RATIONALE: The nurse should assess the client for prolonged bleeding time. von Willebrand disease is a congenital bleeding disorder, inherited as an autosomal dominant trait, that is characterized by a prolonged bleeding time, a deficiency of von Willebrand factor, and impairment of

platelet adhesion. A fever of 100.4° F after the first 24 hours following childbirth and presence of foul-smelling vaginal discharge indicate infection. A client with a postpartum fundal height that is higher than expected may have subinvolution of the uterus.

6. **Answer: d**
   RATIONALE: The nurse should assess for calf tenderness in the client to verify the diagnosis of a DVT. Other signs and symptoms of DVT include calf swelling, erythema, warmth and tenderness, and pedal edema. Sudden chest pain, dyspnea, and tachypnea are signs and symptoms associated with pulmonary embolism and not DVT.

7. **Answer: d**
   RATIONALE: The presence of a large uterus with painless dark-red blood mixed with clots indicates retained placental fragments in the uterus. This cause of hemorrhage can be prevented by carefully inspecting the placenta for intactness. A firm uterus with a trickle or steady stream of bright-red blood in the perineum indicates bleeding from trauma. A soft and boggy uterus that deviates from the midline indicates a full bladder, interfering with uterine involution.

8. **Answer: a**
   RATIONALE: The nurse can identify whether the bleeding is from lacerations by looking for a well-contracted uterus with bright-red vaginal bleeding. Lacerations commonly occur during forceps delivery. In subinvolution of the uterus, there is inadequate contraction, resulting in bleeding. A boggy uterus with vaginal bleeding is seen in uterine atony. An inverted uterus with vaginal bleeding is seen in uterine inversion.

9. **Answer: c**
   RATIONALE: Early postpartal hemorrhage can be assessed within the first few hours following delivery. Postpartal infection may be noticed as a rise in temperature after the first 24 hours following childbirth. Postpartal blues and postpartum depression are emotional disorders noticed much later, in the days to weeks following delivery.

10. **Answer: c**
    RATIONALE: To help prevent the occurrence of postpartum thromboembolic complications, the nurse should instruct the client to avoid sitting or standing in one position for long periods of time. This prevents venous pooling. The nurse should instruct the client to perform postoperative deep-breathing exercises to improve venous

return by relieving the negative thoracic pressure on leg veins. The nurse should instruct the client to prevent venous pooling by avoiding the use of pillows under the knees. Elevating the legs above heart level promotes venous return, and therefore the nurse should encourage it.

11. **Answer: c**
    RATIONALE: A nurse should monitor for decreased blood pressure when evaluating the client for signs of hemorrhage. A falling blood pressure along with increased heart rate and decreased urinary output are the typical signs of severe hemorrhage. The client will also experience reduced, not increased, body temperature during hemorrhage.

12. **Answer: b**
    RATIONALE: The nurse should educate the client to perform hand-washing before and after breast-feeding to prevent mastitis. Discontinuing breast-feeding to allow time for healing, avoiding hot or cold compresses on the breast, and discouraging manual compression of breast for expressing milk are inappropriate interventions. The nurse should educate the client to continue breastfeeding, because it reverses milk stasis, and to manually compress the breast to express excess milk. Hot and cold compresses can be applied for comfort.

13. **Answer: b, c, & d**
    RATIONALE: The nurse should monitor for bleeding gums, tachycardia, and acute renal failure to assess for an increased risk of disseminated intravascular coagulation in the client. The other clinical manifestations of this condition include petechiae, ecchymosis, and uncontrolled bleeding during birth. Hypotension and amount of lochia greater than usual are findings that might suggest a coagulopathy or hypovolemic shock.

14. **Answer: a, b, & d**
    RATIONALE: The nurse should monitor the client for symptoms such as inability to concentrate, loss of confidence, and decreased interest in life to verify the presence of postpartum depression. Manifestations of mania and bizarre behavior are noted in clients with postpartum psychosis.

15. **Answer: a, b, & d**
    RATIONALE: A nurse should evaluate the efficacy of IV oxytocin therapy by assessing the uterine tone, monitoring vital signs, and getting a pad count. Assessing the skin turgor and assessing deep tendon reflexes are not interventions applicable to administration of oxytocin.

Answers

CHAPTER 23

SECTION I: ASSESSING YOUR UNDERSTANDING

Activity A FILL IN THE BLANKS

1. Polycythemia
2. Gavage
3. asphyxia
4. preterm
5. atelectasis
6. term
7. Retinopathy
8. Pain
9. inversely
10. genetic

Activity B LABELING

1. The figure displays a low-birth-weight newborn (or a newborn) in an Isolette.
2. An Isolette keeps the newborn warm to conserve energy and prevent cold stress. The Isolette may be warmed or may have an overhead radiant warmer.

Activity C MATCHING

1. c   2. a   3. b   4. d

Activity D SEQUENCING

1.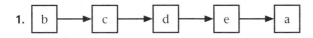

Activity E SHORT ANSWERS

1. The common physical characteristics of preterm newborns include:
   - Birth weight of less than 5.5 lb
   - Scrawny appearance
   - Head disproportionately larger than chest circumference
   - Poor muscle tone
   - Minimal subcutaneous fat
   - Undescended testes
   - Plentiful lanugo (a soft downy hair), especially over the face and back
   - Poorly formed ear pinna with soft, pliable cartilage
   - Fused eyelids

   - Soft and spongy skull bones, especially along suture lines
   - Matted scalp hair, wooly in appearance
   - Absent or only a few creases in the soles and palms
   - Minimal scrotal rugae in male infants; prominent labia and clitoris in female infants
   - Thin, transparent skin with visible veins
   - Breast and nipples not clearly delineated
   - Abundant vernix caseosa

2. The clinical signs of hypoglycemia in the newborn are often subtle and include lethargy, apathy, drowsiness, irritability, tachypnea, weak cry, temperature instability, jitteriness, seizures, apnea, bradycardia, cyanosis or pallor, feeble suck and poor feeding, hypotonia, and coma. Blood glucose level below 40 mg per dL in term newborns and below 20 mg per dL in preterm newborns is indicative of hypoglycemia in the newborn.

3. Developmentally supportive care is defined as care of a newborn or an infant to support growth and development. Developmental care focuses on what newborns or infants can do at that stage of development; it uses therapeutic interventions only to the point that they are beneficial; and it provides for the development of the newborn–family unit.

4. Preterm infants are at a high risk for neurodevelopmental disorders such as cerebral palsy or intellectual disability, intraventricular hemorrhage, congenital anomalies, neurosensory impairment, behavioral disadaptation, and chronic lung disease.

5. The characteristics of large-for-gestational-age newborns are as follows:
   - Large body; appears plump and full faced
   - Increase in body size is proportional
   - Head circumference and body length in upper limits of intrauterine growth
   - Poor motor skills
   - Difficulty in regulating behavioral states
   - More difficult to arouse to a quiet alert state

6. Postterm newborns typically exhibit the following characteristics:
   - Dry, cracked, wrinkled skin
   - Long, thin extremities
   - Creases that cover the entire soles of the feet

- Wide-eyed, alert expression
- Abundant hair on scalp
- Thin umbilical cord
- Limited vernix and lanugo
- Meconium-stained skin
- Long nails

SECTION II: APPLYING YOUR KNOWLEDGE

Activity F   CASE STUDY

1. A nurse can help the parents in the detachment process in the following ways:
   - To see their newborn through the maze of equipment
   - Explain the various procedures and equipment
   - Encourage them to express their feelings about the fragile newborn's status
   - Provide the parents time to spend with their dying newborn

2. The nursing interventions when caring for a family experiencing a perinatal loss are as follows:
   - Help the family to accept the reality of death by using the word "died."
   - Acknowledge their grief and the fact that their newborn has died.
   - Help the family to work through their grief by validating and listening.
   - Provide the family with realistic information about the causes of death.
   - Offer condolences to the family in a sincere manner.
   - Initiate spiritual comfort by calling the hospital clergy if needed.
   - Acknowledge variations in spiritual needs and readiness.
   - Encourage the parents to have a funeral or memorial service to bring closure.
   - Encourage the parents to take photographs, make memory boxes, and record their thoughts in a journal.
   - Suggest that the parents plant a tree or flowers to remember the infant.
   - Explore with family members how they dealt with previous losses.
   - Discuss meditation and relaxation techniques to reduce stress.
   - Provide opportunities for the family to hold the newborn if they choose to do so.
   - Assess the family's support network.
   - Address attachment issues concerning subsequent pregnancies.
   - Reassure the family that their feelings and grieving responses are normal.
   - Provide information about local support groups.
   - Provide anticipatory guidance regarding the grieving process.
   - Recommend that family members maintain a healthy diet and get adequate rest and exercise to preserve their health.

SECTION III: PRACTICING FOR NCLEX

Activity G   NCLEX-STYLE QUESTIONS

1. **Answer: a**
   RATIONALE: The nurse should focus on decreasing blood viscosity by increasing fluid volume in the newborn with polycythemia. Checking blood glucose within 2 hours of birth by a reagent test strip and screening every 2 to 3 hours or before feeds are not interventions that will alleviate the condition of an infant with polycythemia. The nurse should monitor and maintain blood glucose levels when caring for a newborn with hypoglycemia, not polycythemia.

2. **Answer: a, c, & e**
   RATIONALE: To minimize the risk of infections, the nurse should avoid coming to work when ill, use sterile gloves for an invasive procedure, and monitor laboratory test results for changes. The nurse should remove all jewelry before washing hands, not cover the jewelry. The nurse should use disposable equipment rather than avoid it.

3. **Answer: a**
   RATIONALE: When preterm infants receive sensorimotor interventions such as rocking, massaging, holding, or sleeping on waterbeds, they gain weight faster, progress in feeding abilities more quickly, and show improved interactive behavior. Interventions such as swaddling and positioning, use of minimal amount of tape, and use of distraction through objects are related to pain management.

4. **Answer: c**
   RATIONALE: The nurse should identify acute respiratory complication as the risk to the newborn that results from meconium in the amniotic fluid. Bradycardia, perinatal asphyxia, and polycythemia are some of the common problems faced by an SGA newborn, but are not related to meconium in the amniotic fluid.

5. **Answer: d**
   RATIONALE: A good cry or good breathing efforts are signs that the resuscitation has been successful. A pulse above 100 bpm, not 80 bpm, is an indication of a successful resuscitation. Pink tongue, not blue, indicates a good oxygen supply to the brain. Tremors are associated with the signs of hypothermia; this is not a sign of successful resuscitation.

6. **Answer: c**
   RATIONALE: The nurse should observe for clinical signs of cold stress, such as respiratory distress, central cyanosis, hypoglycemia, lethargy, weak cry, abdominal distention, apnea, bradycardia, and acidosis. The temperature of the radiant warmer should not be set at a fixed level and should be adjusted to the newborn's temperature. The nurse need not check the blood pressure of the infant every 2 hours. The infant's temperature should be measured more often than every 5 hours.

7. **Answer: b**
   RATIONALE: The nurse should administer 0.5 to 1 mL/kg/h of breast milk enterally to induce surges in gut hormones that enhance maturation of the intestine. Administering vitamin D supplements, iron supplements, or intravenous dextrose will not significantly help the preterm newborn's gut overcome feeding difficulties.

8. **Answer: a**
   RATIONALE: The nurse should maintain the fluid and electrolyte balance of an infant born with hypoglycemia. Dextrose should be given intravenously only if the infant refuses oral feedings, not before offering the infant oral feedings. Placing the infant on a radiant warmer will not help maintain blood glucose levels. The nurse should focus on decreasing blood viscosity in an infant who is at risk for polycythemia, not hypoglycemia.

9. **Answer: c**
   RATIONALE: The nurse should assess for a decrease in urinary output and fluid balance in the preterm or postterm newborn. Weight of the newborn should be measured daily, not once every 2 days. Increased muscle tone does not indicate nutrition and fluid imbalance. A rise, not fall, in temperature indicates dehydration.

10. **Answer: a, b, & d**
    RATIONALE: Diabetes mellitus, postdates gestation, and glucose intolerance are the maternal factors the nurse should consider that could lead to a newborn being large for gestational age. Renal condition and maternal alcohol use are not factors associated with a newborn's being large for gestational age.

11. **Answer: a**
    RATIONALE: Jaundice is a sign of polycythemia. Restlessness, temperature instability, and wheezing are not fetal distress signs; they are the signs of a newborn with hypothermia.

12. **Answer: a**
    RATIONALE: The infant is demonstrating signs and symptoms of hypoglycemia. IV dextrose should be administered to the term newborn intravenously when the blood glucose level is less than 40 mg per dL, and the newborn is symptomatic for hypoglycemia. Administration of IV glucose assists in stabilizing blood glucose levels. Placing the infant on a radiant warmer will not help maintain the glucose level. Monitoring the infant's hematocrit level is not a priority.

13. **Answer: a, c, & e**
    RATIONALE: Hydration, early feedings, and phototherapy are measures that the nurse should take to reduce bilirubin levels in the newborn. Increasing the infant's water intake or administering vitamin supplements will not help reduce bilirubin levels in the infant.

14. **Answer: c**
    RATIONALE: A stained umbilical cord indicates a possibility of meconium aspiration, and the nurse should inform the primary care provider immediately. Listlessness or lethargy by themselves does not indicate meconium aspiration. Bluish skin discoloration is normal in infants, and so is pink discoloration of the tongue.

15. **Answer: a, c, & d**
    RATIONALE: The nurse should be alert to the possibility of an SGA newborn if the history of the mother reveals smoking, chronic medical conditions (such as asthma), and drug abuse. Additional maternal factors that increase the risk for an SGA newborn include hypertension, genetic disorders, and multiple gestations.

CHAPTER 24

SECTION I: ASSESSING YOUR UNDERSTANDING

Activity A FILL IN THE BLANKS

1. omphalocele
2. Cephalohematoma
3. Hyperbilirubinemia
4. sepsis
5. Methadone
6. hemolytic
7. phototherapy
8. Gastroschisis
9. asphyxia
10. Kernicterus
11. inflammatory
12. ventriculoperitoneal

Activity B MATCHING

I.
1. a   2. d   3. b   4. c   5. e

II.
1. d   2. b   3. c   4. a

Activity C SHORT ANSWERS

1. The characteristics of an infant born to a diabetic mother are as follows:
   - Full rosy cheeks with a ruddy skin color
   - Short neck with a buffalo hump over the nape of the neck
   - Massive shoulders showing full intrascapular area
   - Distended upper abdomen resulting from organ overgrowth
   - Excessive subcutaneous fat tissue, producing fat extremities
2. The most common types of malformations in infants of diabetic mothers involve anomalies in the following systems:
   - Cardiovascular
   - Skeletal
   - Central nervous system
   - Gastrointestinal
   - Genitourinary

3. The treatment of infants born to diabetic mothers focuses on correcting hypoglycemia, hypocalcemia, hypomagnesemia, dehydration, and jaundice. Oxygenation and ventilation for the newborn are supported as necessary.
4. Birth trauma may result from the pressure of birth, especially in a prolonged or abrupt labor, abnormal or difficult presentation, cephalopelvic disproportion, or mechanical forces such as a forceps or vacuum used during delivery.
5. Meconium aspiration syndrome occurs when the newborn inhales particulate meconium mixed with amniotic fluid into the lungs while still in utero or on taking the first breath after birth. It is a common cause of newborn respiratory distress and can lead to severe illness.
6. PVH/IVH is defined as bleeding that usually originates in the subependymal germinal matrix region of the brain, with extension into the ventricular system. It is a common problem of preterm infants, especially those born before 32 weeks.
7. The goals of therapy include restoring urinary continence, preserving renal function, and reconstructing functional and cosmetically acceptable genitalia.
8. Encourage the parents to express their feelings about this highly visible anomaly. Emphasize the newborn's positive features and role model nurturing behaviors when interacting with the infant. Encourage parental interaction and involvement with the newborn. Provide support to the parents, especially related to feeding difficulties. Allow them to vent their frustrations. Offer practical suggestions and continued encouragement for their efforts.

SECTION II: APPLYING YOUR KNOWLEDGE

Activity D CASE STUDY

1. The role of the nurse in handling substance-abusing mothers includes:
   - Being knowledgeable about issues of substance abuse
   - Being alert for opportunities to identify, prevent, manage, and educate clients and families about this key public health issue

2. The nurse can use the "5 As" approach in the following way:
   - Ask: Ask the client if she smokes and if she would like to quit.
   - Advise: Encourage the use of clinically proved treatment plans.
   - Assess: Provide motivation by discussing the 5 Rs:
     - Relevance of quitting to the client
     - Risk of continued smoking to the fetus
     - Rewards of quitting for both
     - Roadblocks to quitting
     - Repeat at every visit
   - Assist: Help the client to protect her fetus and newborn from the negative effects of smoking.
   - Arrange: Schedule follow-up visits to reinforce the client's commitment to quit.

SECTION III: PRACTICING FOR NCLEX

Activity E NCLEX-STYLE QUESTIONS

1. **Answer: d**
   RATIONALE: End-expiratory grunting, a barrel-shaped chest with an increased anterior–posterior chest diameter, prolonged tachypnea, progression from mild-to-severe respiratory distress, intercostal retractions, cyanosis, surfactant dysfunction, airway obstruction, hypoxia, and chemical pneumonitis with inflammation of pulmonary tissues are seen in a newborn with meconium aspiration syndrome. A high-pitched cry may be noted in PVH/IVH. Bile-stained emesis occurs in necrotizing enterocolitis. Increased intracranial pressure occurs in cases of hydrocephalus.

2. **Answer: a**
   RATIONALE: The nurse should assess for systolic ejection murmur. Respiratory alkalosis, rhinorrhea, and lacrimation may be symptoms of neonatal abstinence syndrome.

3. **Answer: d**
   RATIONALE: Noting any absence of or decrease in deep tendon reflexes is a nursing intervention when assessing a newborn with a risk of trauma. The nurse should examine the skin for cyanosis, should be alert for signs of apathy and listlessness, and should assess for any temperature instability when caring for a newborn born to a diabetic mother. These interventions are not required to assess for trauma or birth injuries in a newborn.

4. **Answer: b**
   RATIONALE: The nurse should know that the infant's mother must have been a diabetic. The large size of the infant born to a diabetic mother is secondary to exposure to high levels of maternal glucose crossing the placenta into the fetal circulation. Common problems among infants of diabetic mothers include macrosomia, respiratory distress syndrome (RDS), birth trauma, hypoglycemia, hypocalcemia and hypomagnesemia, polycythemia, hyperbilirubinemia, and congenital anomalies. Listlessness is also a common symptom noted in these infants. Infants born to clients who have abused alcohol, infants who have experienced birth traumas, or infants whose mothers have had a low birth weight are not known to exhibit these particular characteristics, although these conditions do not produce very positive pregnancy outcomes.

5. **Answer: a, d, & e**
   RATIONALE: A nurse should associate obstructive hydrocephalus, vision or hearing defects, and cerebral palsy with newborns having PVH/IVH. Acid–base imbalances are complications occurring during exchange transfusion for lowering serum bilirubin levels. Pneumonitis is a complication associated with esophageal atresia.

6. **Answer: c**
   RATIONALE: The nurse should assess for meconium aspiration syndrome in the newborn. Meconium aspiration involves patchy, fluffy infiltrates unevenly distributed throughout the lungs and marked hyperaeration mixed with areas of atelectasis that can be seen through chest X-rays. Direct visualization of the vocal cords for meconium staining using a laryngoscope can confirm aspiration. Lung auscultation typically reveals coarse crackles and rhonchi. Arterial blood gas analysis will indicate metabolic acidosis with a low blood pH, decreased PaO_2, and increased $PaCO_2$. Newborns with choanal atresia, necrotizing enterocolitis, and hyperbilirubinemia are not known to exhibit these manifestations.

7. **Answer: a**
   RATIONALE: The nurse should administer IV fluids and gavage feedings until the respiratory rate decreases enough to allow oral feedings when caring for a newborn with transient tachypnea. Maintaining adequate hydration and performing gentle suctioning are relevant nursing interventions when caring for a newborn with respiratory distress syndrome. The nurse need not monitor the newborn for signs and symptoms of hypotonia because hypotonia is not known to occur as a result of transient tachypnea. Hypotonia is observed in newborns with inborn errors of metabolism or in cases of PVH/IVH.

8. **Answer: b**
   RATIONALE: Ensuring effective resuscitation measures is the nursing intervention involved when treating a newborn for asphyxia. Ensuring adequate tissue perfusion and administering surfactant are nursing interventions involved in the care of newborns with meconium aspiration syndrome. Similarly, administering IV fluids is a nursing intervention involved in the care of newborns with transient tachypnea.

9. **Answer: c**
   RATIONALE: The preoperative nursing care focuses on preventing aspiration by elevating the head

of the bed 30° to 45° to prevent reflux. Providing colostomy care is a part of postoperative nursing care for the newborn. Documenting the amount and color of drainage is the postoperative nursing care for a newborn with omphalocele. Administering antibiotics and total parenteral nutrition is a postoperative nursing intervention when caring for a newborn with esophageal atresia.

10. **Answer: d**
    RATIONALE: When caring for a substance-exposed newborn, the nurse should check the newborn's skin turgor and fontanels. Encouraging early initiation of feedings and monitoring the newborn's cardiovascular status are nursing interventions involved when caring for a newborn with pathologic jaundice. In cases of pathologic jaundice, the nurse also encourages supplementing breast milk with formula to supply protein if bilirubin levels continue to increase with breast-feeding only.

11. **Answer: b**
    RATIONALE: The nurse should shield the newborn's eyes and cover the genitals to protect these areas from becoming irritated or burned when using direct lights and to ensure exposure of the greatest surface area. The nurse should place the newborn under the lights or on the fiberoptic blanket, exposing as much skin as possible. Breast or bottle feedings should be encouraged every 2 to 3 hours. Loose, green, and frequent stools indicate the presence of unconjugated bilirubin in the feces. This is normal; therefore, there is no need for therapy to be discontinued. Lack of frequent green stools is a cause for concern.

12. **Answer: b, d, & e**
    RATIONALE: When caring for a newborn with meconium aspiration syndrome, the nurse should place the newborn under a radiant warmer or in a warmed Isolette, administer oxygen therapy as ordered via a nasal cannula or with positive pressure ventilation, and administer broad-spectrum antibiotics to treat bacterial pneumonia. Repeated suctioning and stimulation should be limited to prevent overstimulation and further depression in the newborn. The nurse should also ensure minimal handling to reduce energy expenditure and oxygen consumption that could lead to further hypoxemia and acidosis. Handling and rubbing the newborn with a dry towel is needed to stimulate the onset of breathing in a newborn with asphyxia.

13. **Answer: a**
    RATIONALE: The nurse should know that gastroschisis is a herniation of abdominal contents in which there is no peritoneal sac protecting herniated organs. A peritoneal sac is present in omphalocele. In gastroschisis, the herniated organs are not normal; they are unprotected and become thickened, edematous, and inflamed because of

exposure to amniotic fluid. Gastroschisis is not a defect of the umbilical ring; it is a herniation of abdominal contents through an abdominal wall defect. Despite surgical correction, feeding intolerance, failure to thrive, and prolonged hospital stays occur in nearly all newborns with gastroschisis.

14. **Answer: c**
    RATIONALE: The nurse should inform the parents that surgery for necrotizing enterocolitis requires the placement of a proximal enterostomy and ostomy care. Surgically treated NEC is a lengthy process, and the amount of bowel that has necrosed, as determined during the bowel resection, significantly increases the likelihood that infants requiring surgery for NEC may have long-term medical problems. If surgery for NEC is required, antibiotics may be needed for an extended period.

15. **Answer: a**
    RATIONALE: BPD can be prevented by administering steroids to the mother in the antepartal period and exogenous surfactant to the newborn to aid in reducing the development of RDS and its severity. A high oxygen content can cause damage to the neonatal lung. Steroid injections for newborns at risk for BPD do not help the lungs mature. Giving exogenous surfactant to the mother does not increase the level of surfactant in the infant.

16. **Answer: b**
    RATIONALE: After birth, carefully assess the newborn's cardiovascular and respiratory systems, looking for signs and symptoms of respiratory distress, cyanosis, or congestive heart failure that might indicate a cardiac anomaly. Assess rate, rhythm, and heart sounds, reporting any abnormalities immediately. Note any signs of heart failure, including edema, diminished peripheral pulses, hepatomegaly, tachycardia, diaphoresis, respiratory distress with tachypnea, peripheral pallor, and irritability (Kenner & Lott, 2007). Capillary refill time and the color of the infant's hands and feet are important to note, but do not indicate possible heart failure. Neither does the blood glucose level.

17. **Answer: c**
    RATIONALE: Provide comfort measures to the newborn who will be subjected to a variety of painful procedures. Be vigilant in ensuring the newborn's comfort, since it cannot report or describe pain. Assist in preventing pain as much as possible; interpret the newborn's cues suggesting pain and manage it appropriately.

18. **Answer: d**
    RATIONALE: A myelomeningocele is a more severe form of spina bifida cystica, in which the spinal cord and nerve roots herniate into the sac through an opening in the spine, compromising the meninges. A meningocele includes the

meninges and spinal fluid only. Spina bifida occulta is a defect in the vertebrae only. Spina bifida cystica is a generalized term that includes both a meningocele and a myelomeningocele.

19. **Answer: c**
    RATIONALE: Measure head circumference daily to observe for hydrocephalus. Level of irritability is a much later sign of hydrocephalus in an infant. Weight and movement of the legs are not assessments that would indicate hydrocephalus.

20. **Answer: a, b & c**
    RATIONALE: Administer prescribed medications as ordered. For example, give inotropics to support systemic blood pressure. Administer surfactant, steroids, and inhaled nitric oxide as ordered to correct hypoxia and acid–base imbalance.

21. **Answer: b**
    RATIONALE: Repairing the facial anomaly as soon as possible is important to facilitate bonding between the newborn and the parents and to improve nutritional status. Treatment of cleft lip is surgical repair between the ages of 6 and 12 weeks. More extensive corrective surgery may occur later, often around the age of 6 to 18 months.

22. **Answer: a**
    RATIONALE: The degree of hypospadias depends on the location of the opening. It is often accompanied by a downward bowing of the penis (chordee), which can lead to urination and erection problems in adulthood. Prepuce is the foreskin of the penis. Priapism is an abnormally prolonged erection of the penis. Cholangi is a bile duct.

23. **Answer: d**
    RATIONALE: Treatment for either type starts with serial casting, which is needed because of the rapid growth of the newborn. Surgery, braces, and physical therapy all have their place in the treatment of one or the other type of club foot, but they follow the initial treatment of serial casting.

24. **Answer: a**
    RATIONALE: Ortolani maneuver elicits the sensation of the dislocated hip reducing. Barlow maneuver detects the hip dislocating from the acetabulum. Pavlik maneuver is a harness, not a maneuver. Bill maneuver is an obstetric procedure of using forceps to turn the baby's head before birth.

25. **Answer: b, c & e**
    RATIONALE: Retinopathy of the preterm newborn typically develops in both the eyes secondary to an injury such as hyperoxemia resulting from prolonged assistive ventilation and high oxygen exposure, acidosis, and shock.

CHAPTER 25

SECTION I: ASSESSING YOUR UNDERSTANDING

Activity A FILL IN THE BLANKS

1. Colic
2. Anticipatory
3. Prolactin
4. Colostrums
5. Separate
6. Development
7. 12 to 18

Activity B LABELING

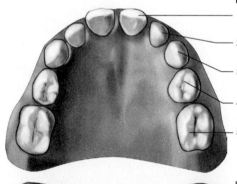

UPPER

1 Central incisor
  8-12 months
2 Lateral incisor
  9-13 months
3 Cuspid
  16-22 months
4 First molar
  13-19 months
5 Second molar
  25-33 months

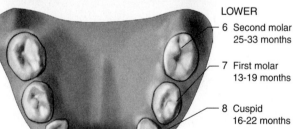

LOWER

6 Second molar
  25-33 months
7 First molar
  13-19 months
8 Cuspid
  16-22 months
9 Lateral incisor
  9-13 months
10 Central incisor
  8-12 months

Activity C MATCHING

Question 1

1. f   **2.** a   **3.** b   **4.** e   **5.** d   **6.** c

Question 2

1. b   **2.** a   **3.** d   **4.** c   **5.** e

Activity D SEQUENCING

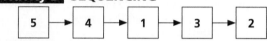

5 → 4 → 1 → 3 → 2

Activity E SHORT ANSWERS

1. Encourage breastfeeding in all mothers beginning with the prenatal visit if applicable. Provide accurate education related to breastfeeding.

   Be available for questions or problems related to initiation and continuation of breastfeeding. Consult lactation consultant as needed or available.

   Encourage pumping of breast milk when mother returns to work in order to continue breastfeeding.

   Refer to local breastfeeding support groups such as La Leche League.

2. Breastfeeding or feeding of expressed human milk is recommended for all infants, including sick or premature newborns (with rare exceptions). The exceptions include infants with galactosemia, maternal use of illicit drugs and a few prescription medications, maternal untreated active tuberculosis, and maternal human immunodeficiency virus (HIV) infection in developed countries.

3. Early cues of hunger in a baby include making sucking motions, sucking on hands, or putting the fist to the chin.

4. When assessing the growth and development of a premature infant, use the infant's adjusted age to determine expected outcomes. To determine adjusted age, subtract the number of weeks that the infant was premature from the infant's chronological age.

5. Primitive reflexes are subcortical and involve a whole-body response. Selected primitive reflexes present at birth include Moro root, suck, asymmetric tonic neck, plantar and palmar grasp, step, and Babinski. Except for the Babinski, which disappears around 1 year of age, these primitive reflexes diminish over the first few months of life, giving way to protective reflexes.

6. The heart doubles in size over the first year of life. As the cardiovascular system matures, the average pulse rate decreases from 120 to 140 in the newborn to about 100 in the 1-year-old. Blood pressure steadily increases over the first 12 months of life, from an average of 60/40 in the newborn to 100/50 in the 12-month-old. The peripheral capillaries are closer to the surface of the skin, thus making the newborn and young infant more susceptible to heat loss. Over the first year of life, thermoregulation (the body's ability to stabilize body temperature) becomes more effective: the peripheral capillaries constrict in response to a cold environment and dilate in response to heat.

SECTION II: APPLYING YOUR KNOWLEDGE
Activity F CASE STUDY

1. The discussion should include the following points:

    Play is the work of children and is the natural way they learn. It is critical to their development. It allows them to explore their environment, practice new skills, and problem solve. They practice gross, fine motor and language skills through play. Young infants love to watch people's faces and will often appear to mimic the expressions they see. Parents can talk to and sing to their child while participating in the daily activities that infants need such as feeding, bathing, and changing. As infants become older, toys may be geared toward the motor skills or language skills that are developing currently. Appropriate toys for this age group include: fabric or board books, different types of music, easy to hold toys that do things or make noise (fancy rattles), floating, squirting bath toys, and soft dolls or animals. Books are also very important toys for infants. Reading aloud and sharing books during early infancy are critical to the development of neural networks that are important in the later tasks of reading and word recognition. Reading books increases listening comprehension. Infants demonstrate their excitement about picture books by kicking and waving their arms and babbling when looking at them. Reading to all ages of infants is appropriate and the older infant develops fine motor skills as he learns to turn book pages. Reading picture books and simple stories to infants starts a good habit that should be continued throughout childhood.

2. The discussion should include the following points:

    Erikson's stage of psychosocial development is trust versus mistrust. Development of a sense of trust is crucial in the first year, as it serves as the foundation for later psychosocial tasks. The parent or primary caregiver is in a position to significantly impact the infant's development of a sense of trust. When the infant's needs are consistently met, the infant develops this sense of trust. Caregivers respond to these basic needs by feeding, changing diapers, and cleaning, touching, holding, and talking to infants. If the parent or caregiver is inconsistent in meeting the infant's needs in a timely manner, then over time the infant develops a sense of mistrust. As the infant gets older, the nervous system matures. The infant begins to realize a separation between self and caregivers. The infant learns to tolerate small amounts of frustration, and learns to trust the caregivers even if gratification is delayed, because the infant understands that needs will eventually be provided.

    The first stage of Jean Piaget's theory of cognitive development is referred to as the sensorimotor stage (birth to 2 years). Infants learn about themselves and the world around them through developing sensory and motor capacities. Infants between 4 and 8 months repeat actions to achieve wanted results, such as shaking a rattle to hear the noise it makes. At this age their actions are purposeful, though do not always have an end goal in mind.

3. The discussion should include the following points:

    Inability to sit with assistance, does not turn to locate sound, crosses eyes most of the time, does not laugh or squeal, does not smile or seem to enjoy people.

SECTION III: PRACTICING FOR NCLEX
Activity G NCLEX-STYLE QUESTIONS

1. **Answer: c**
   The child's head size is large for his adjusted age of 4 months which would be cause for concern. Normal growth would be 3.6 inches. At 10 pounds, 2 ounces, the child is the right weight for a 4-month-old adjusted age. Palmar grasp reflex disappears between 4 and 6 months adjusted age, so this would not be a concern yet. The child is of average weight for a 4-month-old adjusted age.

2. **Answer: a**
   Urging the parents to get time away from the child would be most helpful in the short term, particularly if the parents are stressed. Educating the parents about when colic stops would help them see an end to the stress. Observing how the parents respond to the child helps to determine if the parent/child relationship was altered. Assessing the parents' care and feeding skills may identify other causes for the crying.

3. **Answer: d**
   The normal newborn may lose up to 10% of their birth weight. The baby in question has lost just

below this amount. This will likely not require hospitalization. Expressing to the mother that her baby will likely be hospitalized is rash and will most likely not occur.

4. **Answer: b**

The nurse will warn against putting the child to bed with a bottle of milk or juice because this allows the sugar content of these fluids to pool around the child's teeth at night. Not cleaning a neonate's gums when he is done eating will have minimal impact on the development of dental caries, as will using a cloth instead of a brush for cleaning teeth when they erupt. Failure to clean the teeth with fluoridated toothpaste is not a problem if the water supply is fluoridated.

5. **Answer: b**

If the parents are keeping the child up until she falls asleep, they are not creating a bedtime routine for her. Infants need a transition to sleep at this age. If the parents are singing to her before she goes to bed, if she has a regular, scheduled bedtime, and if they check on her safety when she wakes at night, then lie her down and leave, they are using good sleep practices.

6. **Answer: c**

The nurse would advise the mother to watch for increased biting and sucking. Mild fever, vomiting, and diarrhea are signs of infection. The child would more likely seek out hard foods or objects to bite on.

7. **Answer: d**

When introducing a new food to an infant, it may take multiple attempts before the child will accept it. Parents must demonstrate patience. Letting the child eat only the foods she prefers, forcing her to eat foods she does not want, or actively urging the child to eat new foods can negatively affect eating patterns.

8. **Answer: a**

The best way to ensure effective feeding is by maintaining a feed-on-demand approach rather than a set schedule. Applying warm compresses to the breast helps engorgement. Encouraging the infant to latch on properly helps prevent sore nipples. Maintaining proper diet and fluid intake for the mother helps ensure an adequate milk supply.

9. **Answer: b**

If the child's rectal temperature is greater than 100.4° F, the parents should call their care provider. Infants are very susceptible to infection. If the dried umbilical cord stump falls off, or the child wets her diaper 8 times per day, this is normal. In the first 5 to 10 days of life, it is also normal for the child to eat but still lose weight.

10. **Answer: c**

At 6 months of age, the child is able to put down one toy to pick up another. He will be able to shift a toy to his left hand to reach for another with his right hand by 7 months. He will pick up an object with his thumb and finger tips at 8 months, and he will enjoy hitting a plastic bowl with a large spoon at 9 months.

11. **Answer: b**

The average infant's weight doubles at 6 months and will triple at 1 year of life. The rate of increase for the infant's length is an increase of 1 inch per month for the first 6 months.

12. **Answer: b**

The normal respiratory rate for a 1-month-old infant is 30 to 60 breaths per minute. By 1 year of age the rate will be 20 to 30 breaths per minute. The respiratory patterns of the 1-month-old infant are irregular. There may normally be periodic pauses in the rhythm.

13. **Answer: b**

Normally infants are not born with teeth. Occasionally there are one or more teeth at birth. These are termed natal teeth and are often associated with anomalies. The first primary teeth typically erupt between the ages of 6 and 8 months.

14. **Answer: c**

The capacity of the normal newborn's stomach is between one-half and one ounce. The recommended feeding plan is to use a demand schedule. Newborns may eat as often as 1½ to 3 hours. Demand scheduled feedings are not associated with problems sleeping at night.

Answers

CHAPTER 26

SECTION I: ASSESSING YOUR UNDERSTANDING

Activity A FILL IN THE BLANKS

1. Myelinization
2. Drowning
3. Receptive
4. Urethra
5. Preoperational

Activity B MATCHING

Question 1

1. d   **2.** f   **3.** e   **4.** b   **5.** a   **6.** c

Question 2

1. c   **2.** a   **3.** b   **4.** e   **5.** d

Activity C SEQUENCING

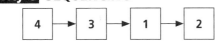

$$4 \rightarrow 3 \rightarrow 1 \rightarrow 2$$

Activity D SHORT ANSWERS

1. Prevention is best concerning temper tantrums. Fatigue or hunger may limit the toddler's coping abilities, so adhering to reasonable food and sleep schedules help prevent tantrums. When parents note the beginnings of frustrations during activities, friendly warnings, distractions, refocusing or removal from the situation may prevent the tantrum.
2. Toddler discipline should focus on clear limits, consistency, not involve spanking, and be balanced with a caring and nurturing environment along with frequent praise for appropriate behavior.
3. At the age of 1, every child should have an initial dental visit. To prevent the development of dental caries children should be weaned by 15 months of age. In addition, the use of sippy cups should be limited. Cleaning of the toddler's teeth should progress from brushing simply with water to using a very small pea-sized amount of fluoridated toothpaste with brushing beginning at age 2.
4. Changes in the anatomy of the toddler's genitourinary system make toilet training possible. The kidney functions reach adult levels between 16 and 24 months of age. The bladder is able to hold urine for increased periods of time.
5. The abdominal musculature is weak in the young toddler. This causes a pot-bellied appearance. In addition the child appears sway backed. As the muscles mature this resolves.

SECTION II: APPLYING YOUR KNOWLEDGE

Activity E CASE STUDY

The potentially bilingual child may blend two languages, that is, parts of the word in both languages are blended into one word or may language mix within a sentence; he will combine languages or grammar within a sentence. The assessment of adequate language development is more complicated in bilingual children. Due to the possible language mixing the bilingual child may be more difficult to assess for speech delay.

The bilingual child should have command of 20 words (between both languages) by 20 months of age and be making word combinations; if this is not the case, then further investigation may be warranted.

1. Talking and singing to the toddler during routine activities such as feeding and dressing provides an environment that encourages conversation. Frequent, repetitive naming helps the toddler learn appropriate words for objects. Be attentive to what the toddler is saying as well as to his moods. Listen to and answer the toddler's questions. Encouragement and elaboration convey confidence and interest to the toddler. Give the toddler time to complete his or her thoughts without interrupting or rushing. Remember that the toddler is just starting to be able to make the connections necessary to transfer thoughts and feelings into language.

Do not over-react to the child's use of the word "no." Give the toddler opportunities to appropriately use the word "no" with silly questions such as "Can a cat drive a car?" Teach the toddler appropriate words for body parts and objects. Help the toddler choose appropriate words to label feelings and emotions. Toddlers' receptive language and interpretation of body language and subtle signs far surpasses their expressive language especially at a younger age.

Encourage the use of both English and Spanish in the home.

Reading to the toddler everyday is one of the best ways to promote language and cognitive development. Toddlers particularly enjoy books about feelings, family, friends, everyday life, animals and nature, and fun and fantasy. Board books have thick pages that are easier for young toddlers to turn. The toddler may also enjoy "reading" the story to the parent.

2. Erikson defines the toddler period as a time of autonomy versus shame and doubt. It is a time of exerting independence. Exertion of independence often results in the toddler's favorite response, "No." The toddler will often answer "no" even when he or she really means "yes." Always saying "no," referred to as negativism, is a normal part of healthy development.

    If there is no option of avoiding an action, do not ask toddlers if they want to do something. Avoid closed ended yes–no questions, as the toddler's usual response is "No," whether he means it or not. Offer the child simple choices such as "Do you want to use the red cup or the blue cup." This helps give the toddler a sense of control. When getting ready to leave, do not ask the child if he wants to put his shoes on. Simply state in a matter of fact tone that shoes must be worn outside and give the toddler a choice on type of shoe or color of socks. If the child continues with negative answers, then the parent should remain calm and make the decision for the child.

3. Does not use 2-word sentences, does not imitate actions, does not follow basic instructions, and cannot push a toy with wheels.

SECTION III: PRACTICING FOR NCLEX

Activity F NCLEX-STYLE QUESTIONS

1. **Answer: c**
   Suggesting that the parents transition the child to a healthier diet by serving him more healthy choices along with smaller portions of junk food will reassure them that they are not starving their child. The parents would have less success with an abrupt change to healthy foods. Explaining calorie requirements and the time line for acceptance of a new food do not offer a practical reason for making a change in diet.

2. **Answer: a**
   This child has most recently acquired the ability to undress himself. Pushing a toy lawnmower and kicking a ball are things he learned at about 24 months. He was able to pull a toy while walking at about 18 months.

3. **Answer: d**
   Stopping the child when she is misbehaving and describing proper behavior sets limits and models good behavior and will be the most helpful advice to the parents. The child is too young to use time out or extinction as discipline. Slapping her hand, even done carefully with two fingers, is corporal punishment, which has been found to have negative effects on child development.

4. **Answer: b**
   Because they are curious and mobile, toddlers require direct observation and cannot be trusted to be left alone. The priority guidance is to never let the child be out of sight. Gating stairways, locking up chemicals, and not smoking around the child are excellent, but specific, safety interventions.

5. **Answer: b**
   The nurse would be concerned if the child is babbling to herself rather than using real words. By this age, she should be using simple sentences with a vocabulary of 150 to 300 words. Being unwilling to share toys, playing parallel with other children, and moving to different toys frequently are typical toddler behaviors.

6. **Answer: c**
   The fact that the child does not respond when the mother waves to him suggests he may have a vision problem. The toddler's sense of smell is still developing, so he may not be affected by odors. Their sense of taste is not well developed either, and this allows him to eat or drink poisons without concern. The child's crying at a sudden noise assures the nurse that his hearing is adequate.

7. **Answer: c**
   If the child is still speaking telegraphically in only 2- to 3-word sentences, it suggests there is a language development problem. If the child makes simple conversation, tells about something that happened in the past, or tells the nurse her name she is meeting developmental milestones for language.

8. **Answer: a**
   Separation anxiety should have disappeared or be subsiding by 3 years of age. The fact that it is persistent suggests there might an emotional problem. Emotional lability, self soothing by thumb sucking, or the inability to share are common for this age.

9. **Answer: b**

The nurse would be sure to tell the mother to feed her child iron-fortified cereal and other iron-rich foods when she weans her child off the breast or formula. Weaning from the breast is dependent upon the mother's need and desires with no set time. Weaning from the bottle is recommended at 1 year of age in order to prevent dental caries. Use of a no-spill sippy cup is not recommended because it too is associated with dental caries.

10. **Answer: d**

The nurse would recommend a preschool where the staff is trained in early childhood development and cardiopulmonary resuscitation. Cleanliness and a loving staff are not enough without competence. Good hygiene procedures require that a sick child not be allowed to attend. It is also important that parents are allowed to visit any time without an appointment.

11. **Answer: b**

The Erickson stage of development for the toddler is autonomy versus shame and doubt. During this period of time the child works to establish independence. Trust versus mistrust is the stage of infancy. Initiative versus guilt is the stage for the preschooler. Industry versus inferiority is the stage for school-aged children.

12. **Answer: a**

The ability to have object permanence is consistent with the phase of tertiary circular reactions.

13. **Answer: d**

The 20-month-old toddler should have a vocabulary greater than 75 to 100 words. A toddler at this age should comprehend approximately 200 words. The ability to point to named body points, discuss past events, and point to pictures in a book when asked are communication skills associated with an older child.

14. **Answer: a**

The social skills of the toddler at this age include parallel play. During parallel play children will play alongside each other not cooperatively. There is no indication that the aggression levels of the child need to be investigated. There is no indication the child needs increased socialization with other children.

Answers

CHAPTER 27

SECTION I: ASSESSING YOUR UNDERSTANDING

Activity A FILL IN THE BLANKS

1. Iron
2. Concrete
3. Urethra
4. Terror
5. Dense

Activity B MATCHING

Question 1

1. d **2.** a **3.** b **4.** f **5.** c **6.** e

Activity C SEQUENCING

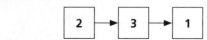

Activity D SHORT ANSWERS

1. The child in the intuitive phase can count 10 or more objects, correctly name at least 4 colors, can understand the concept of time, and knows about things that are used in everyday life such as appliances, money, and food.
2. A nightmare is a scary or bad dream. After a nightmare, the child is aroused and interactive. Night terrors are different. A short time after falling asleep, the child seems to awaken and is screaming. The child usually does not respond much to the parent's soothing, eventually stops screaming, and goes back to sleep. Night terrors are often frightening for parents, because the child does not seem to be responding to them.
3. The preschooler should have his or her teeth brushed and flossed daily with a pea-sized amount of toothpaste. Cariogenic foods should continue to be avoided. If sugary foods are consumed, the mouth should be rinsed with water if it is not possible to brush the teeth directly after their consumption. The preschool-age child should visit the dentist every 6 months.
4. The parent should ascertain the reason for the lie before punishing the child. If the child has broken a rule and fears punishment, then the parent must determine the truth. The child needs to learn that lying is usually far worse than the misbehavior itself. The punishment for the misbehavior should be lessened if the child admits the truth. The parent should remain calm and serve as a role model of an even temper.
5. The primary psychosocial task of the preschool period is developing a sense of initiative.

SECTION II: APPLYING YOUR KNOWLEDGE

Activity E CASE STUDY

1. Magical thinking and playing make believe are a normal part of preschool development. The preschool age child believes her thoughts to be all-powerful. The fantasy experienced through magical thinking and make believe allows the preschooler to make room in his world for the actual or the real and to satisfy her curiosity about differences in the world around her. Encouraging pretend play and providing props for dress-up stimulate and develop curiosity and creativity. Fantasy play is usually cooperative in nature and encourages the preschooler to develop social skills like turn-taking, communication, paying attention, and responding to one another's words and actions. Fantasy play also allows preschoolers to explore complex social ideas such as power, compassion, and cruelty.
2. Kindergarten may be a significant change for some children. The hours are usually longer than preschool and it is usually held 5 days per week. The setting and personnel are new and rules and expectations are often very different. When talking about starting kindergarten with Nila do so using an enthusiastic approach. Keep the conversation light and positive. Meet with Nila's teacher prior to the start of school and discuss any specific needs or concerns you may have. A tour of the school and attending the school's open house can help ease the transition also. Incorporate and practice the new daily routine prior to school starting. This can help the child adjust to the changes that are occurring.

3. The discussion should include the following points:
   - Cannot jump in place or ride a tricycle
   - Cannot stack four blocks
   - Cannot throw ball overhand
   - Does not grasp crayon with thumb and fingers
   - Difficulty with scribbling
   - Cannot copy a circle
   - Does not use sentences with three or more words
   - Cannot use the words "me" and "you" appropriately
   - Ignores other children or does not show interest in interactive games
   - Will not respond to people outside the family, still clings or cries if parents leave

SECTION III: PRACTICING FOR NCLEX

Activity F NCLEX-STYLE QUESTIONS

1. **Answer: b**
   The presence of only 10 deciduous teeth would warrant further investigation. The preschooler should have 20 deciduous teeth present. The absence of dental caries or presence of 19 teeth does not warrant further investigation.

2. **Answer: b**
   The nurse should encourage the mother to schedule a meeting with the teacher prior to school's start date and set up a time to tour the classroom and school so the boy knows what to expect. The other statements are not helpful and do not address the mother's or boy's concerns.

3. **Answer: c**
   The average preschool child will grow 2½ to 3 inches per year. The nurse would expect that the child's height would have increased 2½ to 3 inches since last year's well child examination.

4. **Answer: b**
   By the age of 5, persons outside of the family should be able to understand most of the child's speech without the parents "translation." The other statements would not warrant additional referral or follow-up. A child of 5 years should be able to count to at least 10, know his or her address, and participate in long detailed conversations.

5. **Answer: a**
   During a night terror, a child is typically unaware of the parent's presence and may scream and thrash more if restrained. During a nightmare, a child is responsive to the parent's soothing and reassurances. The other statements are indicative of a nightmare.

6. **Answer: d**
   The preschooler is not mature enough to ride a bicycle in the street even if riding with adults, so the nurse should emphasize that the girl should always ride on the sidewalk even if the mother is riding with her daughter. The other statements are correct.

7. **Answer: c**
   The nurse needs to emphasize that there are number of reasons that a parent should not choose a preschool that utilizes corporal punishment. It may negatively affect a child's self-esteem as well as ability to achieve in school. It may also lead to disruptive and violent behavior in the classroom and should be discouraged. The other statements would not warrant further discussion or intervention.

8. **Answer: b**
   The nurse should explain to the parents that attributing life-like qualities to inanimate objects is quite normal. Telling the parents that their daughter is demonstrating animism is correct, but it would be better to explain what animism is and then remind them that it is developmentally appropriate. Asking whether they think their daughter is hallucinating or whether there is a family history of mental history is inappropriate and does not teach.

9. **Answer: a**
   The nurse needs to remind the parents that the girl should use a helmet when riding any wheeled toy, not just her bicycle. The other statements are correct.

10. **Answer: c**
    It is important to remind the parents that they should perform flossing in the preschool period because the child is unable to perform this task. The other statements are correct.

11. **Answer: d**
    The average 4-year-old child is 40.5 inches. The average rate of growth per year is between 2.5 and 3 inches. The child in the scenario demonstrates normal stature and growth patterns.

12. **Answer: c**
    Preschool-aged children may become occupied with activities around them and not remember to void. Reminding them to void is helpful. Discipline should not be applied to infrequent episodes of incontinence. There is no indication the child has an infection.

13. **Answer: d**
    Preschool-aged children often interact with imaginary friends. The nurse should recognize this as normal for the age group. No special actions are needed.

14. **Answer: c**
    Sexual curiosity is normal in the preschool-aged child. The parents should be encouraged to provide brief, honest answers to the child. The parents must also determine the type of curiosity the child has. Explanations should be within the level of understanding of the child.

15. **Answer: a**
    Fears are normal in the preschool-aged child. Some children are afraid of the dark. The parents should be advised to show patience with their child as he works through this fear. Refusing a night light will further increase the stress of the child. Turning out the light may have the child waking up in darkness and becoming further afraid.

CHAPTER 28

SECTION I: ASSESSING YOUR UNDERSTANDING

Activity A FILL IN THE BLANKS

1. 8
2. 2
3. 10th
4. Energy
5. Injury
6. Stress
7. Industry
8. Peers
9. Lower
10. 12

Activity B MATCHING

Question 1

1. c   2. a   3. e   4. b   5. f   6. d

Question 2

1. c   2. b   3. a

Question 3

1. b   2. c   3. d   4. a

Activity C SEQUENCING

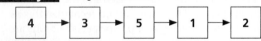

4 → 3 → 5 → 1 → 2

Activity D SHORT ANSWERS

1. Children aged 6 to 8 enjoy bicycling, skating, and swimming. Children between 8 and 10 years of age have greater rhythm and gracefulness of muscular movements; they enjoy activities such as sports. Those aged 10 to 12 years, especially girls, are more controlled and focused, similar to adults.
2. The child typically feels discomfort in new situations, requires additional time to adjust, and exhibits frustration with tears or somatic complaints. Also described as irritable and moody, the child could benefit from patience, firmness, and understanding when faced with new situations.

3. The nurse's role includes promotion of healthy growth and development through anticipatory guidance, goal attainment, playing, learning, education, and reading. The nurse's role also includes addressing common developmental concerns, assessing the individual child, and recommending intervention or referral where needed.
4. Children between ages 6 and 8 years require approximately 12 hours of sleep per night; those between 8 and 10 years of age require 10 to 12 hours of sleep per night. Children between 10 and 12 years of age require 9 to 10 hours of sleep per night. Some children, regardless of their age group, may need an occasional nap.
5. Body image refers to the perception of one's body. During the school-age period there is a strong interest on the clothing and appearance of others. It is important not to be teased or ridiculed.

SECTION II: APPLYING YOUR KNOWLEDGE

Activity E CASE STUDY

1. The discussion should include the following points:

    The role of the family in promoting healthy growth and development is critical. Respectful interchange of communication between the parent and child will foster self-esteem and self-confidence. This respect will give the child confidence in achieving personal, educational, and social goals appropriate for his or her age. During your exam, model appropriate behaviors by listening to the child and making appropriate responses. Serve as a resource for parents and as an advocate for the child in promoting healthy growth and development. Negative comments to the child concerning her appearance may be counterproductive and harm her self-esteem.

2. The discussion should include the following points:

    The school-age child is able to see how her actions affect others and to realize that her behaviors can have consequences. Therefore, discipline techniques with consequences often work well. For example, the child refuses to put away his or her toys, so the parent forbids him or her to play with those toys. Parents need to teach children the rules established by the family, values, and social rules of conduct. This will help give the child guidelines to what behaviors are acceptable and unacceptable. Parents need to be role models and demonstrate appropriate expressions of feelings and emotions and allow the child to express emotions and feelings. They should never belittle the child, and they need to preserve the child's self-esteem and dignity. Parents should be encouraged to discipline with praise. This positive acknowledgment can encourage appropriate behavior.

When misbehaviors occur, the type and amount of discipline should be based upon the developmental level of the child and the parents, severity of misbehavior, established roles of the family, temperament of the child, and response of the child to rewards. The child should participate in developing a plan of action for his or her misbehavior. Consistency in discipline, along with providing it in a nurturing environment, is essential.

3. The discussion should include the following points:

Although some television shows and video games can have positive influences on children, guidelines on the use of television and video games are important. Research has shown that the amount of time watching television or playing video games can lead to aggressive behavior, less physical activity, and altered body image.

Parents should set limits on how much television the child is allowed to watch. The Academy of Pediatrics recommends 2 hours or less of television viewing per day. The parent should establish guidelines on when the child can watch television, and television watching should not be used as a reward. The parents should monitor what the child is watching, and they should watch the programs together and use that opportunity to discuss the subject matter with the child.

Parents should also prohibit television or video games with violence. There should be no television during dinner and no television in the child's room. The parents need to set examples for the child and encourage sports, interactive play, and reading. They should encourage their child to read instead of watching television or to do a physical activity together as a family. If the television causes fights
or arguments, it should be turned off for a period of time.

SECTION III: PRACTICING FOR NCLEX
Activity F NCLEX-STYLE QUESTIONS

1. **Answer: a**
The child will be able to consider an action and its consequences in Piaget's period of concrete operational thought. However, she is now able to

empathize with others. She is more adept at classifying and dividing things into sets. Defining lying as bad because she gets punished for it is a Kohlberg characteristic.

2. **Answer: b**
The child with an easy temperament will adapt to school with only minor stresses. The slow-to-warm child will experience frustration. The difficult child will be moody and irritable and may benefit from a preschool visit.

3. **Answer: b**
It is very important to get a bike of the proper size for the child. Getting a bike that the child can "grow into" is dangerous. Training wheels and grass to fall on are not acceptable substitutes for the proper protective gear. The child should already demonstrate good coordination in other playing skills before attempting to ride a bike.

4. **Answer: c**
Asking how often the family eats together is an appropriate question for the girl. All the others should be directed to the parents.

5. **Answer: c**
The nurse would have found that the child still has a leaner body mass than girls at this age. Both boys and girls increase body fat at this age. Food preferences will be highly influenced by those of her parents. Although caloric intake may diminish; appetite will increase.

6. **Answer: d**
Parents are major influences on school-age children and should discuss the dangers of tobacco and alcohol use with the child. Not smoking in the house and hiding alcohol send mixed messages to the child. Open and honest discussion is the best approach rather than forbidding the child to make friends with kids that use tobacco or alcohol.

7. **Answer: b**
The girl would need approximately 2,065 calories per day. (65 lbs = 29.5 kg $\times$ 70 calories per day per kg = 2,065 calories per day).

8. **Answer: b**
Because they are role models for their children, parents must first realize the importance of their own behaviors. It is possible that the parents are pressuring the child, but that is not the primary message. Punishment should be appropriate, consistent, and not too severe.

9. **Answer: b**
Lymphatic tissue growth is complete by age 9 better helping to localize infections and produce antibody–antigen responses. Brain growth will be complete by age 10. Frontal sinuses are developed at age 7. Third molars do not erupt until the teen years.

10. **Answer: d**
The nurse would recommend that the parents be good role models and quit smoking. Locking up or hiding your cigarettes and going outside to

smoke is not as effective as having a tobacco-free environment in the home.

11. **Answer: c**
Self-esteem is developed early in childhood. The feedback a child receives from those perceived in authority such as parents and educators impact the child's sense of self-worth. As the child ages, the influences of peers and their treatment of the child begin to have an increasing influence on self-esteem.

12. **Answer: b**
The child can be permanently scarred by negative experiences such a bullying. Activities such as self-defense and sports can promote a sense of accomplishment but are not most import option. There is no indication the child in the scenario will become a bully.

13. **Answer: d**
School-aged children are often preoccupied with thoughts of death and dying. There is no indica-tion these thoughts will lead to mental health issues or the development of depression.

14. **Answer: b**
The values of a child are determined largely by the influences of their parents. As the child ages the impact of peers does begin to enter the pic-ture. Children may also begin to test the values with their actions. In most cases the values of the family will prevail.

15. **Answer: a, d**
During hospitalization the school-aged child may exhibit increased clinging behaviors. The child may also demonstrate regression. It will be helpful to promote the child be able to make some decisions or have some age appropriate sense
of control. Ignoring the behaviors may be counterproductive.

Answers

CHAPTER 29

SECTION I: ASSESSING YOUR UNDERSTANDING

Activity A FILL IN THE BLANKS

1. Psychosocial
2. Infancy
3. Abstract
4. Positive
5. Hispanic
6. Crisis
7. Identity
8. Ossification
9. Coordination
10. Socioeconomics

Activity B MATCHING

Question 1

1. c   2. f   3. a   4. e   5. b   6. d

Question 2

1. e   2. c   3. a   4. d   5. f   6. b

Question 3

1. c   2. a   3. d   4. b   5. e

Activity C SEQUENCING

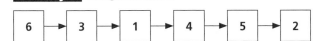

Activity D SHORT ANSWERS

1. Ambivalence, 10% wanted to become pregnant, 40% did not mind being pregnant, escape from home life, rite of passage to adulthood, peer pressure, confrontation of parental authority, ignorance.
2. The adolescent tries out various roles when interacting with peers, family, community, and society; this strengthens his or her sense of self. Past stages revisited tend to be those of trust (who/what to believe in), autonomy (expression of individuality), initiative (vision for what he or she might become), and industry (choices in school, community, church, and at work).

3. Completing school prepares the adolescent for college and/or employment. Schools that support peer bonds, promote health and fitness, encourage parental involvement, and strengthen community relationships lead to better student outcomes. Teachers, coaches, and counselors provide guidance and support to the adolescent.
4. The nurse should encourage parents and teens to have sexuality discussions. Sexuality discussions increase the teen's knowledge and strengthen his or her ability to make responsible decisions about sexual behavior.
5. Diet, exercise, and hereditary factors influence the height, weight, and body build of the adolescent. Over the past three decades, adolescents have become taller and heavier than their ancestors and the beginning of puberty is earlier. During the early adolescent period, there is an increase in the percentage of body fat and the head, neck, and hands reach adult proportions.
6. According to Piaget, the adolescent progresses from a concrete framework of thinking to an abstract one. It is the formal operational period. During this period, the adolescent develops the ability to think outside of the present; that is, he or she can incorporate into thinking concepts that do exist as well as concepts that might exist. Her thinking becomes logical, organized, and consistent. She is able to think about a problem from all points of view, ranking the possible solutions while solving the problem. Not all adolescents achieve formal operational reasoning at the same time.

SECTION II: APPLYING YOUR KNOWLEDGE

Activity E CASE STUDY

1. The discussion should include the following points:

   Today, piercing of the tongue, lip, eyebrow, naval, and nipple are common. Generally, body piercing is harmless, but Cho should be cautioned about receiving these procedures under nonsterile conditions and about the risk of complications. Qualified personnel using sterile needles should perform the procedure, and proper cleansing of the area at least twice a day is important. Although body piercing is common and considered relatively harmless, complications can occur. The complications of body piercing vary by site. Infections from body piercing usually result from unclean tools of the trade. Some of the infections that may occur as a result of unclean tools include hepatitis, tetanus, tuberculosis, and HIV. These complications may not become evident for some time after the piercing has been performed. Also, keloid formation and allergies to metal may occur. The naval is an area prone for infection since it is a moist area that endures friction from clothing. Once a naval infection occurs, it may take up to a year to heal.

2. The discussion should include the following points:

Be open and respectful of the teen's decision about sexual activity. Discuss contraceptive options and a referral to a teen clinic may be appropriate. Provide education and information on abstinence, contraception, and the reality of caring for an infant. Reinforce that pregnancy and STIs, including HIV, can occur with any sexual encounter without the use of contraception. Stress the importance of the use of contraception.

Identify if Cho is at risk for STIs and pregnancy based on her sexual practices. Encourage frequent and ongoing follow-ups. Encourage discussion with her parents about sexuality. Reinforce that engaging in sexual relations should be her choice and should not be influenced by peers. It is her right to say no. Reinforce that sexual activity in mature relationships should be respectful to both parties.

3. The discussion should include the following points:

Families and parents of adolescents experience changes and conflicts that require adjustments and understanding of the development of the adolescent. The adolescent is striving for self-identity and increased independence. Maintaining open lines of communication is essential but often difficult during this time. Parents sense that they have less influence on the adolescent as they spend more time with peers, questions family values, and become more mobile.

To help improve communication, encourage Cho's mother to set aside an appropriate amount of time to discuss matters without interruptions. Encourage her to talk face-to-face with Cho and to be aware of both her and Cho's body language. Suggest that she ask questions about what Cho is feeling and offer Cho suggestions and advice. Cho's mother should choose her words carefully and be aware of her tone of voice and body language. Cho's mother should listen to what Cho has to say and should speak to her as an equal. It is important that her mother does not pretend to know all the answers and admits her mistakes. The

mother should be reminded to give praise and approval to Cho often and to ensure rules and limits are set fairly and discussed.

SECTION III: PRACTICING FOR NCLEX

Activity F NCLEX-STYLE QUESTIONS

1. **Answer: c**
Asking broad, unanswerable questions, such as what the meaning of life is, is a Kohlberg activity for early adolescence. An example of Piaget activities for middle adolescence is wondering why things can't change (like wishing her parents were more understanding) and assuming everyone shares her interests. Comparing morals with those of peers is a Kohlberg activity for middle adolescence.

2. **Answer: b**
Since most contraception methods are designed for females, it is important to teach the boy that contraception is a shared responsibility. Statistics about adolescent cases of STIs and warnings about getting the girl pregnant can easily be ignored by the child's sense of invulnerability. The fact that girls are more susceptible to STIs may give the boy a false sense of security.

3. **Answer: d**
Cheese, yogurt, white beans, milk, and broccoli are good sources of calcium. Strawberries, watermelon, raisins, peanut butter, tomato juice, and whole grain bread are all foods high in iron. Beans, poultry, fish, meats, and dairy products are foods high in protein.

4. **Answer: a**
Peers serve as role models for social behaviors, so their impact on an adolescent can be negative if the group is using drugs, or the group leader is in trouble. Sharing problems with peers helps the adolescent work through conflicts with parents. The desire to be part of the group teaches the child to negotiate differences and develop loyalties.

5. **Answer: c**
Amphetamine use manifests as euphoria with rapid talking and dilated pupils. Signs of opiate use are drowsiness and constricted pupils. Barbiturates typically cause a sense of euphoria followed by depression. Marijuana users are typically relaxed and uninhibited.

6. **Answer: b**
Checking for signs of depression or lack of friends would be most effective for preventing suicide. All other choices are more effective for preventing violence to others.

7. **Answer: a**
The best approach is to describe the proper care using frequent cleansing with antibacterial soap. This is too late for warnings about the dangers of

piercing such as skin- or blood-borne infections, or disease from unclean needles.

8. **Answer: c**

   If the boy has entered adolescence, he would also have frequent mood changes. A growing interest in attracting girls' attention and understanding that actions have consequences are typical of the middle stage of adolescence. Feeling secure with his body image does not occur until late adolescence.

9. **Answer: d**

   Increased blood pressure to adult levels indicates the child is in the early stage of adolescence. Increased shoulder, chest, and hip widths and muscle mass increase occurs in mid-adolescence. Eruption of the last four molars occurs in late adolescence.

10. **Answer: b**

    Whole grain bread contains high amounts of iron and is a type of food the child would not have an aversion to. Milk is a good source of vitamin D. Carrots are high in vitamin A. Orange juice is a good source for vitamin C.

11. **Answer: c**

    Teen age boys can experience growth in height until age 17.5. The nurse should reassure the teen that this may happen for him. Telling the client not to be ashamed, or assuring him it is not as short as his peers fails to provide information or support. Determining the height of the other men

in the family may be indicated at a later time but is not the most appropriate initial comment.

12. **Answer: c**

    The dietary intake for active teen females should include be approximately 2,200 calories daily.

13. **Answer: c**

    Piaget's developmental theories focus on the cognitive maturation of the child. The ability to critically think is a sign of successful cognitive maturation. A sense of internal identity is consistent with Erikson's theories of development. Kohlberg's theories development focus on morals and values.

14. **Answer: c**

    The sedentary teen needs to consume approximately 1,600 calories each day. The recommended numbers of servings of fruit needed daily are two. A balanced diet includes a small amount of fat. To avoid all fat could place the child's health at risk. Protein intake is important for the development of tissue. The teen will need about 5 ounces of protein daily.

15. **Answer: b**

    The teenaged male has pubic hair that is beginning to curl. This takes place between ages 11 and 14. Absent or sparse pubic hair is consistent with a younger child. Coarse pubic hair is seen in older teens and adult men.

Answers

CHAPTER 30

SECTION I: ASSESSING YOUR UNDERSTANDING

Activity A FILL IN THE BLANKS

1. Atraumatic
2. Therapeutic
3. Nonverbal
4. Child life
5. Verbal
6. Active
7. Interpreter

Activity B MATCHING

1. e   2. a   3. d   4. c   5. b

Activity C SEQUENCING

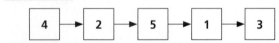

Activity D SHORT ANSWERS

1. Therapeutic hugging is a method of safely preventing a child from harm during a painful or uncomfortable procedure that decreases fear and anxiety. The parent or caregiver holds the child in a position that promotes close physical contact in a way that restrains the child as necessary for the procedure to be performed successfully. This technique provides atraumatic care during procedures such as injections, venipunctures, and other invasive procedures.
2. The child or family will be able to demonstrate a skill, repeat information in their own words, answer open-ended questions, and act out the proper care procedure.
3. Signs exhibited by families or children that should alert the nurse of problems with health literacy include: difficulty completing registration forms or health care forms that are incomplete; frequently missed appointments; noncompliance with prescribed treatment; history of medication errors; claiming to have forgotten glasses or asking to take forms home to complete in regards to reading material or filling out forms; inability to answer questions about health care or avoiding asking questions regarding health care.
4. Draw pictures or use medical illustrations, use videos, color-code medications or steps of a procedure, record an audio tape, repeat verbal information often and "chunk" it into small bites, and teach a "back-up" family member.
5. The nurse should be an advocate of family-centered care in order to prevent separation, resulting in anxiety of both the family and child during hospitalization. The nurse can provide comfortable accommodations for the family and allow the family to choose if they want to be present for procedures that are uncomfortable for their child.

SECTION II: APPLYING YOUR KNOWLEDGE

Activity E CASE STUDY

1. The discussion should include the following:
   The nurse should avoid using terms that Emma may not understand or interpret differently from the intended meaning. The nurse could tell Emma that she will be taken to another room on a "special bed with wheels" rather than on a "stretcher." When describing the CT equipment the nurse could use an explanation such as, "there will be a big machine in the room that works like a camera. It will take pictures of your head since you hurt it when you fell. Your mommy and daddy will be able to go to this room with you and they will stand right outside the room when the camera takes the pictures."
2. The discussion should include the following:
   Therapeutic hugging should be utilized since this will allow Emma's parents to provide a comforting way of safely holding her so that the stitches can
   be placed with decreased trauma. The nurse should be sure that the parents understand how to hold Emma properly so that the procedure can be performed successfully while maintaining safety and security.

SECTION III: PRACTICING FOR NCLEX
Activity F NCLEX-STYLE QUESTIONS

1. **Answer: c**
   Nodding the head while the other person speaks indicates interest in what they are saying. When children and parents feel they are being heard, it builds trust. Sitting straight with feet flat on the floor, looking away from the speaker, and keeping distance from the family may send a message of disinterest.

2. **Answer: a**
   Having a child life specialist play with the child would provide the greatest support for the child and make the greatest contribution to atraumatic care. It is important to explain the procedure to the child and parents, let the child have a favorite toy and keep the parents calm, but these interventions are not as effective for atraumatic care.

3. **Answer: c**
   Since the child has just been diagnosed, concerns about postoperative home care would be least important. Arranging an additional meeting with the specialist and discussing treatment options may be necessary at some point, but involving the child and family in decision making is always a goal and is a part of family-centered care.

4. **Answer: b**
   Asking questions is a valid way to evaluate learning. However, it is far more effective to ask open-ended questions because they will better expose missing or incorrect information. As with teaching, evaluation of learning that involves active participation is more effective. This includes the child and family demonstrating skills, teaching skills to each other, and acting out scenarios.

5. **Answer: d**
   Recognizing the parents' and child's desire regarding treatment options is part of family-centered care. Presenting options for treatment is vague. Informing the child in terms that she can understand is the best example of therapeutic communication, which is goal, focused, purposeful communication.

6. **Answer: c**
   The nurse is responsible for determining that the parents or legal guardians understand teaching that has been provided, as well as what they are signing, by asking pertinent questions of them. The physician or advanced practitioner is responsible for informing the child and family about the treatment, the potential risks and benefits, and alternative methods available; simply presenting this information does not ensure understanding. Witnessing the signing of the consent form should not occur until the nurse is sure the family understands teaching.

7. **Answer: c**
   While it is important that the nurse recognizes and show respect for the parents' beliefs, and communicates in appropriate terms that they will understand, educating them carefully about the procedure and prognosis is vitally important in ensuring the child receives appropriate care. Assuring the competency of the surgeon is not therapeutic.

8. **Answer: a**
   Missing appointments is one of the red flags to health literacy problems as the parents may not have understood the importance of the appointment or may not have been able to read or understand appointment reminders. Being bi-lingual does not indicate health literacy issues. Taking notes or one-parent being the primary leader of the child's health care are not unusual practices.

9. **Answer: a, c, d**
   School age children better understand about and participate in their own care than preschoolers and toddlers. They need time to prepare themselves mentally for the procedure and should be given 3 to 7 days. Plays and puppets are more appropriate for preschoolers. Active involvement in self-care will help them adjust and learn. Giving them choices to make allows them control and involvement in the process.

10. **Answer: c**
    Asking questions or having private conversations with the interpreter may make the family uncomfortable and destroy the child/nurse relationship. Translation takes longer than a same-language appointment, and must be considered so that the family is not rushed. Using a nonprofessional runs the risk that they won't be able to adequately translate medical terminology. Using an older sibling can upset the family relationships or cause legal problems.

11. **Answer: a, d, e**
    RATIONALE: The child life specialist commonly assists with nonmedical preparation for diagnostic testing, provides tours, assists in play therapy, and is the child's advocate. The child's nurse gives medication, vaccines, and starts intravenous lines.

12. **Answer: a, c, d, e**
    RATIONALE: Taking notes is an indicator that the mother is literate. All of the other options are "red flags" that indicate the mother may not be literate.

13. **Answers: a, c, d**
    RATIONALE: The nurse should position himself or herself at the child's level. The nurse should speak in an unhurried manner. The nurse should ensure that the child's parents are present during education. It is appropriate to use words that the child will understand. It is appropriate to show patience during the interaction and look for nonverbal cues that indicate understanding or confusion.

14. **Answers: a, d, e**
    RATIONALE: It is appropriate to use the word "tube" and not a "catheter." It is appropriate to call a "gurney" a "rolling bed." It is better to call "dye" special medicine. Terms used in the other options may be misunderstood by the child.

15. **Answers: b, c, d, e**
    RATIONALE: When following the principles of atraumatic care, it is appropriate to apply numbing cream prior to starting the child's intravenous line. It is appropriate to empower the child with choices about care, if possible. It is appropriate for the child to have a security item present in the hospital. It is helpful for the family if the parent is able to stay with the child because it helps make the environment less stressful. The nurse should avoid using the phrase "holding the child down" and replace this with "therapeutic hugging."

Answers

CHAPTER 31

SECTION I: ASSESSING YOUR UNDERSTANDING

Activity A FILL IN THE BLANKS

1. Development
2. In-utero
3. Community
4. Prevention
5. When
6. Coronary
7. Bone
8. Immunosuppression
9. Fixate
10. Active

Activity B MATCHING

Question 1

1. b   2. e   3. c   4. f   5. d   6. a

Question 2

1. c   2. a   3. b   4. e   5. d

Question 3

1. b   2. d   3. a   4. e   5. c

Activity C SEQUENCING

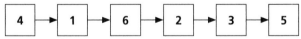

Activity D SHORT ANSWERS

1. Place a vibrating tuning fork in the middle of the top of the head. Ask if the sound is in one ear or both ears. The sound should be heard in both ears.
2. Conditions in parents or grandparents what would suggest screening for hyperlipidemia in children includes coronary atherosclerosis, myocardial infarction, angina pectoris, peripheral vascular disease, cerebrovascular disease, and sudden cardiac death.
3. If problems are noted in the provided history, objective audiometry should be performed. When the child is capable of following simple commands, the nurse can perform basic procedures to screen

for hearing loss. The "whisper," Weber, and Rinne tests can be used to screen for sensorineural or conductive hearing loss.

4. Iron deficiency is the leading nutritional deficiency in the United States. Iron deficiency can cause cognitive and motor deficits resulting in developmental delays and behavioral disturbances. The increased incidence of iron deficiency anemia is directly associated with periods of diminished iron stores, rapid growth, and high metabolic demands. At 6 months of age, the in utero iron stores of a full-term infant are almost depleted. The adolescent growth spurt warrants constant iron replacement. Pregnant adolescents are at even higher risk for iron deficiency due to the demands of the mother's growth spurt and the needs of the developing fetus.
5. Universal hypertension screening for children beginning at 3 years of age is recommended. If the child has risk factors for systemic hypertension, such as preterm birth, very low birth weight, renal disease, organ transplant, congenital heart disease or other illnesses associated with hypertension, then screening begins when the risk factor becomes apparent.

SECTION II: APPLYING YOUR KNOWLEDGE

Activity E CASE STUDY

Case Study 1

1. The discussion should include the following points:

   Nutritional history should be collected directly from Jasmine. There must be a discussion of her activity levels. Her height and weight should be plotted on a growth chart to observe trends.
2. The discussion should include the following points:

   Screening for iron deficiency is warranted for Jasmine. Iron deficiency is the leading nutritional deficiency in the United States. The increased incidence of iron deficiency anemia is directly associated with periods of rapid growth and high metabolic demands. The adolescent growth spurt warrants constant iron replacement. The Centers for Disease Control and Prevention recommends universal screening of high-risk children at various age intervals. Jasmine demonstrates risk factors for iron deficiency anemia, including the rapid growth spurt of adolescence, meal skipping and dieting, and low intake of fish, meat, and poultry. The American Academy of Pediatrics (AAP) recommends universal screening of all adolescent females during all routine physical examinations, therefore placing Jasmine in this category.

3. The discussion should include the following points:

Your focus of healthy weight promotions should be health-centered, not weight-centered. Emphasize the benefits of health through an active lifestyle and nutritious eating pattern. Gear the education to focus on Jasmine's growing autonomy in making self-care decisions. Encourage healthy eating habits and healthy activity. Limit sedentary activities such as television viewing, computer usage, and video games.

Case Study 2

1. The discussion should include the following points:

Children with chronic illnesses require repeated assessments to determine their health maintenance needs. How their illnesses impact their functional health patterns determines if standard health supervision visits need to be augmented to meet the individual child's situation.

Nurses need to ensure comprehensive health supervision with frequent repeated assessments that include psychosocial assessments. The assessments should cover issues such as health insurance coverage, availability of transportation, financial stressors, family coping, and school personnel response to the child's chronic illness. The nurse needs to help develop an effective partnership between the child's medical home, family, and community.

Coordination of care and access to resources is vital and enhances the quality of life for children with chronic illnesses. Nurses need to assist families in finding support groups and community-based resources, as well as financial and medical assistance programs. The nurse can also educate school personnel about the child's illness and assist them in maximizing the child's potential for academic success.

SECTION III: PRACTICING FOR NCLEX

Activity F NCLEX-STYLE QUESTIONS

1. **Answer: d**
Congenital facial malformations are developmental warning signs. Neonatal conjunctivitis, when properly treated, has no long-term effects on development. Parents who are college students are not risk factors as would be high school dropouts. A 36-week birth is not a warning sign, but 33 weeks or less is.

2. **Answer: b**
Asking what activities that promote exercise for the child is best for several reasons. It provides assessment of the child's activity preferences, whether health-centered (positive) or weight centered (negative), and it offers variety. If on option doesn't work, others might. Emphasizing appropriate weight or dietary shortcomings can lead to eating disorders or body hatred. Suggesting only softball limits the success of the healthy weight promotion.

3. **Answer: c**
The most compelling argument for vaccinating for Varicella is that children not immunized are at risk if exposed to the disease. The mother needs to know about the chance of her child contracting the illness if not immunized. The contagious nature of the disease, low risk of the vaccine, or the low incidence of reactions is not appropriate explanations for why the child should have the vaccine.

4. **Answer: c**
Iron deficiency anemia could be present because the iron stores in the boy's body may have diminished by the adolescent's growth spurt. This would be checked for by blood work. Developmental problems are not caused by the adolescent's growth spurt. Hyperlipidemia could be possible if the child's diet included an excessive amount of fat. Hypertension might be a problem if a family member had the condition in early adulthood or if many family members had this condition.

5. **Answer: d**
The nurse will provide information to prevent injury or disease such as discussing the hazards of putting the baby to sleep with a bottle. Assessing for an infection and taking a health history for an injury are not part of a health supervision visit. Administering a vaccination for Varicella would not occur until 12 months of age.

6. **Answer: a**
The nurse will advise the mother that poor oral health can have significant negative effects on systemic health. Discussing fluoridation and community health may have little interest to the mother. Placing the hands in the mouth exposes the child to pathogens and is appropriate for personal hygiene promotion. Soft drink consumption is better covered during healthy diet promotion.

7. **Answer: b**
Maintaining proper therapy for eczema can be exhausting both physically and mentally. Therefore it is essential that the nurse assess parents' ability to cope with this stress. Changing a bandage is not part of a health supervision visit. Skin hydration is important for a child with eczema;

however, fluid volume is not a concern. Systemic corticosteroid therapy is very rarely used and the success of the current therapy needs to be assessed first.

8. **Answer: c**
The Ishihara chart is best for the 6-year-old because the child will know numbers. CVTME charts are designed to assess color vision discrimination for preschoolers. The Allen figures chart and the Snellen charts are for assessing visual acuity.

9. **Answer: d**
Neighborhoods with high crime, high poverty, and lack of resources may contribute to poor health care and illness. If the aged grandparents have healthy lifestyles, they would be positive partners. Developmentally appropriate chores and responsibilities could be positive signs of parental guidance. The doting mother could make a strong health supervision partner.

10. **Answer: a**
The Rinne test compares air conduction of sound with bone conduction of sound and can be performed in the office. The Whisper test requires a quiet room with no distractions. Auditory Brainstem Response (ABR) and the Evoked Otoacoustic Emissions (EOAE) are indicated for newborns and are usually done by an audiologist.

11. **Answer: c**
A 3-year-old child should have the ability to copy a circle. Stacking five blocks, grasping a crayon, and throwing a ball overhand are not reasonable accomplishments for a 3-year-old child.

12. **Answer: a, c, d**
The Denver II screening test is used on children from birth to age 6 months. It is used to assess personal–social, fine motor–adaptive, language, and gross motor skills. The test employs props. These include dolls, crayons, and balls.

13. **Answer: c**
In the absence of risk factors vision screening should begin in children once they reach the age of 3.

14. **Answer: b**
Passive immunity results when immunoglobulins are passed from one person to another. This immunity is temporary. This is the type of immunity that takes place when a mother breastfeeds her child. Active immunity results when an individual's own immunity generates an immune response.

15. **Answer: d**
Populations at an increased risk for elevated blood lead levels include immigrants, refugees, or international adoptees.

Answers

CHAPTER 32

SECTION I: ASSESSING YOUR UNDERSTANDING

Activity A FILL IN THE BLANKS

1. PERRLA
2. BMI
3. Fontanel
4. Stethoscope
5. Stridor
6. Milia
7. Auscultation

Activity B LABELING

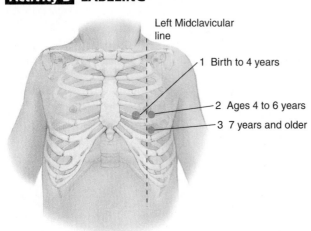

Left Midclavicular line

1 Birth to 4 years

2 Ages 4 to 6 years

3 7 years and older

Activity C MATCHING

1. c   2. e   3. a   4. d   5. b

Activity D SEQUENCING

2 → 3 → 4 → 1

Activity E SHORT ANSWERS

1. Grade one is barely audible, sometimes heard, sometimes not. Grade two is quiet, yet heard each time the chest is auscultated. Grade three and four are audible with grade three having an intermediate intensity and grade four having a palpable thrill. Grade five is loud and is audible with the edge of stethoscope lifted off the chest. Grade six is very loud and audible with the stethoscope placed near but not touching the chest.

2. Ecchymosis is a purplish discoloration (bruise) that changes from blue, to brown to black. It is common on the lower extremities in young children.

    Petechiae are pinpoint reddish purple macules that do not blanch when pressed. They are broken tiny blood vessels that occur with coughing, bleeding disorders and meningococcemia.

    Purpura is purple larger macules caused by bleeding under the skin and occurs with bleeding disorders and meningococcemia.

3. The canal should be pink, have tiny hairs, and be free from scratches, drainage, foreign bodies, and edema. The tympanic membrane should appear pearly pink or gray and be translucent allowing visualization of the bony landmarks.

4. The heart rate of the child gradually decreases from infancy to adolescence. The infant's normal heart rate ranges from 80 to 150 beats per minute, with the toddlers heart rate decreasing slightly to 70 to 120 beats per minute. The preschooler and school-age child have similar normal heart rates at 65 to 110 and 60 to 100, respectively. The adolescent's normal heart rate drops to 55 to 95 beats per minute.

5. Inaccurate pulse oximetry readings may result from the child having a low hemoglobin value, hypotension, hypothermia, hypovolemia, skin breakdown, carbon monoxide poisoning, interference with the ambient light, and movement of the extremity.

6. Possible risk factors that indicate the need for BP measurement of children under the age of 3 years include: history of prematurity, very low birth weight, or other neonatal complications; congenital heart disease; recurrent urinary tract infections or any other renal complication; any malignancy or transplant; any treatment that causes the BP to increase; systemic illnesses that affect the BP; and increased intracranial pressure.

SECTION II: APPLYING YOUR KNOWLEDGE

Activity F CASE STUDY

The discussion should include the following points:

FIRST PRIORITY: A 7-month-old hospitalized with pneumonia. Vital signs are heart rate of 165 with brief episodes of dropping into the 60's during the previous shift, respiratory rate of 78, blood pressure 112/72, and axillary temperature of 99.5 F.

RATIONALE: This child is the most unstable. The tachypnea, tachycardia with bradycardic episodes can be indicative of a potentially unstable airway. The increased blood pressure may also indicate acute distress.

SECOND PRIORITY: A 3-month-old hospitalized for rule out sepsis secondary to fever. Vital signs are heart rate of 165, respiratory rate of 34, blood pressure 108/64, rectal temperature of 102.5 F taken immediately before report. No intervention was initiated.

RATIONALE: This child is potentially unstable. The tachycardia and increased blood pressure are most likely due to fever and stress. The increased temperature (without intervention) is a concern but overall this child's vital signs are less life-threatening than the tachypnea and bradycardia present in the first priority child.

THIRD PRIORITY: A 5-year-old hospitalized with an acute asthma attack. Vital signs are heart rate 124, respiratory rate 28 to 30, blood pressure 93/48, and axillary temperature of 98.6 F.

RATIONALE: This child has an acute illness and may be potentially unstable due to slightly increased respiratory rate and mild tachycardia. This child warrants close monitoring but at this time is more stable than either of the other two children.

SECTION III: PRACTICING FOR NCLEX

Activity G NCLEX-STYLE QUESTIONS

1. **Answer: a**
   RATIONALE: The newborn's labia minora is typically swollen from the effects of maternal estrogen. The minora will decrease in size and be hidden by the labia majora within the first weeks. Lesions on the external genitalia are indicative of sexually transmitted infection. Labial adhesions are not a normal finding for a healthy newborn. Swollen labia majora is not a normal finding.

2. **Answer: c**
   RATIONALE: The nurse should first begin with open-ended questions regarding work, hobbies, activities, and friendship in order to make the teen feel comfortable. Once a trusting rapport has been established, the nurse should move on to the more emotionally charged questions. While it is important to assure confidentiality, the nurse should first establish rapport.

3. **Answer: c**
   RATIONALE: A good health history includes open-ended questions that allow the child to narrate their experience. The other questions would most likely elicit a yes or no response.

4. **Answer: c**
   RATIONALE: It is best to approach a shy 4-year-old by introducing the equipment slowly and demonstrating the process on the girl's doll first. Toddlers are egocentric; referring to how another child performed probably will not be helpful in gaining the child's cooperation. The other questions would most likely elicit a "no" response.

5. **Answer: b**
   RATIONALE: Asking "What can I help you with?" is very welcoming and allows for a variety of responses that may include functional problems, developmental concerns, or disease. Asking about the chief complaint may not be clear to all parents. Asking if the child feels sick will most likely elicit a yes or no answer and no other helpful details. Asking whether the child has been exposed to infectious agents is unclear and would not open a dialogue.

6. **Answer: c**
   RATIONALE: Preschoolers like to play games. To encourage deep breathing, the nurse should elicit the child's cooperation by engaging the child in a game to blow out the light bulb on the penlight. Telling the child that he or she may not leave or must breathe deeply would not engage the child. Asking whether the child would allow his or her caregiver to listen would most likely elicit a no.

7. **Answer: a**
   RATIONALE: The physical examination of children, just as for adults always begins with a systematic inspection, followed by palpation or percussion, then by auscultation.

8. **Answer: b**
   RATIONALE: Touching the thumb to the ball of the infant's foot would elicit the plantar grasp reflex. The other reflexes are not elicited by this method.

9. **Answer: c**
   RATIONALE: The nurse knows that some of the history must be delayed until after the child is stabilized. After the child is stabilized the nurse can take a detailed history. The child who has received routine health care and presents with a mild illness would need only a problem-focused history. The nurse should be sensitive to repetitive interviews in hospital situations but should not assume that the child's history can be obtained from other providers. A complete and detailed

history would be in order if physicians rarely see the child or if the child is critically ill.

10. **Answer: b**
    RATIONALE: This indicates a positive Romberg test which warrants further testing for possible cerebellar dysfunction.

11. **Answer: 21**
    RATIONALE: Using the metric method, the formula is:

    weight in kilograms divided by height in meters squared

    weight (kg)/height (m)^2
    42 kg/1.42^2
    42/2.0164 = 20.8292 = 21

12. **Answer: b, c, a, d**
    RATIONALE: The proper order of the assessment of the thorax is to inspect, palpate, percuss, and auscultate.

Answers

CHAPTER 33

SECTION I: ASSESSING YOUR UNDERSTANDING

Activity A FILL IN THE BLANKS

1. Hugging
2. 15
3. Bath
4. Eat
5. Therapeutic
6. Individualized Health Plans (IHPs)
7. Health department

Activity B MATCHING

1. b   2. e   3. a   4. c   5. d

Activity C SEQUENCING

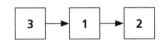

Activity D SHORT ANSWERS

1. The nurse can address and minimize separation anxiety by:

    Understanding the stages of separation anxiety and be able to recognize them in children; realizing that behaviors demonstrated during the first stage do not indicate that the child is "bad"; encouraging the family to stay with the child when appropriate; helping the family deal with various reactions and intervene before the behaviors of detachment occur; using guided imagery based on the use of the child's imagination and enjoyment of play in order to help the child relax.

2. Discharge planning actually begins upon admission. The nurse should assess the family's resources and knowledge level upon admission to determine the need for education and possible referrals.

3. Some common coping behaviors/methods include: stoicism, ignoring or negating problem, acting out, anger, withdrawal, rejection, and intellectualizing.

4. Under the age of 5 years, children are most commonly admitted to the hospital for respiratory issues. Older children are typically hospitalized for issues such as diseases of the respiratory system,

mental health problems, injuries, and gastrointestinal disorders. In regards to adolescents, problems related to pregnancy, childbearing, mental health, and injury account for the majority of hospitalizations.

5. The home care nurse should be sure to include the child in the conversation; address the caregivers formally unless asked to address them otherwise; be friendly and respectful, and use a soft, calm voice; use good listening skills; and be sure to schedule the first visit when the primary caregiver is present.

SECTION II: APPLYING YOUR KNOWLEDGE

Activity E CASE STUDY

The discussion should include the following points:

1. **INTERVENTIONS:** Assess if irritability is related to surgical intervention, including pain.

    RATIONALE: The irritability could be related to the surgery, especially pain, resulting from the procedure. Once this is ruled out address the infant's basic needs (trust versus mistrust).

    INTERVENTIONS: Encourage and facilitate family presence at the bedside and rooming-in. Provide consistent nursing staff. Arrange to have a volunteer hold and rock the baby when family is not present at bedside. Place the baby in a room near the nurse's station.

    RATIONALE: Infants gain a sense of trust in the world through reciprocal patterns of contact. Crying without comfort and lack of stimulation can lead to distress in the infant. By 5 to 6 months infants are acutely aware of the absence of their primary caregiver and may be fearful of unfamiliar persons. Providing caregivers who will address the comfort and care needs of the infant consistently is important for the developing infant. Response time to crying may be reduced by placing the infant near the nurse's station.

2. **INTERVENTIONS:** Address discomfort or pain that may be associated with disease process. Promote home routine related to bedtime and naptime. Provide a quiet, darkened room. Allow the parent to

lie in bed or crib next to toddler if possible. Group care activities and allow undisturbed periods of rest during designated nap/sleep times.

RATIONALE: Pain and discomfort could be contributing to lack of rest. Once ruled out, address the toddler's developmental needs. The change in routine caused by the hospitalization could be contributing to the lack of rest. Maintaining home rituals can help to normalize naptime and bedtime. Toddlers have a need of familiarity and the closeness of a primary caregiver. Providing parental comfort can help to minimize the toddler's distress. Allowing undisturbed times for naps can also help promote adequate rest.

3. **INTERVENTIONS:** Address pain management needs. Explain procedures honestly, using concrete terms. Encourage expression of feelings using therapeutic play. Consult child life physician if available. Encourage family member to room in. Leave a small light on at night.

RATIONALES: Fantasy and magical thinking may be heightened when pain and discomfort are experienced. Once ruled out address the preschoolers developmental needs. Preschoolers fear mutilation and are afraid of intrusive procedures. They interpret words literally and have an active imagination. Explaining procedures in terms the child can understand can help allay fears. Therapeutic play can help the child express and work through fears. Child life physician are excellent resources to encourage medical play and assist with preparation of the child. Presence of family provides comfort and security. Simply having a small amount of light in the room can help prevent fantasies and fears related to darkness leading to nightmares.

4. **INTERVENTIONS:** Talk to the child about the reasons for his lack of eating. Provide the child's favorite foods and allow the child to choose his meals (allow foods from home, if possible allow child to go to cafeteria to pick out food).

RATIONALE: The refusal to eat may be related to a lack of appetite due to disease process. Once ruled out, focus on the school-age child's developmental needs. Lack of eating may be a reaction to the hospitalization or a dislike of the foods provided. Offering favorite foods and asking the child the reasons he is not eating may help determine the cause of the lack of appetite. School-age children are accustomed to controlling self-care and they like being involved. They are used to making decisions about their meals and activities. By allowing them to pick their food you give them the opportunity to maintain independence, retain self-control, enhance self-esteem, and continue to work toward achieving a sense of industry.

5. **INTERVENTIONS:** Establish rapport with the adolescent. Encourage her to discuss her feelings. Provide a phone at her bedside. Encourage her to call her friends and family. Encourage her friends to visit.

Encourage use of a journal. Collaborate with a psychologist if appropriate.

RATIONALE: Adolescents typically do not experience separation anxiety from being away from their parents; instead, their anxiety comes from separation from their friends. They typically do not like to be different than their peers and appearance is an important factor for them. Adolescents with a chronic illness may become depressed due to prolonged separation from peers, altered body image, lack of self-esteem, and feeling different. Loss of control may lead to behaviors of anger, withdrawing, and general uncooperativeness. Developing rapport with the adolescent and encouraging discussion and expression of her feelings can help the adolescent cope. Also connecting the adolescent with her peers can be an important factor in improving coping. Collaboration with a psychologist may be appropriate if depression seems severe.

SECTION III: PRACTICING FOR NCLEX

Activity F NCLEX-STYLE QUESTIONS

1. **Answer: a**
   RATIONALE: Children in the first phase, protest, react aggressively to this separation, and reject others who attempt to comfort the child. The other behaviors are indicators of the second phase, despair.

2. **Answer: d**
   RATIONALE: It is best to include the families whenever possible so they can assist the child in coping with their fears. Preschoolers fear mutilation and are afraid of intrusive procedures. Their magical thinking limits their ability to understand everything, requiring communication and intervention to be on their level. Telling the child that we need to put a little hole in their arm might scare the child. Talking about taking or removing blood might be interpreted literally.

3. **Answer: a**
   RATIONALE: Previous experience with hospitalization can either add to the positive aspects of preparation or distract if the experiences were perceived as negative. If the child associates the hospital with the death of a relative, the experience is likely viewed as negative. The other statements would most likely indicate that the child's previous experiences were viewed as positive.

4. **Answer: c**
   RATIONALE: Distraction with books or games would be the best remedy to provide an outlet to distract him from his restricted activity. The other responses would be unlikely to affect a change in the behavior of a 6-year-old.

5. **Answer: a**
   RATIONALE: Parents who do not tell children the truth or do not answer their questions confuse, frighten, and may weaken the children's trust in

the parent. The other statements are effective forms of communication.

6. **Answer: d**

   RATIONALE: The nurse should start the initial contact with children and their families as a foundation for developing a trusting relationship. Asking about a favorite toy would be a good starting point. The nurse should allow the child to participate in the conversation without the pressure of having to comply with a request or undergo any procedures.

7. **Answer: c**

   RATIONALE: The nurse needs to describe the procedure and equipment in terms the child can understand. For a 4-year-old, a simple explanation along with the chance to touch and feel the tiny tubes would be best. Using the term tympanostomy tubes is not age-appropriate and does not teach. Telling the child that he or she will be asleep the whole time might increase their fears. Showing the child the operating room might increase fear with all of the strange and imposing equipment.

8. **Answer: b**

   RATIONALE: The nurse understands that a toddler is most likely to develop anxiety and fears due to separation from the parents. Separation from friends, loss of control, and loss of independence are fears typically experienced by an adolescent.

9. **Answer: c**

   RATIONALE: It is important to be honest and encourage the child to ask questions rather than wait for the child to speak up. The other statements are correct.

10. **Answer: c**

    RATIONALE: The best approach would be to write the name of his nurse on a small board and then identify all staff members working with the child (each shift and each day). Reminding the boy he

will be going home soon or telling him not to worry does not address his concerns or provide solutions. Encouraging the boy's parents to stay with him at all times may be unrealistic and may place undue stress on the family.

11. **Answer: d, a, c, b**

    RATIONALE: Nursing care for a hospitalized child typically occurs in four phases: introduction, building a trusting relationship, decision-making phase, and providing comfort and reassurance.

12. **Answer: a, b, d**

    RATIONALE: It is important to assess the child's peripheral vascular circulation especially when the child has a restraint placed on an extremity. Capillary refill, color, temperature, and pulses are appropriate to assess to ensure that the child's peripheral vascular circulation has not been compromised.

13. **Answers: b, c, d**

    RATIONALE: Even minor nursing interventions should not be performed in the playroom. The playroom should be referred to as the "activity room" or "social room" instead of "playroom" when speaking with adolescent children. It is inappropriate to perform procedures in the child's crib. It is better to perform procedures in the treatment room. It is important to give anti-emetics prior to mealtimes. Parents can be encouraged to bring in security items to help reduce the child's level of stress.

14. **Answer: 2 cups of fluid**

    RATIONALE: Ice is approximately equivalent to half the same amount of water.

Answers

CHAPTER 34

SECTION I: ASSESSING YOUR UNDERSTANDING

Activity A FILL IN THE BLANKS

1. 3
2. Respite
3. Family
4. Cancer
5. Written
6. Palliative
7. Hospice

Activity B MATCHING

1. e   2. a   3. b   4. c   5. d

Activity C SEQUENCING

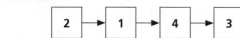

Activity D SHORT ANSWERS

1. Answers may include homeopathic and herbal medicine, pet therapy, hippotherapy, massage or music. Discharge planning actually begins upon admission. The nurse should assess the family's resources and knowledge level upon admission to determine the need for education and possible referrals.
2. Formerly premature infants need extra calories for growth. They also need extra calcium and phosphorus for adequate bone mineralization. Their diet consists of breast milk fortified with additional nutrients or a commercially prepared formula specific for premature infants.
3. The nurse should explain that DNR (do not resuscitate) refers to withholding cardiopulmonary resuscitation should the child's heart stop beating. It is important to ensure that this does not mean they are giving up on their child. Nurses must educate families that resuscitation may be inappropriate and lead to more suffering than if death were allowed to occur naturally. Families may wish to specify a certain extent of resuscitation that they feel more comfortable with (e.g., allowing

supplemental oxygen but not providing chest compressions). Some institutions are now replacing the DNR terminology with "allow natural death" (AND), which may be more acceptable to families facing the decision to withhold resuscitation.
4. Respecting the child and family's goals, preferences, and choices; comprehensive caring; using the strengths of interdisciplinary resources; acknowledging and addressing caregivers' concerns; building systems and mechanisms of support (Association of Pediatric Oncology Nurses, 2003).
5. Do not excessively try to get the child to eat or drink; offer small frequent meals or snacks, such as soups or shakes; provide the child with foods they request; administer anti-emetics as needed; provide good mouth care; ensure environment is free of odors and is conducive to eating.

SECTION II: APPLYING YOUR KNOWLEDGE

Activity E

The discussion should include the following points:

Children with special health care needs require comprehensive and coordinated care from multiple health care professionals. The nurse can facilitate communication and help to ensure collaboration to address the child's health, educational, psychological, and social service needs. The nurse needs to promote family-centered care and work with the parents as a team. Include both parents and other caregivers in learning skills needed to care for this child. The nurse can assist the family to incorporate the child's medical needs into daily life and to minimize the child's self perception of being different. Developing a trusting and permanent relationship with the family will allow the nurse to identify the family's changing needs and will allow better two-way communication. The nurse should support and empower the family and assist parents and families to find support systems and resources.

The nurse needs to be attuned to the entire family's needs and emotions and be fully present with the child and family. Listen to the child and family and foster respect for the whole child. Respect the parents and help them to honor the commitments they have made to their child. Work collaboratively with the family and health care team. Acknowledge that the parents have diverse needs for information and encourage participation in decision making. The school-age child has a concrete understanding of death. Give Georgia specific honest details when they are requested. Encourage participation in decision making and help the child to establish a sense of control.

SECTION III: PRACTICING FOR NCLEX

Activity F NCLEX-STYLE QUESTIONS

1. **Answer: c**
    RATIONALE: A good therapeutic relationship is built on trust and communication. It is strengthened by listening to the parents, acknowledging their triumphs, and supporting them when they fail. Continuing to educate them, helping them access resources, and helping them to save money on medications are good interventions, but not as effective at building a trusting relationship.

2. **Answer: a**
    RATIONALE: Providing full participation in decision making gives the adolescent a sense of worth and builds his self-esteem. The adolescent may have difficulty initiating conversation, but wants and needs to voice his fears and concerns. He also requires direct, honest answers to his questions. However, these needs are not as effective in meeting his need for sense of self-worth or self-esteem.

3. **Answer: d**
    RATIONALE: School-age children need specific details about procedures related to dying. Explaining how a morphine drip keeps her sister comfortable would best minimize the child's anxiety. Saying her sister won't need food any more when she dies is more appropriate for a younger child. School-age children are curious about death and may deny that it is impending. These behaviors should be handled with understanding and patience.

4. **Answer: b**
    RATIONALE: Serving on his individualized education plan committee will be most beneficial to his education because this plan is designed to meet his individual educational needs. Collaborating with the school nurse and assessing the health effects of attending school, and getting a motorized wheel chair do not address his educational needs.

5. **Answer: b**
    RATIONALE: Watching the interaction between mother and child to see if the child maintains eye contact may indicate that the child is being neglected which is an inorganic cause for failure to thrive. Refusing the nipple is a sign of organic cause for failure to thrive. Prematurity is a risk factor for failure to thrive. Checking the health history may disclose other organic causes for failure to thrive.

6. **Answer: c**
    RATIONALE: Communication can best be improved if the nurse uses reflective listening techniques to show the parents that their input is heard and valued. Giving direct, understandable answers and saying the same thing different ways helps ensure effective communication with the parents but does nothing to build communication between the nurse and family. Sharing cell phone numbers only allows the nurse and family to talk to each other.

7. **Answer: d**
    RATIONALE: A good way to involve the father and gain his input regarding in the child's care is to schedule education sessions in the evening when he can get away from the office. Leaving voice mails and sending email reports leave him isolated from care group. Lunchtime visits are not long enough for him to focus on the situation.

8. **Answer: a**
    RATIONALE: Nurses can help parents build on their strengths and empower them to care for their child by educating them about the course of treatment and the child's expected outcome. Evaluating emotional strength, assessing the home, and preparing a list of supplies do not empower the parents for the task ahead of them.

9. **Answer: b**
    RATIONALE: Young adolescents require time with their peers. Encouraging her to have visitors would best meet this need. Assuring her illness is not her fault and acting as her personal confidant are interventions suited to school-age children. Explaining her condition in detail meets the needs of an older adolescent.

10. **Answer: c**
    RATIONALE: The child may be struggling to fit in with his peers by avoiding his treatment regimen in an effort to hide his illness. Monitoring his compliance would disclose this risky behavior. Assessing for depression, encouraging participation in activities, and joining a support group would not address risky behavior.

11. **Answers: b, c**
    RATIONALE: Hearing deficits and strabismus are associated with prematurity.

12. **Answer: 7-month-old**
    RATIONALE: When assessing growth and development of the infant or child who was born prematurely, determine the child's adjusted or corrected age so that you can perform an accurate assessment. 40 weeks–32 weeks is 8 weeks or 2 months. The child was born 2 months early.

13. **Answer: 2,784 kilocalories**
    RATIONALE: 23.2 kilograms × 120 kilocalories/ 1 kilogram = 2,784 kilocalories

14. **Answer: d, b, a, c**
    RATIONALE: The proper order of occurrence is trust, autonomy, initiative, and industry.

15. **Answer: c, d, e**
    RATIONALE: Risk factors for the development of vulnerable child syndrome include newborn jaundice, an illness that the child was not expected to recover from, and congenital anomalies.

CHAPTER 35

SECTION I: ASSESSING YOUR UNDERSTANDING

Activity A FILL IN THE BLANKS

1. Implanted
2. Pharmacodynamics
3. Distraction
4. Fifth
5. Hypoglycemia
6. Nasogastric
7. Ophthalmic

Activity B LABELING

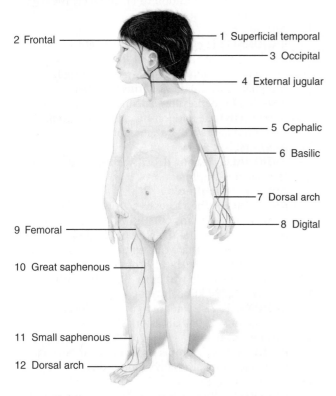

2 Frontal

1 Superficial temporal

3 Occipital

4 External jugular

5 Cephalic

6 Basilic

7 Dorsal arch

8 Digital

9 Femoral

10 Great saphenous

11 Small saphenous

12 Dorsal arch

Activity C MATCHING

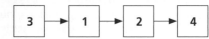

1. e   2. a   3. b   4. c   5. d

Activity D SEQUENCING

3 → 1 → 2 → 4

Activity E SHORT ANSWERS

1. The child's room should remain a safe and secure area. In the hospital, all invasive procedures should be performed in the treatment room.
2. Check identification since children may deny their identity in attempt to avoid unpleasant situations, play in another child's bed, or remove ID bracelet; confirm identity each time medication is given; verify the child's name with the caregiver to provide additional assurance of identification.
3. Monitor the child's vital signs closely for changes; adhere to strict aseptic technique when caring for the catheter and administering TPN; ensure that the system remains a closed system at all times, including securing all connections, using occlusive dressings, and clamping catheter or having child perform the Valsalva maneuver during tubing and cap changes; follow agency policy for flushing of catheter and maintaining catheter patency; assess intake and output frequently; monitor blood glucose levels and obtain laboratory tests as ordered to evaluate for changes in fluid and electrolytes.
4. The eight rights of medication administration for children are the right: medication, patient, time, route of administration, dose, documentation, to be educated, and to refuse.
5. A feeding tube can be checked for placement by checking the pH (results vary between gastric and intestinal tubes); observing the appearance of the fluid removed from the tube upon aspiration; instilling air and performing gastric auscultation; checking external markings on tube and external tube length; assessing for signs indicative of feeding tube misplacement; and reviewing any chest or abdominal X-rays for placement.

SECTION II: APPLYING YOUR KNOWLEDGE
Activity F CASE STUDY
The discussion should include the following points:

1. **a.** Identify the need for the PRN medication based on the order. Rationale: Identification of the child's condition that warrants the medication is the first step in administering a PRN medication. Jennifer's rectal temperature of 102.5 F demonstrates a need for acetaminophen for fever (per the order).
   b. Verify medication order. Rationale: To ensure appropriate medication will be administered.
   c. Calculate the correct dose. Rationale: To ensure that the amount of medication is appropriate for the child based on weight.
   d. Calculate amount to be drawn up from the bottle of acetaminophen. Rationale: To ensure the appropriate amount of medication is given based on the available medication concentration.
   e. Wash hands. Rationale: To prevent infection
   f. Verify correct medication and expiration date of medication. Verify time of last dose given and ensure at least 4 hours ago. Verify oral route is the ordered route of administration. Draw up acetaminophen from the bottle using an oral syringe. Rationale: Right medication, right time, and right route of administration are three of the 8 right parts of medication administration. A syringe is the best way to accurately measure the liquid medication. It is also the best way to administer medicine to an infant.
   g. Prepare a bottle of juice, formula, or breastmilk. Rationale: It is recommended to have a "chaser" for the infant to drink immediately after the medication is given.
   h. Educate Jennifer's parents at the bedside regarding why the medicine is needed, what the child will experience and the desired effect of the medication, what is expected of the child and how the parents can participate and support their child. Rationale: Parent teaching is an important part of medication administration. Involvement of parents in medication administration can reduce stress for the infant.
   i. Invite the parents to assist and/or give suggestions for techniques. Rationale: The parents may have helpful suggestions for how their child best takes medications. Involvement of parents in medication administration can reduce stress for the infant, validates their roles as caregivers, and may increase the likelihood of successful medication administration.
   j. Check identification of the child. Rationale: To ensure medicine is given to correct child.
   k. Administer the medication into the back of the infant's mouth between the teeth and gums. Give small amounts and allow the child to swallow before more medicine is placed in the mouth. Have the child upright or at least 45 degree angle. Rationale: Allows infant to swallow the medication and decreases the likelihood of spitting, coughing up, or aspirating the medication.
   l. Offer the infant a sip from the prepared bottle. Rationale: The juice can help rinse the medication taste from the mouth and sucking on the bottle often will help soothe and calm the infant.
   m. Document the medication administration and within 30 to 60 minutes document the child's response (recheck temperature). Rationale: Documentation should be done after the medication is administered. Since this is a PRN medication the infant's response should be noted.

2. Dosing for acetaminophen is 10 to 15 mg/kg every 4 to 6 hours. Convert 15 lbs to kg (1 kg = 2.2 lbs)
   Therefore 15 lb equals 6.8 kg multiplied by 10 = 68 mg; 6.8 multiplied by 15 = 102 mg. The range of acetaminophen Jennifer can receive is 68 mg to 102 mg every 4 to 6 hours; therefore 70 mg every 4 hours po is a safe and therapeutic dose.

3. Ratio method:

   70 mg:x = 80 mg:0.8 mL-multiply means and extremes and get 56 = 80x, solve for x
   x = 0.7 mL

   Proportion method:

   $$\frac{70 \text{ mg}}{x} = \frac{80 \text{ mg}}{0.8 \text{ mL}} \text{ (cross multiply)} = 56 = 80x \text{ solve for x, x} = 0.7 \text{ mL}$$

SECTION III: PRACTICING FOR NCLEX
Activity G NCLEX-STYLE QUESTIONS

1. **Answer: a**
   RATIONALE: The nurse should provide a description of and reason for the procedure in age-appropriate language. The nurse should avoid the use of terms such as culture or strep throat as it is not age appropriate for a 4-year-old. The nurse should also avoid confusing terms like "take your blood" that might be interpreted literally.

2. **Answer: b**
   RATIONALE: Signs of infiltration included cool, puffy, or blanched skin. Warmth, redness, induration, and tender skin are signs of inflammation.

3. **Answer: b**
   RATIONALE: The priority nursing action is to verify the medication ordered. The first step in the eight rights of pediatric medication administration is to ensure that the child is receiving the right medication. After verifying the order, the nurse would then gather the medication, the necessary equipment and supplies, wash hands and put on gloves.

4. **Answer: c**
   RATIONALE: The nurse should emphasize that the parents should never threaten the child in order to make him take his medication. It is more appropriate to develop a cooperative approach that will elicit the child's cooperation since he needs ongoing, daily medication. The other statements are correct.

5. **Answer: d**
   RATIONALE: The preferred injection site for infants is the vastus lateralis muscle. An alternative site is the rectus femoris muscle. The dorsogluteal is not a recommended site for the infant. The deltoid muscle, which is a small muscle mass, is used as an IM injection site in children after the age of 4 to 5 years of age due to the small muscle mass.

6. **Answer: b**
   RATIONALE: The nurse should explain what is to occur and enlist the child's help in the removal of the tape or dressing. This provides the child with a sense of control over the situation and also encourages his or her cooperation. The nurse should avoid using scissors to remove the tape or dressing and the comment regarding cutting may be perceived as threatening and/or frightening. Telling the child to be a big girl is inappropriate and does not teach. Telling the child the procedure will not hurt and using the terms tug and pinch could increase the child's fear and lead to misunderstanding.

7. **Answer: a**
   RATIONALE: A good way to involve the father and gain his input regarding in the child's care is to schedule education sessions in the evening when he can get away from the office. Leaving voice mails and sending email reports leave him isolated from care group. Lunchtime visits are not long enough for him to focus on the situation.

8. **Answer: c**
   RATIONALE: The child's daily intravenous fluid maintenance is 1700 mL. The child requires 100 mL/kg for the first 10 kg plus 50 mL/kg for the next 10 kg plus 20 mL/kg for each kg more than 20 kg equals the number of kg required for 24 hours. (10 × 100) + (10 × 50) + (10 × 20) = 1,700.

9. **Answer: b**
   RATIONALE: Yellow or bile-stained aspirate indicates intestinal placement. Clean, tan, or green aspirate indicates gastric placement.

10. **Answer: a**
    RATIONALE: The nurse should convert the child's weight in pounds to kilograms by dividing the child's weight in pounds by 2.2 (70 pounds divided by 2.2 = 32 kg). The nurse would then multiply the child's weight in kilograms by 3 mg (32 kg × 3 mg = 96 mg) for the low end and then by 4 mg for the high end (32 pounds × 4 mg = 128 mg).

11. **Answer: 21.4 kg**
    RATIONALE: There are 2.2 pounds per kg

    47 pounds × 1 kg/2.2 pounds = 21.363636 kg

    When rounded to the tenth place, the answer is 21.4 kg.

12. **Answer: 1,640 mL**
    RATIONALE:

    (First 10 kg) 10 kg × 100 mL/kg = 1,000 mL
    (Second 10 kg) 10 kg × 50 mL/kg = 500 mL
    (remaining kilograms of body weight) 7 kg × 20 mL/kg = 140 mL
    1,000 + 500 + 140 = 1,640 mL.

13. **Answer: 411 mL**
    RATIONALE: The child weighs 113 pounds. 113 pounds × 1 kg/2.2 pounds = 51.363636 kg

    51.363636 kg × 1 mL/1 kg = 51.363636 mL/hour
    51.363636 × 8 hours = 410.90908

    when rounded to the nearest whole number = 411 mL

14. **Answer: 35 mL**
    RATIONALE: The diaper must be weighed before being placed on the infant and after removal to determine urinary output. For each 1 gram of increased weight, this is the equivalent of 1 mL of fluid.

    75 grams − 40 grams = 35 grams = 35 mL

15. **Answers: a, e**
    RATIONALE: It is true that infants and young children have an increased percentage of water in their bodies. Infants and young children have immature livers.

Answers

CHAPTER 36

SECTION I: ASSESSING YOUR UNDERSTANDING

Activity A FILL IN THE BLANKS

1. Midazolam
2. 60
3. Depressed
4. Morphine
5. Seven
6. Pain threshold
7. OUCHER

Activity B MATCHING

Question 1

1. d   2. a   3. b   4. e   5. c

Question 2

1. b   2. d   3. a   4. d

Activity C SEQUENCING

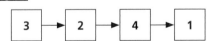

$$3 \rightarrow 2 \rightarrow 4 \rightarrow 1$$

Activity D SHORT ANSWERS

1. Somatic pain refers to pain that develops in the tissues. Superficial somatic pain is also called cutaneous pain. It involves stimulation of nociceptors in the skin, subcutaneous tissue, or mucous membranes. It is typically well localized and described as sharp, pricking, or burning sensation. Tenderness is common. Deep somatic pain typically involves the muscles tendons, joints, fascia, and bones. It can be localized or diffuse and is usually described as dull, aching, or cramping.

2. The three principles that guide pain management in children are:
   - Individualize interventions based on the amount of pain experiences during procedure and the child's personality
   - Use nonpharmacologic approaches to ease or eliminate the pain
   - Use aggressive pharmacologic treatment with the first procedure

3. The situation factors can be changed. They include behavioral, cognitive, and emotional aspects.

4. Conscious sedation utilizes medications to place the child in a depressed state. This is used to allow the physician to perform procedures. Conscious sedation enables the child to retain protective reflexes. The child is then able to maintain a patent airway and respond to verbal and physical stimuli. Medications used to achieve conscious sedation may include morphine, fentanyl, midazolam, chloral hydrate, or diazepam.

5. Epidural anesthesia is administered after the placement of a catheter in the epidural space. The locations used are L 1–2, L 3–4, or L 4–5. Medications used include fentanyl or morphine. The medications enter the cerebrospinal fluid and cross the dura mater to the spinal cord.

SECTION II: APPLYING YOUR KNOWLEDGE

Activity E CASE STUDY

1. The discussion should include the following:
   Recent research supports that infants do feel pain and short- and long-term consequences of inadequately treating their pain do occur. Infants cannot tell us in words that they feel pain like older children or adults but they do give cues with their behaviors, expressions, and vital signs. Infants will act differently when they are in pain than when they are comfortable. Typically, infants respond to pain with irritability, crying, withdrawal, pushing away, restless sleeping, and poor feeding. They may indicate pain by their facial expressions. A facial expression with brows lowered and drawn together, eyes tightly closed, and mouth opened can be a sign of pain. They are preverbal so this facial expression, diffuse body movements and other signs, as indicated above, provide feedback that the infant is in pain. As parents you play an important role in helping us assess Owen's pain and informing us of changes in his behavior that may indicate pain.

2. The discussion should include the following:

The FLACC scale is an appropriate pain assessment tool for an infant. Based on the scale (refer to Table 36-6 in Essentials of Pediatric Nursing textbook) Owen's pain level is a three at this time.

Owen's vital signs including oxygen saturation as well as how well Owen is feeding may be helpful. (Children in acute pain will often have an increased heart rate, respiratory rate, or elevated blood pressure. Decreased oxygen saturation may be seen secondary to pain. Also, infants in pain will often demonstrate poor feeding.)

3. The discussion should include the following:

Parents are important components in both pain assessment and intervention. Many of the non-pharmacologic techniques can be done by parents and are often received better from the parents. Holding the child with as much skin to skin contact as possible, repositioning, rocking, and massaging the child can help decrease pain. Nonnutritive sucking, breastfeeding, or sucrose or other sweet tasting solutions such as glucose water can decrease discomfort. Distracting the infant with a soothing voice, music, stories, and songs can also be helpful.

SECTION III: PRACTICING FOR NCLEX

Activity F NCLEX-STYLE QUESTIONS

1. **Answer: a**

A preschooler may have difficulty distinguishing between the types of pain such as if the pain is sharp or dull. It also limits the information being obtained by the nurse. They can, however, tell someone where it hurts and can use various tools such as the FACES scale (cartoon faces) or the OUCHER scale (photograph and corresponding numbers) to rate their pain.

2. **Answer: a**

When administering parenteral or epidural opioids, the nurse should always have naloxone readily available in order to reverse the opioids effects, should respiratory distress occur. Premedication with acetaminophen is not required with opioids. After administration, the nurse should continually assess for adverse reaction. The nurse should assess bowel sounds for decreased peristalsis after administration.

3. **Answer: d**

Respiratory depression, although rare when epidural analgesia is used, is always a possibility. However, when it does occur it usually occurs gradually over a period of several hours after the medication is initiated. This allows adequate time for early detection and prompt intervention. The nurse should also monitor for pruritus, urinary retention, and nausea and vomiting but the priority is to monitor for respiratory depression.

4. **Answer: c**

EMLA is contraindicated in children less than 12 months who are receiving methemoglobin-inducing agents, such as sulfonamides, phenytoin, phenobarbital, and acetaminophen. Children with darker skin may require longer application times to ensure effectiveness. EMLA is not contraindicated for children less than 6 weeks of age or those undergoing venous cannulation or intramuscular injections.

5. **Answer: b**

When a child is manifesting extreme anxiety and behavioral upset, the priority nursing intervention is to serve as an advocate for the family and ensure that the appropriate pharmacologic agents are chosen to alleviate the child's distress. Ensuring emergency equipment is readily available and lighting is adequate for the procedure is also part of nursing function, but secondary interventions. Conducting an initial assessment of pain is important but would likely be difficult if the child was crying inconsolably or extremely anxious.

6. **Answer: a**

Just because the girl is sleeping does not mean she is not in pain. Sleep may be a coping strategy or reflect excessive exhaustion due to coping with pain. An easy going temperament and the ability to articulate how she feels will be helpful for the nurse to establish a baseline assessment. If the girl had never had surgery before, she is less likely to have previous memories or episodes of prolonged or severe pain.

7. **Answer: b**

The parents must understand that they should begin the technique or method chosen before the child experiences pain or when he first indicates he is anxious about or beginning to experience pain. The other statements are accurate.

8. **Answer: b**

Decreased heart rate is not a physiologic response to pain. Instead, infants demonstrate an increased heart rate, usually averaging approximately 10 beats per minute with possible bradycardia in preterm newborns. Decreased oxygen saturation and palmar and plantar sweating are common physiologic responses to pain in the infant.

9. **Answer: b**

The FLACC behavioral scale is a behavioral assessment tool that is useful in assessing a child's pain when the child is unable to report accurately his or her level of pain or discomfort and is reliable for children from age 2 months to 7 years. The preferred base age for the visual analog and numerical scales is 7 years. The FACES pain rating scale and Oucher pain rating scale are appropriate for children as young as 3; however, in this situation the FLACC is required due to the child's inability to report his level of pain.

10. **Answer: a**

    The nurse should select the pain assessment tool that is appropriate for the child's cognitive abilities. The FACES pain rating scale is designed for use with children ages 3 and up. A child with limited reading skills or vocabulary may have difficulty with some of the words listed to describe pain on the word graphic scale. Some of the concepts might be too difficult on the visual analog and numerical scales for a developmentally disabled child. The base age for the Adolescent pediatric pain tool is 8 years, but would likely be inappropriate for an 8-year-old with cognitive delays.

11. **Answer: d**

    The nervous system structures needed for pain impulse transmission and perception are present by the 23rd week of gestation. Therefore, children of any age, including preterm newborns, are capable of experiencing pain.

12. **Answer: d**

    The epidural is placed at the level of L 1–2, L 3–4, or L 4–5. This is below the area of the spinal cord. Advising the child and family that paralysis is not a serious concern trivializes the concerns and does little to promote therapeutic communication. Nurses have the responsibility to provide education to the child and caregivers. Simply telling them that the cord ends above the area of the epidural does not provide the needed information to promote reassurance. Assuring the child and family that their physician has skills does not meet the needed education.

13. **Answer: c**

    Responsible nursing care requires the nurse administer pain medication as needed. The nurse has the authority to discuss the child's pain control needs with the parents. There is no need to discuss the reduction of medications with the physician. Family history of drug abuse is not a factor in the care of this child. Young children can become addicted to analgesics. There is, however, no indication that addiction is a valid concern with this child.

14. **Answer: c**

    Children may underreport feelings of pain. They may assume that adults know how they are feeling or they may feel worried about spearing to lose control. The nurse should assess for the presence of behavioral cues that might be consistent with pain. The nurse should not simply administer analgesics without cause.

15. **Answer: c**

    Toradol (ketorolac) is an NSAID medication. It is associated with gastrointestinal upset. To reduce this side effect the nurse may administer the medication with food.

CHAPTER 37

SECTION I: ASSESSING YOUR UNDERSTANDING

Activity A FILL IN THE BLANKS

1. Pyrogens
2. Phagocytosis
3. Antibodies
4. Neutrophils
5. Ibuprofen

Activity B MATCHING

Question 1

1. b   2. e   3. f   4. c   5. d   6. a

Question 2

1. b   2. c   3. a   4. e   5. d

Activity C SEQUENCING

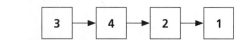

Activity D SHORT ANSWERS

1. Risk factors for sepsis associated with pregnancy include:
   - premature or prolonged rupture of membranes
   - difficult delivery
   - maternal infection or fever, including sexually transmitted infections
   - resuscitation and other invasive procedures
   - positive maternal group beta streptococcal vaginosis

2. The nurse primarily manages the patient's symptoms. Acetaminophen may be given for fever management. Narcotic analgesics may be required for pain management. Oral fluids prevent dehydration. If orchitis is present, ice packs and gentle support for the testicles may be necessitated. Hospitalized children should be confined to respiratory isolation. Children are considered to no longer be contagious after 9 days following the onset of parotid swelling.

3. Concurrent use of passive and active immunoprophylaxis is recommended. It consists of a regimen of one dose of immune globulin and five doses of human rabies vaccine over a 28-day period. Rabies immune globulin and the first dose of rabies vaccine should be given as soon as possible after exposure, ideally within 24 hours. Additional doses of rabies vaccine should be given on days 3, 7, 14, and 28 after the first vaccination. Rabies immune globulin is infiltrated into and around the wound with any remaining volume administered intramuscularly at a site distant from the vaccine inoculation. Human rabies vaccine is administered intramuscularly into the anterolateral thigh or deltoid depending on the age and size of the child.

4. Fever is a protective mechanism the body uses to fight infection. Evidence exists that an elevated body temperature actually enhances various components of the immune response. Fever can slow the growth of bacteria and viruses and increase neutrophil production and T-cell proliferation (Crocetti & Serwint, 2005). Studies have shown that the use of antipyretics may prolong illness. Another concern is that reducing fever may hide signs of serious bacterial illness.

5. Sepsis is a systemic over response to infection resulting from bacteria (most common), fungi, viruses, or parasites. It can lead to septic shock, which results in hypotension, low blood flow, and multi-system organ failure. Septic shock is a medical emergency and children are usually admitted to an intensive care unit. The cause of sepsis may not be known, but common causative organisms in children include *Neisseria meningitidis, Streptococcus pneumoniae,* and *Haemophilus influenzae.* Sepsis can affect any age group but is more common in neonates and young infants. Neonates and young infants have a higher susceptibility due to their immature immune system, inability to localize infections, and lack of IgM immunoglobulin, which is necessary to protect against bacterial infections.

SECTION II: APPLYING YOUR KNOWLEDGE
Activity E CASE STUDY

1. The discussion should include the following points:

   Continue attempting to open dialogue with Jennifer. Make sure your style, content, and message are appropriate to her developmental level. Do not talk down to her and approach her in a direct and nonjudgmental manner. Work on identifying risk factors and risk behaviors.

2. The discussion should include the following points:

   Encourage completion of antibiotic prescription. Encourage sexual partners to get an evaluation, testing, and treatment.

   Once risk factors and risk behaviors have been identified, guide Jennifer to develop specific individualized actions of prevention. You can encourage abstinence at this point along with encouraging Jennifer to minimize her lifetime number of sexual partners, to use barrier methods consistently and correctly, and to be aware of the connection between drug and alcohol use and the incorrect use of barrier methods.

3. The discussion should include the following points:

   Reinforce the risk she is putting herself at and continue to guide her to develop individualized actions of prevention. For possible discussion about other STI's common in adolescents refer to Table 37.9). Discuss barriers to condom use and ways to overcome them (refer Table 37.10).

   To address specific concerns – condoms are uncomfortable and sex with condoms is not as exciting or as good.

   Encourage Jennifer and her boyfriend to try condoms and provide suggestions such as trying smaller or larger condom sizes, placing a drop of water based lubricant or salvia inside the tip of the condom or on the glans of the penis prior to putting on the condom. Try a thinner latex condom or a different brand or more lubrication. Encourage the incorporation of condom use during foreplay. Remind Jennifer that peace of mind may enhance pleasure for herself and her partner.

   Instruct Jennifer on proper condom use (refer to teaching guideline 37.3).

   The discussion should include the following points:
   - Use latex condoms
   - Use a new condom with each sexual act of intercourse and never reuse a condom
   - Handle condoms with care to prevent damage from sharp objects such as nails and teeth
   - Ensure condom has been stored in a cool, dry place away from direct sunlight. Do not store condoms in wallet or automobile or any place where they are exposed to extreme temperatures
   - Do not use a condom if it appears brittle, sticky, or discolored. These are signs of aging.
   - Place condom on before any genital contact
   - Place condom on when penis is erect and ensure it is placed so it will readily unroll.
   - Hold the tip of the condom while unrolling. Ensure there is a space at the tip for semen to collect but make sure no air is trapped in the tip
   - Ensure adequate lubrication during intercourse. If external lubricants are used only use water-based lubricants such as KY jelly with latex condoms. Oil-based or petroleum-based lubricants, such as body lotion, massage oil, or cooking oil, can weaken latex condoms
   - Withdraw while penis is still erect and hold condom firmly against base of pen

SECTION III: PRACTICING FOR NCLEX
Activity F NCLEX-STYLE QUESTIONS

1. **Answer: c**

   If the family had been camping or in a wooded area, the girl could have been bitten by a tick which would not be easy to discover because of her long hair. Ticks like dark, hair-covered areas and the signs and symptoms presented are neurological, with a rapid onset, which can be characteristic of a tick bite. The other questions are important but are not focusing on the causative agent.

2. **Answer: b**

   Recurrent arthritis in large joints, such as the knees, is an indication of late-stage Lyme disease. The appearance of erythema migrans would suggest early-localized stage of the disease. Facial palsy or conjunctivitis would suggest the child is in the early disseminated stage of the disease.

3. **Answer: c**

   It is very important to ensure that the proper dose is given at the proper interval because an overdose can be toxic to the child. Concerns with allergies and taking the entire, prescribed dose are precaution when administering antibiotics and all medications. Drowsiness is not a side effect of antipyretics.

4. **Answer: d**

   In order to ensure a successful culture, the nurse must determine if the child is taking antibiotics. Throat cultures require specimens taken from the pharyngeal or tonsillar area. Stool cultures may require three specimens, each on a different day. The nurse would use aseptic technique when getting a blood specimen as well as the urine, but antibiotics cannot be received by the child prior to the test being done.

5. **Answer: a**

The usual sites for obtaining blood specimens are veins on the dorsal side of the hand or the antecubital fossa. Administration of sucrose prior to beginning helps control pain for young infants. Accessing an indwelling venous access device may be appropriate if the child is in an acute care setting. An automatic lancet device is used for capillary puncture of an infant's heel.

6. **Answer: a**

The presence of petechiae can indicate serious infection in an infant. Grunting is abnormal, indicating respiratory difficulty. The behavior of the 2-month-old is normal after immunizations. The 4-month-old needs to be watched but is adequately hydrated and the 8-month-old also needs to be watched. What the 8-month-old is experiencing is common in infants who are teething and is not indicative of illness.

7. **Answer: a**

Varicella zoster results in a life-long latent infection. It can reactivate later in life resulting in shingles. The American Academy of Pediatrics recommends consideration of Vitamin A supplementation in children 6 months to 2 years hospitalized for measles. Dehydration caused by mouth lesions is a concern with foot and mouth disease. Avoiding exposure to pregnant women is a concern with Rubella, Rubeola, and erythema infectiosum.

8. **Answer: a**

Infants and young children are more susceptible to infection due to the immature responses of their immune systems. Cellular immunity is generally functional at birth; humoral immunity develops after the child is born. Newborns have a decreased inflammatory response. Young infants lose the passive immunity from their mothers, but disease protection from immunizations is not complete.

9. **Answer: b**

The use of immunosuppression drugs is a risk factor for the hospitalized child. Maternal infection or fever and resuscitation or invasive procedures are sepsis risk factors related to pregnancy and labor. Lack of juvenile immunizations is a risk factor affecting the overall health of the child but does not impact the chance of sepsis.

10. **Answer: d**

Penicillin V or erythromycin is the preferred antibiotic for treatment of scarlet fever. Scarlet fever transmission is airborne, not via droplet. Lymphadenopathy occurs with cat scratch disease and diphtheria. Close monitoring of airway status is critical with diphtheria because the upper airway becomes swollen.

11. **Answer: c**

Pruritus may be managed by pressing on the area instead of scratching. Increases in temperature will result in vasodilation and increase the pruritus. Warm baths and hot compresses should be avoided. Rubbing may result in increased itching.

12. **Answer: a**

When treating a child suspected of having an infection the blood cultures must be obtained first. The administration of antibiotics may impact the culture's results. A urine specimen may be obtained but is not the priority action. Intravenous fluids will likely be included in the plan of care but are not the priority action.

13. **Answer: d**

Sepsis may be associated with lethargy, irritability, or changes in level of consciousness. The septic child will likely not be anxious to have a high activity level and would prefer to remain in bed. The temperature elevation of 98.8 °F is not significant and does not confirm the presence of sepsis. Hypotension is a late manifestation of sepsis.

14. **Answer: b**

Pressing the tube against the skin may result in the contamination of the specimen with bacteria from the skin. The remaining options are correct.

15. **Answers: b, c, d**

Aspirin should be avoided in children with fever. It may be associated with Reyes Syndrome. Activities that result in over-cooling or chilling such as using fans and cold baths should be avoided.

Answers

CHAPTER 38

SECTION I: ASSESSING YOUR UNDERSTANDING

Activity A FILL IN THE BLANKS

1. Kernig
2. Painful
3. Circumference
4. Gait
5. Doll's eye
6. Touch
7. Intracranial
8. Bruit

Activity B LABELING

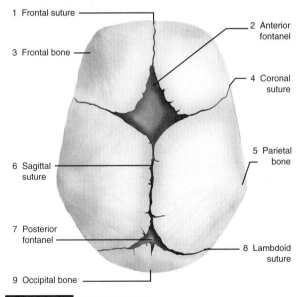

1 Frontal suture
2 Anterior fontanel
3 Frontal bone
4 Coronal suture
5 Parietal bone
6 Sagittal suture
7 Posterior fontanel
8 Lambdoid suture
9 Occipital bone

Activity C MATCHING

1. d **2.** e **3.** c **4.** a **5.** b

Activity D SEQUENCING

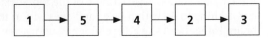

1 → 5 → 4 → 2 → 3

Activity E SHORT ANSWERS

1. Kernig sign is tested by flexing the legs at the hip and knee, then extending the knee. A positive report of pain along the vertebral column is a positive sign and indicates irritation of the meninges, or the presence of meningitis.
2. An infant will hyperextend its head and neck assuming an opisthotonic position in order to relieve discomfort due to bacterial meningitis.
3. Proper positioning for newborns is upright with the head flexed forward. An older infant or child is positioned on its side with head flexed forward and knees flexed toward the abdomen.
4. A ventriculoperitoneal (VP) shunt is designed to relieve the buildup of CSF in hydrocephalus children and maintain proper intracranial pressure. Malfunctions may be due to kinking, clogging, or separation of the tubing. The most common malfunction, however, is due to blockage. Signs and symptoms include vomiting, lethargy, headache in the older child, and altered, diminished, or change in the level of consciousness.
5. The Glasgow Coma scale is a tool used to standardize the degree of consciousness in the child. It consists of three parts: eye opening, verbal response, and motor response. A low score indicates a decreased level of consciousness or responsiveness.

SECTION II: APPLYING YOUR KNOWLEDGE

Activity F CASE STUDY

The discussion should include the following points:

1. The nurse should anticipate the following diagnostic and laboratory tests: Complete blood count (CBC); electrolytes; culture (if febrile); phenobarbital level; toxicology if ingestion of medicine or chemicals is suspected; lumbar puncture (LP) if signs of central nervous system infection are present; and imaging studies, such as CT or MRI, if head injury is suspected.
2. Interventions should include:
   - If child is standing or sitting ease child to the ground if possible, cradle head, place on soft area. Do not attempt to restrain. Place child on one side and open airway if possible.

- Place blow-by oxygen by child and have suction ready if needed.
- Remove any sharp or potentially dangerous objects. Tight clothing and jewelry around the neck should be loosened if possible.
- Observe length of seizure and activity such as movements noted, as well as cyanosis or loss of bladder or bowel control, and any other characteristics about the child's condition during the seizure.
- If child's condition deteriorates or seizures persist, call for help.
- Report seizures to physician promptly.
- Administer anticonvulsants as ordered.
- Remain with child until fully conscious.
- Allow postictal behavior without interfering while providing environmental protection.
- When possible, reorient child.
- Accurately document information in chart, including preseizure activity.
- Provide emotional support and education to family.
- Obtain anticonvulsant levels as ordered.

3. Teaching should include:
    - Discuss seizure warning signs.
    - Teach the family to recognize warning signs and how to care for the child during and after a seizure (refer to Teaching Guidelines 38.1).
    - Discuss the disease process and prognosis of condition and life-long need for treatment if indicated.
    - Teach parents the need for routine medical care and that it is important for the child to wear a medical bracelet.
    - Review medication regimen and the importance of maintaining a therapeutic medication level and administering all prescribed doses.
    - Encourage parents to discuss with the child why she does not want to take the medicine.
    - Explain to the child in simple terms why the medicine is needed and how it will help her. Encourage participation from physician and parents.
    - Discuss alternative ways to administer phenobarbital, such as crushed tablets or elixir, with the physician and family.
    - Explain to the family to use an understanding and gentle yet firm approach with medication administration.
    - Encourage the family to give medicine at same time and place, which helps create a routine.
    - Help the family to identify creative strategies to gain the child's cooperation, such as using a sticker chart and allowing child to do more, such as administering the medication.
    - Offer choices when possible, such as "Do you want your medicine before or after your bath, and would you like to have apple or grape juice after your medicine?"
    - Praise the child's improvements.

SECTION III: PRACTICING FOR NCLEX

Activity G NCLEX-STYLE QUESTIONS

1. **Answer: a**
    RATIONALE: Always start by assessing the family's knowledge. Ask them what they need to know. Knowing when to clamp the drain is important, but they might not be listening if they have another question on their minds. Autoregulation is too technical. Teaching should be based on the parents' level of understanding. Keeping her head elevated is not part of the information which would be taught regarding the drainage system.

2. **Answer: c**
    RATIONALE: Horizontal nystagmus is a symptom of lesions on the brain stem. A sudden increase in head circumference is a symptom of hydrocephalus suggesting that there is a build up of fluid in the brain. An intracranial mass would cause only one eye to be dilated and reactive. A closed posterior fontanel is not unusual at 2 months of age.

3. **Answer: a**
    RATIONALE: The fact that swelling did not cross the midline or suture lines suggests cephalohematoma. Swelling that crosses the midline of the infant's scalp indicates caput succedaneum which is common. Low birth weight is not an accompanying factor for cephalohematoma. Facial abnormalities may accompany encephalocele, not cephalohematoma.

4. **Answer: a**
    RATIONALE: Signs and symptoms for cerebral contusions include disturbances to vision, strength, and sensation. A child suffering a concussion will be distracted and unable to concentrate. Vomiting is a sign of a subdural hematoma. Bleeding from the ear is a sign of a basilar skull fracture.

5. **Answer: a**
    RATIONALE: Positional plagiocephaly can occur because the infant's head is allowed to stay in one position for too long. Because the bones of the skull are soft and moldable, they can become flattened if the head is allowed to remain in the same position for a long period of time. Massaging the scalp will not affect the skull. Measuring the intake and output is important but has no effect on the skull bones. Small feedings are indicated whenever an infant has increased intracranial pressure, but feeding an infant each time he fusses is inappropriate care.

6. **Answer: d**
    RATIONALE: Fragile capillaries in the periventricular area of the brain put preterm infants at risk for intracranial hemorrhage. Closure of the fontanels has nothing to do with fragile capillaries within the brain. Larger head size gives children a higher center of gravity which causes them to hit their head more readily. Congenital hydrocephalus may be caused by abnormal intrauterine development or infection.

7. **Answer: c**
   RATIONALE: Folic acid supplementation has been found to reduce the incidence of neural tube defects by 50%. The fact that the mother has not used folic acid supplements puts her baby at risk for spina bifida occulta, one type of neural tube defect. Neonatal conjunctivitis can occur in any newborn during birth and is caused by virus, bacteria, or chemicals. Facial deformities are typical of babies of alcoholic mothers. Incomplete myelinization is present in all newborns.

8. **Answer: c**
   RATIONALE: A video electroencephalogram can determine the precise localization of the seizure area in the brain. Cerebral angiography is used to diagnose vessel defects or space-occupying lesions. Lumbar puncture is used to diagnose hemorrhage, infection, or obstruction in the spinal canal. Computed tomography is used to diagnose congenital abnormalities such as neural tube defects.

9. **Answer: c**
   RATIONALE: Brain and spinal cord development occur during the first 3 to 4 weeks of gestation. Infection, trauma, teratogens (any environmental substance that can cause physical defects in the developing embryo and fetus), and malnutrition during this period can result in malformations in brain and spinal cord development and may affect normal central nervous system (CNS) development. Good health before becoming pregnant is important but must continue into the pregnancy. Hardening of bones occurs during 13 to 16 weeks gestation, and the respiratory system begins maturing around 23 weeks gestation.

10. **Answer: b**
    RATIONALE: Educating parents how to properly give the antibiotics would be the priority intervention because the child's shunt has become infected. Maintaining cerebral perfusion is important for a child with hydrocephalus, but the priority intervention for the parents at this time is in regards to the infection. Establishing seizure precautions is an intervention for a child with a

seizure disorder. Encouraging development of motor skills would be appropriate for a microcephalic child.

11. **Answer: a, b, c, e**
    RATIONALE: The child with bacterial meningitis should be placed in droplet isolation until 24 hours following the administration of antibiotics. Close contacts of the child should receive antibiotics to prevent them from developing the infection. The nurse should administer antibiotics and initiate seizure precautions. Children with bacterial meningitis have an increased risk of developing problems associated with an increased intracranial pressure.

12. **Answer: a, b, c, d**
    RATIONALE: The following people have an increased risk of becoming infected with meningococcal meningitis: college freshman living in dormitories, children 11 years old or older, children who travel to high risk areas, and children with chronic health conditions.

13. **Answers: a, b, d**
    RATIONALE: A child with Reye's syndrome may require an anti-emetic for severe vomiting. The nurse should monitor the child's intake and output every shift for the development of fluid imbalance. The child may require an anticonvulsant due an increased intracranial pressure that may induce seizures. A distinctive rash is associated with the development of meningococcal meningitis. The nurse should monitor the Reye's syndrome child's laboratory values for indications that the liver is not functioning well.

14. **Answer: 8**
    RATIONALE: The child would be given a score of 2 for best eye response, 2 for best verbal response, and 4 for best motor response. The total score is 8.

15. **Answers: b, d, e**
    RATIONALE: Late signs of increased intracranial pressure are: decerebrate posturing, bradycardia, and pupils that are fixed and dilated. The other options are early signs of increased intracranial pressure.

CHAPTER 39

SECTION I: ASSESSING YOUR UNDERSTANDING

Activity A FILL IN THE BLANKS

1. 3
2. Horizontal
3. Antibiotics
4. Deterioration
5. Developmental
6. Distance

Activity B MATCHING

1. b   2. d   3. a   4. e   5. c

Activity C SEQUENCING

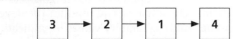

Activity D SHORT ANSWERS

1. Signs and symptoms of children with a hearing loss include:
   a. Infant:
   - Wakes only to touch, not environmental noises
   - Does not startle to loud noises
   - Does not turn to sound by 4 months of age
   - Does not babble at 6 months of age
   - Does not progress with speech development
   b. Young child:
   - Does not speak by 2 years of age
   - Communicates needs through gestures
   - Does not speak distinctly, as appropriate for his or her age
   - Displays developmental (cognitive) delays
   - Prefers solitary play
   - Displays immature emotional behavior
   - Does not respond to ringing of the telephone or doorbell
   - Focuses on facial expressions when communicating
   c. Older child:
   - Often asks for statements to be repeated
   - Is inattentive or daydreams
   - Performs poorly at school
   - Displays monotone or other abnormal speech
   - Gives inappropriate answers to questions except when able to view face of speaker

2. According to the Delta Gamma Center for Children with Visual Impairments, there are several ways to successfully interact with the visually impaired child, including:
   - Use the child's name to gain attention.
   - Identify yourself and let the child know you are there before you touch the child.
   - Encourage the child to be independent while maintaining safety.
   - Name and describe people/objects to make the child more aware of what is happening.
   - Discuss upcoming activities with the child.
   - Explain what other children or individuals are doing.
   - Make directions simple and specific.
   - Allow the child additional time to think about the response to a question or statement.
   - Use touch and tone of voice appropriate to the situation.
   - Use parts of the child's body as reference points for the location of items.
   - Encourage exploration of objects through touch.
   - Describe unfamiliar environments and provide reference points.
   - Use the sighted-guide technique when walking with a visually impaired child.

3. Signs and symptoms that would lead the nurse to suspect that a child was visually impaired include:
   a. Infants:
   - Does not fix and follow
   - Does not make eye contact
   - Unaffected by bright light
   - Does not imitate facial expression
   b. Toddlers and older children:
   - Rubs, shuts, covers eyes
   - Squinting
   - Frequent blinking
   - Holds objects close or sits close to television
   - Bumping into objects
   - Head tilt, or forward thrust

4. Possible risk factors for acute otitis media (AOM) in children include any of the following:
   - Eustachian tube dysfunction
   - Recurrent upper respiratory infection
   - First episode of AOM before 3 months of age
   - Day care attendance (increases exposure to viruses causing upper respiratory infections)
   - Previous episodes of AOM
   - Family history
   - Passive smoking
   - Crowding in the home or large family size
   - Native American, Inuit, or Australian aborigine ethnicity
   - Absence of infant breastfeeding
   - Immunocompromise
   - Poor nutrition
   - Craniofacial anomalies
   - Presence of allergies
5. Children with permanent hearing loss, suspected or diagnosed speech and/or language delay, craniofacial disorders, and pervasive developmental disorders are at risk for difficulty with the development of speech or language, or having learning difficulties. Other children at risk include those with genetic disorders or syndromes, cleft palate, and blindness or significant visual impairment.

SECTION II: APPLYING YOUR KNOWLEDGE

Activity E CASE STUDY

The discussion should include the following points:
1. The nurse should anticipate the following diagnostic and laboratory tests: Complete blood count (CBC); electrolytes; blood culture (if febrile); phenobarbital level; toxicology if ingestion of medicine or chemicals is suspected; lumbar puncture (LP) if signs of central nervous system infection are present; and imaging studies, such as CT or MRI, if head injury is suspected.
2. Interventions should include:
   - If the child is standing or sitting ease the child to the ground if possible, cradle head, place on soft area. Do not attempt to restrain. Place the child on one side and open airway if possible.
   - Place blow-by oxygen by the child and have suction ready if needed.
   - Remove any sharp or potentially dangerous objects. Tight clothing and jewelry around the neck should be loosened if possible.
   - Observe length of seizure and activity such as movements noted, as well as cyanosis or loss of bladder or bowel control, and any other characteristics about the child's condition during the seizure.
   - If the child's condition deteriorates or seizures persist, call for help.
   - Report seizures to physician promptly.
   - Administer anticonvulsants as ordered.
   - Remain with the child until fully conscious.

   - Allow postictal behavior without interfering while providing environmental protection.
   - When possible, reorient child.
   - Accurately document information in chart, including preseizure activity.
   - Provide emotional support and education to family.
   - Obtain anticonvulsant levels as ordered.
3. Teaching should include:
   - Discuss seizure warning signs.
   - Teach the family to recognize warning signs and how to care for the child during and after a seizure (refer to Teaching Guidelines 38.1).
   - Discuss the disease process and prognosis of condition and life-long need for treatment if indicated.
   - Teach parents the need for routine medical care, and that it is important for the child to wear a medical bracelet.
   - Review medication regimen and the importance of maintaining a therapeutic medication level and administering all prescribed doses.
   - Encourage parents to discuss with the child why she does not want to take the medicine.
   - Explain to the child in simple terms why the medicine is needed and how it will help her. Encourage participation from physician and parents.
   - Discuss alternative ways to administer phenobarbital, such as crushed tablets or elixir, with the physician and family.
   - Explain to the family to use an understanding and gentle yet firm approach with medication administration.
   - Encourage the family to give medicine at same time and place, which helps create a routine.
   - Help the family to identify creative strategies to gain the child's cooperation, such as using a sticker chart and allowing child to do more, such as administering the medication.
   - Offer choices when possible, such as "Do you want your medicine before or after your bath, and would you like to have apple or grape juice after your medicine?"
   - Praise the child's improvements.

SECTION III: PRACTICING FOR NCLEX

Activity F NCLEX-STYLE QUESTIONS

1. **Answer: d**
   Reassessing for language acquisition would be most important to the health of the child. There is a risk of otitis media with effusion causing hearing loss, as well as speech, language, and learning problems. Parents should not use over-the-counter drugs to alleviate the child's symptoms, nor should they smoke around her. In addition, proper antibiotic use is important; however, language acquisition is directly related to developmental health.

2. **Answer: c**
The corneal light reflex is extremely helpful in assessment of strabismus. It consists of shining a flashlight into the eyes to see if the light reflects at the same angle in both eyes. Strabismus is present if the reflections are not symmetrical. The visual acuity test measures how well the child sees at various distances. Refractive and ophthalmologic examinations are comprehensive and are performed by optometrists and ophthalmologists.

3. **Answer: b**
Intravenous antibiotics will be the primary therapy for this child, followed by oral antibiotics. Warm compresses will be applied for 20 minutes every 2 to 4 hours. However, narcotic analgesics are not necessary to handle the pain associated with this disorder.

4. **Answer: a**
Assessing for asymmetric corneal light reflex would be the priority intervention as strabismus may develop in the child with regressed retinopathy of prematurity. Observing for signs of visual impairment would not be critical for this child, nor would teaching the parents to check how the glasses fit the child. Referral to Early Intervention would be appropriate if the child was visually impaired.

5. **Answer: c**
Recurrent nasal congestion contributes to the presence of otitis media with effusion. Frequent swimming would put the child at risk for otitis externa. Attendance at school is a risk factor for infective conjunctivitis. Although otitis media is a risk factor for infective conjunctivitis, infective conjunctivitis is not a risk factor for otitis media with effusion.

6. **Answer: d**
Therapeutic management of amblyopia may be achieved by using atropine drops in the better eye. Educating parents on how to use atropine drops would be the most helpful intervention. Explaining postsurgical treatment and discouraging the child from roughhousing would be appropriate only if the amblyopia required surgery. While follow-up visits to the ophthalmologist are important, compliance with treatment is priority.

7. **Answer: d**
Teaching the parents the importance of patching the child's eye as prescribed is most important for the treatment of strabismus. The need for ultraviolet-protective glasses postoperatively is a subject for the treatment of cataracts. The possibility of multiple operations is a teaching subject for infantile glaucoma. Teaching the importance of completing the full course of oral antibiotics is appropriate to periorbital cellulitis.

8. **Answer: c**
Proper hand washing is the single most important factor to reduce the spread of acute infectious conjunctivitis. Proper application of the antibiotic is important for the treatment of the infection, not prevention of transmission; keeping the child home from school until she is no longer infectious and encouraging the child to keep her hands away from her eyes are sound preventative measures, but not as important as frequent hand washing.

9. **Answer: c**
A mixture of ½ rubbing alcohol and ½ vinegar squirted into the canal and then allowed to run out is a good preventative measure, but not when inflammation is present. Cotton swabs should not be placed in the ears to dry them. He can wash his hair as needed. Using a hair dryer on a cool setting to dry the ears works well as long as the vent is clean and free from dust and hair that may have accumulated.

10. **Answer: d**
Encouraging the use of eye protection for sports would be more appropriate if the child was wearing contact lenses that may fall out during athletics. A sport strap would be more appropriate for this child. The child is less likely to wear her glasses if improper fit or incorrect prescription is causing a problem or if the glasses are unattractive. It is important to get scheduled eye examinations on time; watch for signs that the prescription needs changing; and check the condition and fit of glasses monthly.

11. **Answers: a, b**
RATIONALE: Bacterial infections are usually present unilaterally. Drainage from eyes that have been diagnosed with bacterial conjunctivitis is often thick and purulent.

12. **Answers: a, d**
RATIONALE: Visine is not appropriate to use because rebound vasoconstriction may occur and it is not actually treating the infection. The child can go back to school 24 to 48 hours after the mucopurulent drainage is no longer present.

13. **Answers: a, c, e**
RATIONALE: The child with a corneal abrasion may have a normal assessment of the pupils bilaterally. The child may experience photophobia and tearing noted in the eye. The child with a corneal abrasion will typically experience eye pain. The child with a simple contusion of the eye will have bruising and edema around the eye.

14. **Answers: b, c, d, e**
RATIONALE: Children who are 2 years old or younger and have a severe form of acute otitis media with a temperature of 102.2 F or greater (39 °C) will most likely receive antibiotics to treat the infection. Children who are older than 2 years of age with severe otalgia and a fever over 102.2 F (39 °C) typically receive antibiotics. Children who are older than 2 years of age and have mild otalgia and a fever less than 102.2 F have a nonsevere illness. In these cases, the physician may just observe the children to see if their symptoms persist over time or get worse.

Answers

CHAPTER 40

SECTION I: ASSESSING YOUR UNDERSTANDING

Activity A FILL IN THE BLANKS

1. Tracheostomy
2. Atopic
3. Coryza
4. Indirect
5. Wheezes
6. Mantoux
7. Decongestant

Activity B LABELING

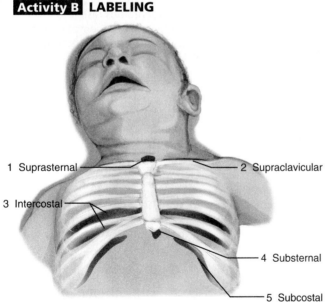

1 Suprasternal
2 Supraclavicular
3 Intercostal
4 Substernal
5 Subcostal

Activity C MATCHING

1. d   **2.** e   **3.** b   **4.** a   **5.** c

Activity D SEQUENCING

8 → 4 → 2 → 5 → 6
1 ← 3 ← 7 ←

Activity E SHORT ANSWERS

1. Signs and symptoms of sinusitis are similar to those found with a cold, with the difference being that sinusitis signs and symptoms are more persistent than with a cold, with nasal discharge lasting more than 7 to 10 days. Common signs and symptoms include cough, fever, halitosis in preschoolers and older children, eyelid edema, irritability, and poor appetite. Facial pain may or may not be present.

2. Laboratory and diagnostic tests typically ordered for the child suspected of having cystic fibrosis and possible findings indicative of cystic fibrosis include the sweat chloride test (above 50mEq/L is considered suspicious levels and above 60mEq is indicative); pulse oximetry (oxygen saturation is usually decreased); chest X-ray (hyperinflation, bronchial wall thickening); and pulmonary function tests (decreased forced vital capacity and forced expiratory volume with increases in residual volume).

3. There is typically no illness that precedes croup or epiglottitis other than possibly mild coryza with croup or a mild upper respiratory infection with epiglottitis. Both have a rapid or sudden onset, with croup frequently occurring at night. Several differences exist between the two illnesses including age groups usually affected (3 months to 3 years with croup and 1 to 8 years for epiglottitis); fever (variable with croup and high with epiglottitis); barking cough and hoarseness with croup; dysphagia and toxic appearance with epiglottitis; lastly, the cause of croup is generally viral whereas the cause of epiglottitis is generally *Haemophilus influenzae* type B.

4. Relief of symptoms is the goal of treatment of the common cold. This may be achieved a number of methods including relief of nasal congestion by providing a humidified environment or using saline nasal sprays or washes. Saline washes are followed by suctioning with a bulb syringe. Over-the-counter cold remedies may reduce the symptoms of the cold, but not the duration and should not be used in children less than 6 years of age due to possible

side effects. Additionally, antihistamines should be avoided as they cause excess drying of secretions.

5. Respiratory syncytial virus (RSV) is the most common cause of bronchiolitis, which is an acute inflammation of the bronchioles. The peak incidence of this disorder occurs in the winter and spring seasons. RSV infection is common in all children, with bronchiolitis RSV occurring most often in infants and toddlers. The severity of the infection typically decreases with age.

SECTION II: APPLYING YOUR KNOWLEDGE

Activity F CASE STUDY

1. The discussion should include the following points:
   - Is there a family history of atopy?
   - Does James have a history of allergic rhinitis or atopic dermatitis?
   - Has James had recurrent episodes diagnosed as wheezing, bronchiolitis, or bronchitis?
   - Has James had these symptoms before?
   - When did James first develop symptoms?
   - Which symptoms developed first?
   - Are there any factors that could have precipitated the attack?
   - Describe James' home environment (include pets, smokers, type of heating use)
   - Does James have any allergies to food or medication?
   - Does James have a seasonal response to environmental pollen or dust allergies?
   - Is James taking any medication?

2. The discussion should include the following points:

   Ineffective airway clearance related to inflammation and increased secretions as evidenced by dyspnea, coughing and wheezing, pallor, tachypnea, tachycardia and bilateral wheezing on auscultation, and c/o chest tightness.

   RATIONALE: Inflammation and increased mucous secretions can contribute to the narrowing of air passages and interfere with airflow during an acute asthma attack. This is the highest priority nursing diagnosis.

   Ineffective breathing pattern related to inflammatory or infectious process as evidenced by dyspnea, coughing and wheezing, pallor, tachypnea, tachycardia and bilateral wheezing on auscultation, and c/o chest tightness.

   RATIONALE: Tachypnea and increased work of breathing can lead to inadequate ventilation.

   Risk for impaired gas exchange related to dyspnea, coughing and wheezing, pallor, tachypnea, tachycardia and bilateral wheezing on auscultation, and c/o chest tightness.

   RATIONALE: Unresolved ineffective airway clearance or ineffective breathing pattern may lead to deficits in oxygenation and carbon dioxide retention and hypoxia.

   Risk for anxiety related to respiratory distress.

RATIONALE: Respiratory distress and related hypoxia may lead to agitation and anxiety as the child struggles to breathe.

Education should include a discussion about the pathophysiology, asthma triggers, and prevention and treatment strategies.

The nurse should explain that asthma is a chronic, inflammatory airway disorder that decreases the size of the airways leading to respiratory distress.

Teaching should include information regarding how attacks of asthma can be prevented by avoiding environmental and emotional triggers (refer to Teaching Guidelines 40.4).

Discussion of appropriate use of medication delivery devices, including the nebulizer and metered-dose inhaler are important. Teaching should include the purposes, functions, and side effects of the prescribed medications. It is essential to require return demonstration of equipment use to ensure that children and families are able to utilize equipment properly. (refer to Teaching Guidelines 40.5).

SECTION III: PRACTICING FOR NCLEX

Activity G NCLEX-STYLE QUESTIONS

1. **Answer: c**
   The 4-year-old with pharyngitis has a sore, swollen throat placing the child at risk for dysphagia (difficulty swallowing). Erythematous rash and mild toxic appearance are typical of influenza. Fever and fatigue are symptoms of a common cold. Influenza and the common cold may cause sore throats but would not be the highest risk for dysphagia.

2. **Answer: a**
   Until the family adjusts to the demands of the disease, they can become overwhelmed and exhausted, leading to noncompliance, resulting in worsening of symptoms. Typical challenges to the family are becoming over vigilant, the child feeling fearful and isolated, and the siblings being jealous or worried.

3. **Answer: d**
   Attending day care is a known risk factor for pneumonia. Being a triplet is a factor for bronchiolitis. Prematurity rather than postmaturity is a risk factor for pneumonia. Diabetes is a risk factor for influenza.

4. **Answer: b**
   A chest X-ray is usually ordered for the assessment of asthma to check for hyperventilation. A sputum culture is indicated for pneumonia, cystic fibrosis, and tuberculosis; fluoroscopy is used to identify masses or abscesses as with pneumonia; and the sweat chloride test is indicated for cystic fibrosis.

5. **Answer: b**
   Oxygen administration is indicated for the treatment of hypoxemia. Suctioning removes excess secretions from the airway caused by colds or flu. Saline lavage loosens mucus that may be blocking the airway so that it may be suctioned out. Saline

gargles are indicated for relieving throat pain as with pharyngitis or tonsillitis.

6. **Answer: c**

Infants consume twice as much oxygen (6 to 8 L) as adults (3 to 4 L). This is due to higher metabolic and resting respiratory rates. Term infants are born with about 50 million alveoli, which is only 17% of the adult number of around 300 million. The tongue of the infant, relative to the oropharynx is larger than adults. Infants and children will develop hypoxemia more rapidly than adults when in respiratory distress.

7. **Answer: d**

If the airway becomes completely occluded due to epiglottitis, respiratory distress may lead to respiratory arrest and death. Aseptic meningitis is a complication of infectious mononucleosis, resulting in nuchal rigidity; acute otitis media resulting in ear pain is a complication of influenza; and children with pneumonia are at risk for pneumothorax.

8. **Answer: a**

A flutter valve device is used to assist with mobilization of secretions for older children and adolescents with cystic fibrosis. Teaching regarding the use of metered dose inhalers, nebulizers, and the peak flow meter is typically for asthma therapy.

9. **Answer: b**

Mucus plugging can occur in the neonate placed on a ventilator after surfactant has been administered; therefore, it is important to monitor for adequate lung expansion for early detection of this complication. Promoting adequate gas exchange, maintaining adequate fluid volume, and preventing infection would be interventions for a neonate on a ventilator, but they are not specific to the complication of mucus plugging.

10. **Answer: a**

Using nasal washes to improve air flow will help prevent secondary bacterial infection by preventing the mucus from becoming thick and immobile. Teaching parents how to avoid allergens such as tobacco smoke, dust mites, and molds helps prevent recurrence of allergic rhinitis. Discussing anti-inflammatory nasal sprays and teaching parents about using oral antihistamines would help in prevention and treatment of the disorder.

11. **Answer: 33%**

RATIONALE: Room air is 21%. Each 1 liter of oxygen flow is equal to an additional 4% of oxygen. The child is receiving 3 liters of oxygen. 21% (room air) + 3(4%) = 33% of oxygen.

12. **Answer: b, d, c, a**

RATIONALE: The first step is to administer a short-acting beta 2-agonist as needed. The second step is to administer a low-dose inhaled corticosteroid. The third step is to administer a medium-dose inhaled corticosteroid. The fourth step is to administer a medium-dose inhaled corticosteroid and a long-acting beta 2-agonist.

13. **Answers: c, d**

RATIONALE: Until 4 weeks of age, newborns are obligatory nose breathers and breathe only through their mouths when they are crying. A newborn's respiratory tract makes very little mucus. Children have an increased risk of developing problems associated with airway edema. Children's tongues are proportionally larger than adults. Children under the age of 6 years have a reduced risk of developing sinus infections.

14. **Answer: 157 mg per dose**

RATIONALE: 23 pounds $\times$ 1 kg/2.2 pounds = 10.4545 kg

10.4545 kg $\times$ 45 g/kg = 470.455 mg
470.455 mg/3 = 156.82 = 157 mg per dose

15. **Answers: b, c, d, e**

RATIONALE: Children with pneumonia may exhibit the following: a chest X-ray with perihilar infiltrates, an elevated leukocyte level, an increased respiratory rate, and a productive cough. The child with pneumonia typically has a fever.

CHAPTER 41

SECTION I: ASSESSING YOUR UNDERSTANDING

Activity A FILL IN THE BLANKS

1. Angiography
2. Electrophysiologic
3. Narrowing
4. Pulmonary
5. 6 months
6. Acquired
7. Rheumatic fever

Activity B MATCHING

1. b **2.** a **3.** d **4.** c **5.** e

Activity C SEQUENCING

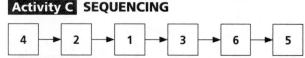

Activity D SHORT ANSWERS

1. Digoxin is prescribed to increase contractility of the heart muscle by decreasing conduction and increasing force. It is commonly indicated for HF, atrial fibrillation, atrial flutters, and supraventricular tachycardia. Digoxin should be given at regular intervals, every 12 hours, such as 8 AM and 8 PM, one hour before or two hours after feeding. If a digoxin dose is missed and more than 4 hours have elapsed, give the missed dose. If the child vomits digoxin, a second dose should not be given. Potassium levels should be carefully monitored as a decrease enhances the effects of digitalis causing toxicity. Digoxin should not be held if the child's heart rate is below or above normal ranges.

2. Heart murmurs must be evaluated on the basis of the following characteristics:
   Location
   Relation to the heart cycle and duration
   Intensity Grades I to VI
   Quality-harsh, musical, or rough in high, medium, or low pitch
   Variation with position (sitting, lying, standing)

3. The three types of ASDs are identified based on the location of the opening:
   Ostium primum (ASD1): the opening is located at the lower portion of the septum.
   Ostium secundum (ASD2): the opening is located near the center of the septum.
   Sinus venosus defect: the opening is located near the junction of the superior vena cava and the right atrium.

4. Ventricular septal defect (VSD) accounts for 30% of all congenital heart defects. By the age of 2 years approximately 50% of small VSD's spontaneously close, and VSD's that require surgical intervention have a high rate of success. Upon assessment, newborns may not exhibit any signs or symptoms. Signs and symptoms of heart failure typically occur at 4 to 6 weeks of age and may include easily tiring and/or color changes and diaphoresis during feeding; lack of thriving; pulmonary infections, tachypnea, or shortness of breath; edema; murmurs; thrill in the chest upon palpation.

5. Risk factors for infective endocarditis include children with:
   Congenital heart defects;
   Prosthetic heart valves;
   Central venous catheters;
   Intravenous drug use.

SECTION II: APPLYING YOUR KNOWLEDGE

Activity E CASE STUDY

1. The discussion should include:
   Prepare the parents and child for the procedure by discussing what the procedure involves, how long it will take, special instructions from the physician, and what to expect after the procedure is complete. Inform the parents of the possible complications that might occur, such as bleeding, low-grade fever, loss of pulse in the extremity used for the catheterization, and arrhythmias. Explain that the child will have a dressing over the catheter site and the leg may need to remain straight for several hours after the procedure. Discuss that frequent monitoring will be required after the procedure. Use a variety of teaching methods such as

videotapes, books, and pamphlets. Discussion with the child should be age appropriate.

Preprocedure care includes a thorough history and physical examination, including vital signs, to establish a baseline. The nurse should obtain height and weight to assist in determining medication dosages. The child should be assessed for allergies, especially iodine or shellfish, because some contrast material contain iodine as a base. The medication history as well as laboratory testing results should be reviewed. The nurse should keep in mind that some medications, such as anticoagulants, are typically held prior to the procedure to reduce the risk of bleeding. Peripheral pulses, including pedal pulses, should be assessed. The location of the child's pedal pulses should be marked in order to facilitate their assessment after the procedure. Ensure informed consent has been obtained and a signed form is in the chart. Premedications ordered should be administered, and the parents should be allowed to accompany the child to the catheterization area if permitted.

2. Discussion should include:

Following the procedure, the child should be monitored for complications of bleeding, arrhythmia, hematoma, and thrombus formation and infection. Assessment includes vital signs, neurovascular status of the lower extremities (pulses, color, temperature, and capillary refill), and the pressure dressing over the catheterization site every 15 minutes for the first hour and then every 30 minutes for 1 hour (depending on hospital policy). Monitoring of cardiac rhythm and oxygen saturation levels for the first few hours after the procedure should occur. Maintain bedrest in the immediate post procedure period. The leg might need to be kept straight for approximately 4 to 8 hours, depending on the approach used and facility policy. Reinforcement of the pressure dressing as necessary should be performed, and any evidence of drainage on the dressing should be noted. The infant's intake and output should be monitored closely. The parents should be provided with post-care and follow-up care education prior to discharge.

SECTION III: PRACTICING FOR NCLEX
Activity F NCLEX-STYLE QUESTIONS

1. **Answer: b**
   Softening of nail beds is the first sign of clubbing due to chronic hypoxia. Rounding of the fingernails is followed by shininess and thickness of nail ends.

2. **Answer: d**
   The normal infant heart rate averages 120 to 130 beats per minute (bpm); the toddler's or preschooler's is 80 to 105, the school-age child's is 70 to 80 bpm, and the adolescent's heart rate average 60 to 68 bpm.

3. **Answer: b**
   The nurse should pay particular attention to assessing the child's peripheral pulses, including pedal pulses. Using an indelible pen, the nurse should mark the location of the child's pedal pulses as well as document the location and quality in the child's medical records.

4. **Answer: c**
   Some medications, like lithium, taken by pregnant women may be linked with the development of congenital heart defects. Reports of nausea during pregnancy and an Apgar score of eight would not trigger further questions. Febrile illness during the first trimester, not the third, may be linked to an increased risk of congenital heart defects.

5. **Answer: a**
   Edema of the lower extremities is characteristic of right ventricular heart failure in older children. In infants, peripheral edema occurs first in the face, then the presacral region, and the extremities.

6. **Answer: b**
   A bounding pulse is characteristic of patent ductus arteriosus or aortic regurgitation. Narrow or thready pulses may occur in children with heart failure or severe aortic stenosis. A normal pulse would not be expected with aortic regurgitation.

7. **Answer: d**
   An accentuated third heart sound is suggestive of sudden ventricular distention. Decreased blood pressure, cool, clammy, and pale extremities, and a heart murmur are all associated with cardiovascular disorders; however, these findings do not specifically indicate sudden ventricular distention.

8. **Answer: d**
   A heart murmur characterized as loud with a precordial thrill is classified as Grade IV. Grade II is soft and easily heard. Grade I is soft and hard to hear. Grade III is loud without thrill.

9. **Answer: d**
   The normal adolescent's blood pressure averages 100 to 120/50 to 70 mm Hg. The normal infant's blood pressure is about 80/40 mm Hg. The toddler or preschoolers blood pressure averages 80 to 100/64 mm Hg. The normal schoolager's blood pressure averages 94 to 112/56 to 60 mm Hg.

10. **Answer: a**
    A mild to late ejection click at the apex is typical of a mitral valve prolapse. Abnormal splitting or intensifying of S2 sounds occurs in children with major heart problems, not mitral valve prolapse. Clicks on the upper left sternal border are related to the pulmonary area.

11. **Answer: 0.7 milligrams**
    RATIONALE: The infant weighs 15.2 pounds (2.2 pounds = 1 kg.)

    15.2 pounds × 1 kg/2.2 pounds = 6.818 kg

The infant weighs 6.818 kg. For each kilogram of body weight, the infant should receive 0.1 mg of morphine sulfate.

6.818 kg × 0.1 mg/ 1 kg = 0.6818 mg, when rounded to the tenth place = 0.7 mg

The infant will receive 0.7 mg of morphine sulfate.

12. **Answers: a, b**
RATIONALE: Abrupt cessation of chest tube output and an increased heart rate are indicators that the child may have developed cardiac tamponade. The child's right atrial filling pressure will increase.

The child may be anxious and their apical heart rate may be faint and difficult to auscultate.

13. **Answers: c, d, e**
RATIONALE: The nurse should not administer digoxin to children with the following issues: The adolescent with an apical pulse under 60 beats per minute, the child with a digoxin level above 2 ng/mL, and the child who exhibiting signs of digoxin toxicity.

14. **Answers: c, d**
RATIONALE: Subcutaneous nodules and carditis are considered major criteria used in the diagnosing process of acute rheumatic fever. The other options are minor criteria.

15. **Answers: b, c, d**
RATIONALE: The following information should be reported to the physician following a cardiac catheterization because they are indicative of possible complications: Negative changes to the child's peripheral vascular circulatory status (cool foot with poor pulse), a fever over 100.4 °F, and nausea or vomiting.

Answers

CHAPTER 42

SECTION I: ASSESSING YOUR UNDERSTANDING

Activity A | FILL IN THE BLANKS

1. Retching
2. Atresia
3. 2
4. Fungal
5. Stones
6. Probiotic
7. Intussusception

Activity B | LABELING

The colostomy is the diagram on the left and the ileostomy is the diagram on the right.

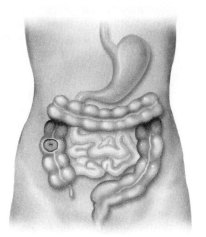
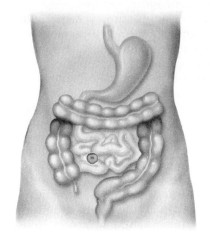

Activity C | MATCHING

1. b   2. c   3. d   4. a   5. e

Activity D | SEQUENCING

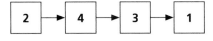

Activity E | SHORT ANSWERS

1. (S) set up equipment, (T) take off the pouch, (O) observe the stoma and surrounding skin, (M) measure the stoma and mark the new pouch backing, (A) apply the new pouch.
2. The mouth is highly vascular making it a common entry point for infectious invaders. This increases the infant's and young child's risk for contraction of infectious agents via the mouth.
3. Acute hepatitis is mainly treated with rest, hydration, and nutrition.
4. Complications of a cleft palate that are of most concern during infancy pertain to feeding. The deformity often prevents the infant from being able to form an adequate seal around a nipple, preventing the ability to suction nutrients and cause excessive air intake. Feeding times are greatly extended, which causes insufficient intake and fatigue – both being precursors to problems with normal growth. Cleft palate during infancy also leads to gagging, choking, and nasal regurgitation of milk during feedings.
5. Data collected during the health history that would indicate pyloric stenosis include forceful, nonbilious vomiting that is not related to the feeding position of the infant, with subsequent weight loss, dehydration, and lethargy. These symptoms most commonly occur 2 to 4 weeks after birth. A positive family history of the disorder also increases the risk for pyloric stenosis.

Physical assessment findings reveal a hard, movable "olive-like" area palpated in the right upper quadrant of the abdomen.

SECTION II: APPLYING YOUR KNOWLEDGE

Activity F CASE STUDY

1. The discussion should include:
   Weight loss of 6 ounces in 2 weeks, sunken anterior fontanel, sticky mucous membranes, and poor skin turgor.

2. The discussion should include the following:
   The nurse should anticipate interventions that are going to rehydrate and restore Nico's fluid volume. Oral rehydration with pedialyte may be sufficient (refer to Teaching Guidelines 42.2). If dehydration appears to be severe, intravenous fluids may be necessary with a bolus of 20 mL/kg of normal saline or lactated ringers. Blood for electrolytes may need to be drawn to assess the extent of dehydration.

3. To evaluate Nico's hydration status the nurse should assess his fontanels, mucous membranes, skin turgor, urine output, pulses, capillary refill, temperature of extremities, and eyes.

4. Medical management of gastroesophageal reflux disease (GERD) usually begins with appropriate positioning such as elevating the head of the crib 30 degrees and keeping the infant or child upright for 30 to 45 minutes after feeding. Smaller more frequent feedings with a nipple that controls flow well may be helpful. Explain to the family to frequently burp the infant during feeds. Thickening of formula or pumped breast milk with products such as rice cereal can help in keeping the feedings and gastric contents down. Positioning of an infant for sleep with GERD is controversial; infants can be positioned safely on their sides or upright in a car seat to minimize the risk of aspiration while on their backs. However, always check with the physician to discuss his or her recommendations regarding sleeping positions for infants with GERD.

   If reflux does not improve with these measures medications are prescribed to decrease acid production and stabilize the pH of the gastric contents. Also, prokinetic agents may be used to help empty the stomach more quickly, minimizing the amount of gastric contents in the stomach that the child can reflux. If prescribed, thoroughly explain medications and their side effects and or adverse reactions. If the GERD cannot be medically managed effectively or requires long-term medication therapy, surgical intervention may be necessary.

   Explain to Nico's parents that reflux is usually limited to the first year of life; though, in some cases, it may persist. Teach Nico's parents and caregivers the signs and symptoms of potential complications. GERD symptoms can often involve the airway. In rare instances, GERD can cause apnea or acute life-threatening events (ALTE). Teach parents how to deal with these episodes, as anxiety is very high. Provide CPR instruction to all parents whose children have had ALTE previously, and use of an apnea or bradycardia monitor may be warranted. The monitor requires a physician's order and can be ordered through a home health company.

SECTION III: PRACTICING FOR NCLEX

Activity G NCLEX-STYLE QUESTIONS

1. **Answer: d**
   Infants are comprised of a high percentage of fluid that can be lost very quickly when vomiting, fever, and diarrhea are all present. This infant needs to be seen by the physician based on her age and symptoms; hospitalization may be necessary for intravenous rehydration depending upon her status when assessed.

2. **Answer: a**
   Anti-nuclear antibodies are one of the diagnostic tests performed to diagnose autoimmune hepatitis. Ultrasound is to assess for liver or spleen abnormalities. Viral studies are performed to screen for viral causes of hepatitis. Ammonia levels may be ordered if hepatic encephalopathy is suspected.

3. **Answer: d**
   If the parent reports that the child passed a meconium plug, the infant should be evaluated for Hirschsprung's disease. Constipation, not diarrhea, is associated with this condition; however, constipation alone would not necessarily warrant further evaluation for Hirschsprung's disease. Passing a meconium stool in the first 24 to 48 hours of life is normal.

4. **Answer: d**
   While most fruits and fruit juices are allowed, the nurse needs to make sure the mother knows that some fruit pie fillings and dried fruit may contain gluten.

5. **Answer: b**
   It is very important to encourage large amounts of water/fluids after this test to avoid barium-induced constipation. It is also important to tell the parents about a possible change in stool color, but the fluids are most important. This procedure is unlikely to cause an infection. Diarrhea is usually not a problem after this examination.

6. **Answer: c**
   The best response would be to remind the boy that there are lots of other children with Crohn's disease that could be found at the local support group. Teenagers do not like to be told that they "have" to do anything. Telling the boy that he will eventually accept his condition or that the disease has periods of remission does not address his concerns.

7. **Answer: c**

   Tenting of skin is an indicator of severe dehydration. Soft and flat fontanels indicate mild dehydration. Pale and slightly dry mucosa indicates mild or moderate dehydration. Blood pressure of 80/42 is a normal finding for an infant.

8. **Answer: d**

   It is best to ask an open-ended question in very specific terms so that the nurse can assess for proper laxative use based on a recent history of stool patterns. Using the term daily stool patterns might be confusing to the parents. Asking the parents whether the laxatives are working may not elicit any helpful information. Asking whether they are giving him the laxatives properly would likely result in a positive response even if this is not accurate.

9. **Answer: a**

   Ulcerative colitis is usually continuous through the colon while the distribution of Crohn's disease is segmental. Crohn's disease affects the full thickness of the intestine while ulcerative colitis is more superficial. Both conditions share age at onset of 10 to 20 years, with abdominal pain and fever in 40 to 50% of cases.

10. **Answer: a**

    A hard, moveable "olive-like mass" in the right upper quadrant is the hypertrophied pylorus. A sausage-shaped mass in the upper mid abdomen is the hallmark of intussusception. Perianal fissures and skin tags are typical with Crohn's disease. Abdominal pain and irritability is common with pyloric stenosis but are seen with many other conditions.

11. **Answer: 48 milliliters**

    RATIONALE: 13.2 pounds $\times$ 1 kg/2.2 pounds = 6 kg
    6 kg $\times$ 1 mL/kg = 6 mL/hour
    6 mL $\times$ 8 hours = 48 mL/8-hour shift

12. **Answers: a, d**

    RATIONALE: Hepatitis A virus is transmitted by contaminated food or water. Hepatitis B virus may be transmitted perinatally from mother to infant, intravenous drug use with contaminated needles, sexual contact with an infected person, and blood transfusions. The mother may have contracted the virus prior to giving birth to the child. Infection with the hepatitis B virus may result in jaundice, fever, and a rash.

13. **Answers: a, b, c**

    RATIONALE: Famotidine may cause fatigue. Omeprazole can cause headaches. Prokinetics use may result in side effects involving the central nervous system. Omeprazole use more likely will result in diarrhea, not constipation. Children with GERD should not lie down after meals.

14. **Answer: 289 milliliters per hour**

    RATIONALE: The child weighs 63.5 pounds.
    63.5 pounds $\times$ 1 kg/2.2 pounds = 577.2727 mL
    577.2727 mL of normal saline/ 2 hours = 288.6364 mL
    When rounded to the nearest whole number = 289 mL/hour

15. **Answers: b, d, e**

    RATIONALE: Newborns with esophageal atresia cough during attempts to feed, may have fluid in their lungs, and X-rays will show that nasogastric tubes just coil in the upper part of the esophagus because the esophagus does not extend to the stomach. They have increased salivation in their mouths and their skin may be dusky or cyanotic.

CHAPTER 43

SECTION I: ASSESSING YOUR UNDERSTANDING

Activity A FILL IN THE BLANKS

1. Suppression
2. Testicular
3. Renal
4. Flow
5. Enuresis
6. 30 mL

Activity B LABELING

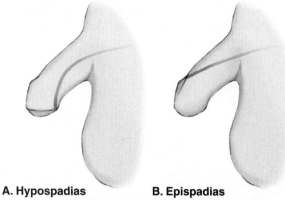

A. Hypospadias   B. Epispadias

A. Hypospadias: shows the urethral opening located on the ventral side of the penis.
B. Epispadias: shows the urethral opening located on the dorsal side of the penis.

Activity C MATCHING

Question 1

1. f   2. d   3. a   4. b   5. c

Question 2

1. c   2. d   3. b   4. a

Activity D SEQUENCING

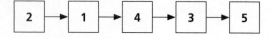

Activity E SHORT ANSWERS

1. After a bladder augmentation the urine may contain mucous.
2. The nurse should encourage fluids and monitor vital signs. The nurse must also be aware that child may feel burning with voiding after the procedure and urine may have a pink tinge because of the irritation of the mucous membrane as a result of the procedure.
3. Medications used in the care and treatment of end-stage renal disease may include:
   - Vitamin D/Calcium to correct hypocalcemia and hyperphosphatemia
   - Ferrous sulfate for anemia
   - Bicitra or sodium bicarbonate tablets to correct acidosis
   - Multivitamins to augment nutrition status
   - Erythropoietin injections to stimulate red blood cell growth
   - Growth hormone injections to stimulate growth in stature
4. A testicle is abnormally attached to the scrotum and twisted. It requires immediate attention because ischemia can result if the torsion is left untreated, leading to infertility. Testicular torsion may occur at any age but most commonly occurs in boys aged 12 to 18 years.
5. Normally both testes are descended at the time of birth. A watch and see approach is taken. If the testes are not descended by 6 months of age surgery is indicated.

SECTION II: APPLYING YOUR KNOWLEDGE

Activity F CASE STUDY

1. The discussion should include the following points:
   Urinary tract infections (UTI) occur most often due to bacteria coming from the urethra and traveling up to the bladder. The most common organism that causes UTI is *Escherichia coli*, which is usually found in the perineal and anal region, close to the urethral opening. UTIs are very common in children, especially infants and

young children and after 1 year of age is more common in females. One explanation for UTI occurring more frequently in females than in males is that the female's shorter urethra allows bacteria to have easier access to the bladder. Additionally, the female urethra is located quite close to the vagina and anus, allowing spread of bacteria such as *Escherichia coli* from those areas.

2. The discussion should include the following points:

Administer oral antibiotics as prescribed and complete the entire course of antibiotics even if Corey is feeling better and is not showing any signs or symptoms any longer. Push oral fluids, which will help flush the bacteria from the bladder. Administer antipyretics, such as acetaminophen or ibuprofen, in order to reduce fever. A heating pad or warm compress may help relieve abdomen or flank pain. If the child is afraid to urinate due to burning or stinging, encourage voiding in a warm sitz or tub bath.

3. The discussion should include the following points:

Encourage Corey and her family to follow-up as the physician has ordered for repeat urine culture after completing the course of antibiotics. Ensure Corey drinks adequate fluid to keep urine flushed through the bladder and prevent urine stasis. A decreased fluid intake can contribute to bacterial growth, as the bacteria become more concentrated. Encourage drinking of juices such as cranberry juice that will acidify the urine. If urine is alkaline, bacteria are better able to flourish. Avoid colas and caffeine which irritate the bladder. Encourage Corey to urinate frequently and avoid holding of urine to avoid urinary stasis which allows bacteria to grow. Avoid bubble baths which can contribute to vulvar and perineal irritation. Teach Corey to wipe front to back after using the restroom, to avoid contamination of the urethra with rectal material. Wearing of cotton underwear can decrease the incidence of perineal irritation. Avoid wearing of tight jeans or pants and wash the perineal area daily with soap and water.

SECTION III: PRACTICING FOR NCLEX
Activity G NCLEX-STYLE QUESTIONS

1. **Answer: c**
   Urinalysis is ordered to reveal preliminary information about the urinary tract. The test evaluates color, pH, specific gravity, and odor of urine. Urinalysis also assesses for presence of protein, glucose, ketones, blood, leukocyte esterase, RBCs, WBCs, bacteria, crystals, and casts. Total protein, globulin, albumin, and creatinine clearance would be ordered for suspected renal failure or renal disease. Urine culture and sensitivity is used to determine the presence of bacteria and determine the best choice of antibiotic.

2. **Answer: c**
   Acute glomerulonephritis often follows a group A streptococcal infection. Strep A infections may manifest as an upper respiratory infection. The history of urinary tract infections, renal disorders, or hypotension are not directly associated with the onset of acute glomerulonephritis.

3. **Answer: b**
   The nurse should weigh the old dialysate to determine the amount of fluid removed from the child. The fluid must be weighed prior to emptying it. The nurse should weigh the new fluid prior to starting the next fill phase. Typically, the exchanges are 3 to 6 hours apart so the nurse would not immediately start the next fill phase.

4. **Answer: d**
   The girl cannot eat whatever she wants on dialysis days. She can eat what she wants during the few hours she is actively undergoing treatment in the hemodialysis unit. The other statements regarding a high sodium diet and potassium intake are correct.

5. **Answer: c**
   It is very important to administer in the morning, encourage large amounts of water/fluids and encourage frequent voiding during and after infusion to decrease the risk of hemorrhagic cystitis

6. **Answer: b**
   The best response would be to include the child in plans for nighttime urinary control. This gives the child a sense of hope and reminds him that there are actions he can take to help achieve dryness. Telling him that he will grow out of this does not offer solutions. Providing statistics can be helpful, but does not offer a solution. Reminding him that pull-ups look just like underwear does not address his concerns.

7. **Answer: c**
   Hemolytic uremic syndrome is defined by all three particular features – hemolytic anemia, thrombocytopenia, and acute renal failure. Dirty green colored urine, elevated erythrocyte sedimentation, and depressed serum complement level are indicative of acute glomerulonephritis. Hypertension, not hypotension would be seen and the child would have decreased urinary output which would not cause nocturia.

8. **Answer: c**
   The nurse should withhold routine medications on the morning that hemodialysis is scheduled since they would be filtered out through the dialysis process. His medications should be administered after he returns from the dialysis unit. A Tenckhoff catheter is used for peritoneal dialysis, not hemodialysis. The nurse should avoid blood pressure measurement in the extremity with the AV fistula as it may cause occlusion.

9. **Answer: c**

The girl's partner should be treated, but she must strongly encourage the girl to require her partner to wear a condom every time they have sex, even after he undergoes antibiotic therapy. The other statements are accurate.

10. **Answer: d**

The nurse should always auscultate the site for presence of a bruit and palpate for presence of a thrill. The nurse should immediately notify the physician if there is an absence of a thrill. Dialysate without fibrin or cloudiness is normal and is used with peritoneal dialysis, not hemodialysis.

11. **Answer: a**

Complications of hydronephrosis include renal insufficiency, hypertension, and eventually renal failure. Hypotension, hypothermia, and tachycardia are not associated with hydronephrosis.

12. **Answer: a, c, e**

A voiding cystourethrogram (VCUG) will be performed to determine the presence of a structural defect that may be causing the hydronephrosis. Other diagnostic tests, such as a renal ultrasound or an intravenous pyelogram, may also be performed to clarify the diagnosis. A urinalysis may be performed to assess the quality and characteristics of the urine but the test will not confirm a diagnosis of hydronephrosis. A complete blood cell count may be used to assess the level of a genitourinary infection but it will not confirm the diagnosis of hydronephrosis.

13. **Answer: c**

Normally both testes will descend prior to birth. In the event this does not happen the child will be observed for the first 6 months of life. If the testicle descends without intervention further treatment will not be needed. Surgical intervention is not needed until after 6 months if the testicle has not descended.

14. **Answer: a**

Epididymitis is caused by a bacterial infection. Treatment may include scrotal elevation, bed rest, and ice packs to the scrotum. Pharmacotherapy may include antibiotics, pain medications, and NSAIDs. Warm compresses would result in vasodilation and do little to relieve the pain and swelling of the condition. Corticosteroid therapy is not included in the plan of care for the condition. Voiding is not impacted by epididymitis. Catheterization is not indicated.

15. **Answer: d**

The discharge instructions for the child who has had a circumcision will include a listing of warning signs to report. Redness or swelling of the penile shaft is not a normal finding and must be reported. Petroleum jelly (Vaseline) is often used for the first 24 hours after the procedure but not for a period of 2 weeks. Small amounts of bleeding may be noted. This bleeding if scant in amount does not warrant reporting to the physician. Reduction of water to impact voiding is inappropriate.

Answers

CHAPTER 44

SECTION I: ASSESSING YOUR UNDERSTANDING

Activity A FILL IN THE BLANKS

1. Autoimmune
2. Clonus
3. Decrease
4. Involuntary
5. Hypotonia
6. Neural tube defects
7. Guillain-Barré

Activity B LABELING

Figure A shows meningocele
Figure B shows myelomeningocele.
Figure C shows normal spine
Figure D shows spina bifida occulta

Activity C MATCHING

1. a **2.** c **3.** d **4.** b **5.** e

Activity D SHORT ANSWERS

1. The four classifications are spastic, athetoid (dyskinetic), ataxic, and mixed. Spastic is the most common form and ataxic is the rarest.
2. Nursing management of a child with myelomeningocele focuses on preventing infection, promoting bowel and urinary elimination, promoting adequate nutrition, and preventing latex allergic reaction. The nurse is also concerned with maintaining the child's skin integrity, providing education and support to the family, and recognizing complications such as hydrocephalus or increased intracranial pressure (ICP) associated with the disorder.
3. Pain in the lower extremities is often one of the first symptoms in children. Additional symptoms include fairly symmetrical flaccid weakness or paralysis. Ataxia and sensory disturbances are commonly seen during the course of the illness.
4. Risk factors for neural tube defects include lack of prenatal care; insufficient intake of folic acid preconception and /or prenatally; previous history of a child born with a neural tube defect or a positive family history of neural tube defects; and certain drugs that antagonize folic acid absorption, such as

anticonvulsants, that are taken by the mother during pregnancy.
5. There are nine types of muscular dystrophy, with Duchenne muscular dystrophy being the most common childhood type. All types of muscular dystrophy result in progressive skeletal (voluntary) muscle wasting and weakness. The disease is inherited, but there are various patterns of inheritance among the various types of muscular dystrophy.

SECTION II: APPLYING YOUR KNOWLEDGE

Activity E CASE STUDY

1. The discussion should include the following points:
   - Cerebral palsy (CP) is a term used to describe a range of nonspecific clinical symptoms characterized by abnormal motor pattern and postures caused by nonprogressive abnormal brain function. The cause of CP generally occurs before or during delivery and is often associated with brain anoxia. Often no specific cause can be identified. Prolonged, complicated difficult delivery and prematurity are risk factors for CP. CP is the most common movement disorder of childhood and is a life-long, nonprogressive condition. It is one of the most common causes of physical disability in children.
   - There is a large variation in symptoms and disability among those with CP. For some children the disability may be as mild as a slight limp and for others it may result in severe motor and neurologic impairments. However, its primary signs include motor impairment such as spasticity, muscle weakness, and ataxia. Complications of CP include mental impairment, seizures, growth problems, impaired vision or hearing, abnormal sensation or perception, and hydrocephalus. Most children can survive into adulthood but may endure substantial effects on function and quality of life.
2. The discussion should include the following points:
   - Earliest signs of cerebral palsy include abnormal muscle tone and developmental delay. Primary signs include spasticity, muscle weakness, and

ataxia. Children with CP may demonstrate abnormal use of muscle groups such as scooting on their back instead of crawling or walking. Hypertonicity with increased resistance to dorsiflexion and passive hip abduction are common early signs. Sustained clonus may be present after forced dorsiflexion. Children with CP will often demonstrate prolonged standing on their toes when supported in an upright standing position.

3. The discussion should include the following points:
   - Nursing management focuses on promoting growth and development through the promotion of mobility and maintenance of optimal nutritional intake. Treatment modalities to promote mobility include physiotherapy, pharmacological management, and surgery. Physical or occupational therapy as well as medications may be used to address musculoskeletal abnormalities, facilitate range of motion, delay or prevent deformities such as contractures, provide joint stability, and to maximize activity and to encourage the use of adaptive devices. The nurse's role in relation to the various therapies is to ensure compliance with prescribed exercises, positioning, or bracing. Children with CP may experience difficulty eating and swallowing due to poor motor control of the throat, mouth, and tongue. This may lead to poor nutrition and problems with growth. The child with CP may require a longer time to feed because of the poor motor control. Special diets, such as soft or pureed, may make swallowing easier. Proper positioning during feeding is essential to facilitate swallowing and reduce the risk of aspiration. Speech or occupational therapists can assist in working on strengthening swallowing muscles as well as assisting in developing accommodations to facilitate nutritional intake. Consult a dietician to ensure adequate nutrition for children with cerebral palsy. In children with severe swallowing problems or malnutrition, a feeding tube such as a gastrostomy tube may be placed.
   - Providing support and education to the child and family is also an important nursing function. From the time of diagnosis, the family should be involved in the child's care. Refer caregivers to local resources including education services and support groups.

SECTION III: PRACTICING FOR NCLEX
Activity F NCLEX-STYLE QUESTIONS

1. **Answer: b**
   The nurse needs to obtain a clear description of weakness. This open-ended question would most likely elicit specific examples of weakness and shed light on whether the boy is simply fatigued.

The other questions would most likely elicit a yes or no answer rather than any specific details about his weakness or development.

2. **Answer: d**
   The persistence of a primitive reflex in a 9-month-old would warrant further evaluation. Symmetrical spontaneous movement and absence of the Moro and tonic neck reflex are expected in a normally developing 9-month-old child.

3. **Answer: b**
   Dimpling and skin discoloration in the child's lumbosacral area can be an indication of spina bifida occulta. It would be best to respond that the dimpling and discoloration is possibly a normal variation with no problems and indicate that the doctor will want to take a closer look; this response will not alarm the parent, but it also does not ignore the findings. Spina bifida is a term that is often used to generalize all neural tube disorders that affect the spinal cord. This can be confusing and a cause of concern for parents. It is probably best to avoid the use of the term initially until a diagnosis is confirmed. Nursing care would then focus on educating the family.

4. **Answer: c**
   Symptoms of constipation and bladder dysfunction may result due to an increasing size of the lesion. Increasing ICP and head circumference would point to hydrocephalus. Leaking cerebrospinal fluid would indicate the sac is leaking.

5. **Answer: b**
   It is very important to remind the parents that they must always wash hands very well with soap and water prior to catheterization to help prevent infection. The other statements are correct.

6. **Answer: c**
   The best response would be to remind the boy that there are many children with muscular dystrophy that could be found at the local support group. Teenagers do not like to be told that they "have" to do anything. Telling the boy that he needs to be active or simply suggesting activities does not address his concerns.

7. **Answer: a**
   A sign of Duchenne muscular dystrophy (DMD) is the walking on the toes or balls of the feet with a rolling or waddling gait. Signs of hydrocephalus are not typically associated with DMD. Kyphosis and scoliosis occur more frequently than lordosis. A child with DMD has an enlarged appearance to their calf muscles due to pseudohypertrophy of the calves.

8. **Answer: d**
   The nurse can offer the child a snack and observe if she has any difficulty chewing, swallowing, or feeding herself. Inquiring about a typical day's diet opens up the conversation to discuss the quantity and quality of food the girl eats. Asking about swallowing or whether the girl feeds herself

would most likely elicit a yes or no response. Checking her hydration status and respiratory system is important, but does not open a dialogue.

9. **Answer: a**
The use of ticking is often a successful technique for assessing the level of paralysis in this age of child, either initially or in the recovery phase. Symmetrical flaccid weakness, ataxia, and sensory disturbances are other symptoms seen during the course of the illness.

10. **Answer: b**
The central nursing priority is to prevent rupture or leaking of cerebrospinal fluid. Keeping infant in prone position will help prevent pressure on lesion. Keeping lesion free from fecal matter or urine is important as well, but the priority is to prevent rupture or leakage. The nurse should consider the lesion first when maintaining the infant's body temperature.

11. **Answers: a, c, d, e**
RATIONALE: Ditropan is used to increase the child's bladder capacity when they have a spastic bladder. The caregivers and the child should be taught about urinary catheterization techniques to allow the bladder to empty. The child and caregivers should be educated about the clinical manifestations associated with a urinary tract infection so that it can be treated promptly. Sometimes surgical interventions such as vesicostomy and the creation of a continent urinary reservoir are used to treat neurogenic bladders.

12. **Answers: a, b, d**
RATIONALE: Significant muscle wasting is associated with this diagnosis. Creatine kinase levels increase with muscle wasting. A muscle biopsy will show an absence of dystrophin. Gowers' sign will be positive. An electromyogram will indicate the problem is with the muscles, not the nerves. Genetic testing will reveal the presence of the gene associated with Duchenne muscular dystrophy.

13. **Answers: a, b, d, e**
RATIONALE: The following are clinical manifestations associated with cholinergic crisis: Sweating, bradycardia, severe muscle weakness, and increased salivation.

14. **Answers: a, b**
RATIONALE: Corticosteroids should be given with food to minimize gastric upset. Corticosteroids can mask infection. This child should avoid large crowds to prevent exposure to infectious organisms. The other parent responses are correct regarding corticosteroids and dermatomyositis.

15. **Answers: d, b, a, c**
RATIONALE: Guillain–Barré syndrome paresthesias and muscle weakness. Classically it initially affects the lower extremities and progresses in an ascending manner to upper extremities and then the facial muscles. Progression is usually complete in 2 to 4 weeks, followed by a stable period leading to the recovery phase.

CHAPTER 45

SECTION I: ASSESSING YOUR UNDERSTANDING

Activity A FILL IN THE BLANKS

1. Convex
2. Epiphysis
3. Fixator
4. Synovitis
5. Bacterial
6. Ossification
7. Adductus

Activity B LABELING

1. Bryant's traction
2. Russell's traction
3. Buck's traction
4. Cervical skin traction
5. Side-arm 90-90
6. Dunlop side-arm 00-90
7. 90-90 traction
8. Cervical skeletal tongs
9. Halo traction
10. Balanced suspension traction

Activity C MATCHING

1. d   2. c   3. e   4. b   5. a

Activity D SEQUENCING

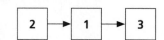

Activity E SHORT ANSWERS

1. In developmental dysplasia of the hip, the femoral head has an abnormal relationship to the acetabulum. Frank dislocation of the hip is complete dislocation. It may occur in which there is no contact between the femoral head and acetabulum. Subluxation is a partial dislocation, meaning that the acetabulum is not fully seated within the hip joint. Dysplasia refers to an acetabulum that is shallow or sloping instead of cup shaped.

2. A plastic or bowing deformity involves significant bending without breaking of the bone. A buckle fracture is a compression injury; the bone "buckles" rather than breaks. A greenstick fracture is an incomplete fracture of the bone. A complete fracture occurs when the bone breaks into two separate pieces.

3. Osteogenesis imperfecta is a genetic disorder that results in instability of joints and fractures. Parent teaching for care of the child with this disorder should include:
   - Never push or pull on the child's arm or leg
   - Do not bend the child's arm or leg into an awkward position
   - Lift a baby by placing one hand under the legs and buttocks and one hand under the shoulders, head, and neck
   - Do not lift a baby's legs by the ankles to change the diaper
   - Do not lift a baby or small child from under the armpits
   - Provide supported positioning
   - If a fracture is suspected, handle the limb as little as possible

4. Instructions for the child and his parents following removal of the cast should include:
   - Soak the arm in warm water daily to help in removing dead skin and secretions that have accumulated under the cast
   - Advise that new skin may be tender
   - Wash the arm with soapy warm water, but avoid excessive rubbing
   - Apply moisturizing lotion to the arm and avoid scratching dry skin
   - Encourage activity to regain strength and motion of the arm

5. Torticollis is a painless muscular condition that is often seen in infants, and sometimes in children with certain syndromes. Tightness of the sternocleidomastoid muscle causes torticollis, resulting in an infant's or child's head being tilted to one side. Passive stretching exercises are included in the treatment of the disorder.

SECTION II: APPLYING YOUR KNOWLEDGE
Activity F CASE STUDY

1. The discussion should include the following points:

   Perform a baseline neurovascular assessment, including color, movement, sensation, edema, and quality of pulses. Enlist the cooperation of the child, show him the cast materials, discuss colors of the cast materials, and have him help choose the color of his cast. Use an age-appropriate approach to describe the cast application process. Premedicate if ordered and provide distraction throughout cast application.

2. The discussion should include the following points:

   Drying time of the cast will vary depending on type of material used. Help the child keep the cast still and position it on pillows. If a plaster cast has been applied, "petal" the cast with moleskin or other soft material that has adhesive backing in order to prevent skin rubbing. Perform frequent neurovascular checks of the casted extremity. Assess for signs of increased pain, edema, pale or blue discoloration, skin coolness, numbness or tingling, prolonged capillary refill, and decreased pulse strength (if able to assess). Notify physician of changes in neurovascular status, persistent complaints of pain, odor, or drainage from the cast. Elevate casted extremity and apply ice if needed.

3. The discussion should include the following points:

   The child can resume increased levels of activity as the pain subsides. The right arm should be elevated above the level of the heart for the first 48 hours. Ice may be applied for 20 to 30 minutes, then off 1 hour and repeat for the first 24 to 48 hours. Check his right fingers for swelling (have him wiggle his fingers) hourly. Check the skin around the cast for irritation daily. If he complains of itching inside the cast blow cool air in from a hair dryer set on the lowest setting. Never insert anything into the cast for scratching and do not use lotions or powders. Keep the cast dry. Apply a plastic bag around the cast and tape securely for bathing or showering. Do not let the child submerge the cast in a bathtub. Call the physician if the casted extremity is cool to touch; inability to move his fingers; severe pain occurs with movement of his fingers; persistent numbness or tingling; drainage or a foul smell comes from the cast; severe itching inside the cast; temperature above 101.5 °F for longer than 24 hours; skin edges are red, swollen, or exhibit breakdown; or the casts gets wet, cracks, splits, or softens. Educate the family on follow-up needs and medications (including pain medication) if ordered.

SECTION III: PRACTICING FOR NCLEX
Activity G NCLEX-STYLE QUESTIONS

1. **Answer: b**

   The baby will most likely wear the harness for 3 months. Telling the parents that the harness does not hurt the baby is appropriate, but stressing the importance of wearing the harness continuously is a higher priority to ensure proper care and effective treatment. Only the physician or nurse practitioner can make adjustments to the harness.

2. **Answer: a**

   Asymmetry of the thigh or gluteal folds is indicative of DDH. Hip and knee joint relationship are not indicative of DDH. The lower extremities of the infant typically have some normal developmental variations due to in utero positioning.

3. **Answer: a**

   It is important to be vigilant in inspecting the child's skin for rashes, redness, and irritation to uncover areas where pressure sores are likely to develop. Applying lotion is part of the routine skin care regimen. Applying lotion, gentle massage, and keeping skin dry and clean are part of the routine skin care regimen.

4. **Answer: c**

   In Type II metatarsus adductus, the forefoot is flexible passively past neutral, but only to midline actively. The forefoot is flexible past neutral actively and passively in Type I. The forefoot is rigid, does not correct to midline even with passive stretching in Type III. An inverted forefoot turned slightly upward is indicative of clubfoot.

5. **Answer: b**

   It is very important to teach parents to identify the signs of neurovascular compromise (pale, cool, or blue skin) and tell them to notify the physician immediately. The other statements are correct.

6. **Answer: c**

   The best response for a 6-year-old is to use distraction throughout the cast application. He is resisting the application of the cast, so the best approach at this point is distraction. Telling him that application will not hurt is not helpful; nor is asking the child whether he wants pain medication. It is helpful to enlist the cooperation of the child by showing the child cast materials before beginning the procedure; but if he is resisting treatment, distraction would be the best approach.

7. **Answer: c**

   The nurse should emphasize that the child should not be allowed to lie on his side for 4 weeks following the surgery to ensure the bar does not shift. The parents should be aware of signs of infection; but the position must be emphasized to protect the bar. The nurse would be expected to monitor the child's vital capacity, not the parents. The prone position is acceptable.

8. **Answer: a**
The Ilizarov fixator uses wires that are thinner than ordinary pins, so simply cleansing by showering is usually sufficient to keep the pin site clean.

9. **Answer: d**
Because the mother is crying and experiencing the initial shock of the diagnosis, the nurse's primary concern is to support the mother and assure her that she is not to blame for the DDH. While education is important, let the mother adjust to the diagnosis and assure her that the baby and her family will be supported now and throughout the treatment period.

10. **Answer: d**
Blue sclera is not diagnostic of osteogenesis imperfecta, but it is a common finding. Foot drawn up and inward (talipes varus) and sole of foot facing backwards (talipes equinus) are associated with clubfoot. Dimpled skin and hair in the lumbar region are common findings with spina bifida occulta.

11. **Answers: a, b**
RATIONALE: This child has taken a benzodiazepine. Common side effects associated with this medication are dizziness and sedation. The skeletal muscle relaxes and the spasms will diminish. Nausea and upper gastrointestinal pain are not common side effects associated with this medication.

12. **Answers: b, c, e**
RATIONALE: The parents should call the physician when the following things occur: The child has
a temperature greater than 101.5F for more than 24 hours, there is drainage from the casted site, the site distal to the casted extremity is cyanotic, or severe edema is present.

13. **Answer: 1 milliliter**
RATIONALE: The supplement has 5 mcg of vitamin D in each 0.5 mL. The child is supposed to receive 10 mcg each day of supplemental vitamin D.

Desired/Have × Quantity = dose
10 mcg/5 mcg × 0.5 mL = 1 mL

Ratio/proportion:
0.5 mL/5 micrograms = x/10 micrograms = 1 mL

14. **Answers: b, c, d, e**
RATIONALE: Slipped capital femoral epiphysis most often occurs in males between the ages of 12 to 15 years. It more commonly affects African American boys. The femoral plate weakens and becomes less resistant to stressors during periods of growth. Boys are more frequently affected. Obese boys are more likely to develop this condition.

15. **Answer: c**
RATIONALE: A greenstick fracture (image C) is an incomplete fracture of the bone. Image A shows a plastic or bowing deformity. Image B shows a buckle fracture (the bone buckles rather than breaks). Image D shows a complete fracture (the bone breaks in two pieces).

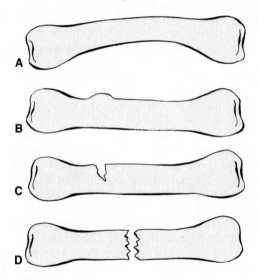

Answers

CHAPTER 46

SECTION I: ASSESSING YOUR UNDERSTANDING

Activity A FILL IN THE BLANKS

1. Decreases
2. IgE
3. Hypersensitivity
4. Cradle cap
5. Androgens

Activity B MATCHING

Question 1

1. b   2. c   3. d   4. a   5. e

Question 2

1. d   2. c   3. a   4. b

Activity C SEQUENCING

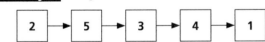

Activity D SHORT ANSWERS

1. Dark-skinned children tend to have more pronounced cutaneous reactions compared to children with lighter skin. Hypopigmentation or hyperpigmentation in the affected area following healing of a dermatologic condition is common.

   Dark-skinned children tend to have more prominent papules, follicular response lichenification, and vesicular or bullous reaction than lighter-skinned children with the same disorder. Additionally, hypertrophic scarring and keloid formation occur more often.

2. Four criteria to describe lesions:
   - Linear refers to lesions in a line
   - Shape: The lesions are round, oval, or annular (ring around central clearing)
   - Morbilliform refers to a rosy, maculopapular rash
   - Target lesions look just like a bull's eye

3. Impetigo is a readily recognizable skin rash. Non-bullous impetigo generally follows some type of skin trauma or may arise as a secondary bacterial infection of another skin disorder, such as atopic dermatitis. Bullous impetigo demonstrates a sporadic occurrence pattern and develops on intact skin resulting from toxin production of *Staphylococcus aureus*.

4. Pressure ulcers develop from a combination of factors, including immobility or decreased activity, decreased sensory perception, increased moisture, impaired nutritional status, inadequate tissue perfusion, and the forces of friction and shear. Common sites of pressure ulcers in hospitalized children include the occipital region and toes, while children who require wheelchairs for mobility have pressure ulcers in the sacral or hip area more frequently.

5. Acne vulgaris affects 50% to 85% of adolescents between the ages of 12 and 16 years. The sebaceous gland produces sebum and is connected by a duct to the follicular canal that opens on the skin's surface. Androgenous hormones stimulate sebaceous gland proliferation and production of sebum. These hormones exhibit increased activity during the pubertal years.

SECTION II: APPLYING YOUR KNOWLEDGE

Activity E CASE STUDY

1. The skin reaction seen in atopic dermatitis is in response to specific allergens (such as food or environmental triggers). So when Eva comes into contact with the triggers it causes her body to respond and her skin starts to feel itchy. This sensation of itchiness comes first and then the rash becomes apparent. Other factors such as high or low temperatures, perspiring, contact with skin irritants (such as fragrance in soaps), scratching, or stress can also trigger the skin to flare up.

2. Management of atopic dermatitis focuses on promoting skin hydration, maintaining skin integrity, and preventing infection. Parents and caregivers need to be instructed to avoid hot water and any skin and hair products that contain perfumes, dyes, or fragrances. Bathing the child twice a day in warm water using a mild soap for sensitive skin is encouraged. Do not rub the child dry but gently pat them

and leave the child moist. Apply prescribed ointments or creams to affected areas. Apply fragrance-free moisturizers. Re-moisturize multiple times throughout the day. Avoid clothing made of synthetic fabrics or wool. Avoid triggers (often food, especially eggs, wheat, milk, and peanut, or environmental triggers such as molds, dust mites, and cat dander) known to exacerbate atopic dermatitis. Cut the child's finger nails short and keep them clean. Avoid tight clothing and heat. Use 100% cotton bed sheets and pajamas. It is very important to stop the child from scratching since this causes the rash to appear and causes trauma to the skin and secondary infection. Antihistamines given at bedtime may sedate the child enough to allow for sleep without awakening because of itching. During the waking hours, behavior modification may help to keep the child from scratching. The parents should keep a diary for 1 week to determine the pattern of scratching. Discuss specific strategies that may raise the child's awareness of scratching such as use of a hand-held clicker or counter to help identify the scratching episode for the child, thus raising awareness. Discuss the use of diversion, imagination, and play to help to detract Eva from scratching. Pressing the skin or fist clenching may replace scratching. Keep the child active and positively reinforce by praising desired behaviors.

SECTION III: PRACTICING FOR NCLEX
Activity F NCLEX-STYLE QUESTIONS

1. **Answer: c**
    Airway injury from burn or smoke inhalation should be suspected if stridor is present. Cervical spine or internal injures would not point to airway injury. Burns on hands would not be indicative of airway injury.

2. **Answer: c**
    Initially, the severely burned child first experiences a decrease in cardiac output with a subsequent hypermetabolic response during which cardiac output increases dramatically. During this heightened metabolic state, the child is a risk for insulin resistance and increased protein catabolism.

3. **Answer: d**
    Staphylococcal scalded skin syndrome results from infection with *S. aureus* that produces a toxin which then causes exfoliation. It is abrupt in onset and results in diffuse erythema and skin tenderness. It is most common in infancy and rare beyond 5 years of age. Bullous impetigo presents with red macules and bullous eruptions on an erythematous base. Nonbullous impetigo presents as papules progressing to vesicles then painless pustules with a narrow erythematous border. Folliculitis presents with red raised hair follicles.

4. **Answer: c**
    The nurse should emphasize that the parents should avoid hot water. The child should be

bathed twice a day in warm water. The other statements are correct.

5. **Answer: a**
    Tinea pedis presents with red scaling rash on soles, and between the toes. Tinea capitis presents with patches of scaling in the scalp with central hair loss and the risk of kerion development (inflamed boggy mass filled with pustules). Tinea cruris presents with erythema, scaling, maceration in the inguinal creases and inner thighs.

6. **Answer: b**
    Small round red circles with scaling, symmetrically located on the girls' inner thighs point to nickel dermatitis that may occur from contact with jewelry, eyeglasses, belts, or clothing snaps. The nurse should inquire about any sleepers or clothing with metal snaps. The girl does not have a rash in her diaper area. It is unlikely that an infant this age would have her inner thighs exposed to a highly allergenic plant. Discussing family allergy history is important, but the nurse should first inquire about any clothing with metal that could have come into contact with the girl's skin when she displays a symmetrical rash.

7. **Answer: a**
    Erythema multiforme typically manifests in lesions over the hands and feet, and extensor surfaces of the extremities with spread to the trunk. Thick or flaky/greasy yellow scales are signs of seborrhea. Silvery or yellow-white scale plaques and sharply demarcated borders define psoriasis. Superficial tan or hypopigmented oval-shaped scaly lesions especially on upper back and chest and proximal arms are indicative of tinea versicolor.

8. **Answer: c**
    The nurse should administer diphenhydramine as soon as possible after the sting in an attempt to minimize a reaction. The other actions are important for an insect sting, but the priority intervention is to administer diphenhydramine.

9. **Answer: b**
    Second degree frostbite demonstrates blistering with erythema and edema. First degree frostbite results in superficial white plaques with surrounding erythema. In third degree frostbite, the nurse would note hemorrhagic blisters that would progress to tissue necrosis and sloughing when the fourth degree is reached.

10. **Answer: a**
    It is important to apply moisture multiply times through the day. Petroleum jelly is a recommended moisturizer that is inexpensive and readily available. The other statements are correct.

11. **Answer: a**
    Impetigo is an infectious bacterial infection. The crusts should be removed after soaking prior to applying topical medications. Leaving the lesions open to air is not contraindicated. Children diagnosed with impetigo may attend school during treatment.

12. **Answer: c**

    Tinea pedis is commonly known as athlete's foot. It is a fungal infection. The fungi are able to readily grow in warm, moist conditions such as shower areas.

13. **Answers: a, b, c**

    The treatment of diaper rash may include topical ointments containing vitamins A and D as well as zinc.

14. **Answer: a**

    Atopic dermatitis is commonly associated allergies to food. Common culprits may include peanuts, eggs, orange juice, and wheat-containing products.

15. **Answers: b, c, e**

    When caring for the child with atopic dermatitis the focus of care will be on the prevention of infection, maintenance of skin integrity, and promotion of skin hydration.

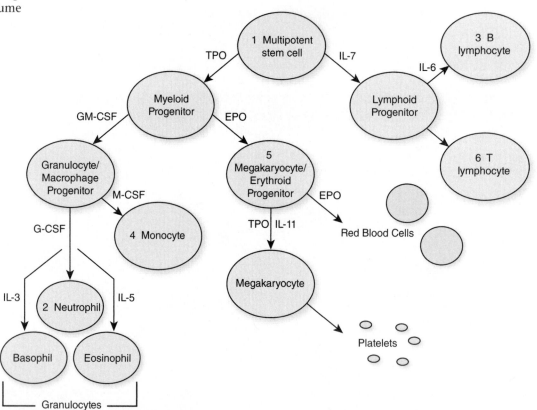

CHAPTER 47

SECTION I: ASSESSING YOUR UNDERSTANDING

Activity A FILL IN THE BLANKS

1. Hemogram
2. Volume
3. Kidneys
4. Size
5. Protoporphyrin
6. Mean platelet volume (MPV)
7. Anemia

Activity B LABELING

Activity C MATCHING

1. e   2. c   3. d   4. b   5. a

Activity D SHORT ANSWERS

1. Folic acid deficiency is caused by a low dietary intake of green leafy vegetables, liver, and citrus. It can also be caused by malabsorption from medication such as Dilantin or parasitic infections. Pernicious anemia is a deficiency of vitamin B12. Management of folic acid deficiency involves insuring compliance with dietary changes. Pernicious anemia is managed with monthly injections of vitamin B12.

2. The recommended action is to confirm the level with a repeat lab within 1 week, as well as educate the caregivers to decrease lead exposure. Refer the

family to the local health department for investigation of the home for lead reduction with referrals for support services.

3. Color changes to the skin such as pallor, bruising, and flushing. Changes in mental status such as lethargy can also indicate a decrease in hemoglobin and decreased oxygenation of the brain.

4. Sickle cell anemia is most commonly seen in persons of African, Mediterranean, Middle Eastern, and Indian decent. In the United States, the number of infants born with sickle cell anemia is approximately 2,000, with 1 in 400 being African American.

5. Iron deficiency anemia occurs when the body does not have enough iron to produce Hgb, often related to dietary issues. Children between the ages of 6 and 20 months, and those at the age of puberty are the periods when iron deficiency anemia is most prevalent.

SECTION II: APPLYING YOUR KNOWLEDGE

Activity E CASE STUDY

1. The discussion should include:
   - How much milk does Jayda drink per day? (excessive cow's milk consumption, greater than 24 ounces a day, leads to an increased risk for iron deficiency anemia)
   - When did Jayda start on cow's milk? (cow's milk consumption before 12 months of age leads to an increased risk for iron deficiency anemia)
   - Was Jayda formula fed? If so, what type (low iron formula can lead to iron deficiency anemia); or breast fed? If so, did she receive iron supplementation (including eating iron-fortified cereal) after 6 months of age?
   - What are Jayda's food preferences and usual eating patterns?
   - Is she on any restricted diet?
   - Is she taking any medications? (certain medications, such as antacids can interfere with iron absorption)

2. The discussion should include:
   - Oral supplements or multivitamin formulas that have iron are often dark in color as the iron is pigmented. Teaching of Jayda's parents should include to precisely measure the amount of iron to be administered and to be sure to place the liquid behind the teeth since iron in liquid form can stain the teeth. Use of straw and brushing her teeth after administration may help. Another problem that frequently occurs is constipation from the iron. In some cases reduction of the amount of iron can resolve this problem, but stool softeners may be necessary to control painful or difficult to pass stools. Encourage parents to increase their child's fluid intake and maintain adequate consumption of fiber to assist in avoiding the development of constipation. Instruct the parents that stools may appear dark in color due to iron administration. Instruct parents to keep iron supplements and all medications in a safe place to avoid accidental overdose.
   - Providing juice enriched with vitamin C can help aid absorption of iron. Limit cow's milk intake to 24 ounces per day. Limit fast food consumption and encourage iron-rich foods such as red meats, tuna, salmon, eggs, tofu, enriched grains, dried beans and peas, dried fruits, leafy green vegetables, and iron-fortified breakfast cereals (iron from red meat is the easiest for the body to absorb). Encourage parents to provide nutritious snacks and finger foods that are developmentally appropriate for Jayda. Toddlers are often picky eaters. This often becomes a means of control for the child, and parents should guard against getting involved in a power struggle with their child. Referring parents to a developmental nurse practitioner that can assist them in their approach to diet with their child may prove beneficial.
   - Encourage appropriate follow-up and review signs and symptoms of anemia.

3. The discussion should include:
   - Low socioeconomic status which can lead to a lack of adequate food supply
   - Recent immigration from a developing country
   - Culturally based food influences that lead to dietary imbalances
   - Child abuse or neglect leading to improper nutrition

SECTION III: PRACTICING FOR NCLEX

Activity F NCLEX-STYLE QUESTIONS

1. **Answer: b**
   If neurological deficits are assessed, immediate reporting of the findings is necessary to begin treatment to prevent permanent damage.

2. **Answer: d**
   A convex shape of the fingernails termed 'spooning' can occur with iron deficiency anemia. Capillary refill in less than 2 seconds, pink palms and nail beds, and absence of bruising are normal findings.

3. **Answer: a**
   When the MCV is elevated, the RBCs are larger and referred to as macrocytic. The WBC count does not affect the MCV. The platelet count and Hgb are within normal ranges for a 7-year-old child.

4. **Answer: d**
   If the screening test result indicates the possibility of SCA or sickle cell trait, hemoglobin (Hgb) electrophoresis is performed promptly to confirm the diagnosis. While Hgb electrophoresis is the only definitive test for diagnosis of the disease, other laboratory testing that assists in the assessment of

the disease include reticulocyte count (greatly elevated), peripheral blood smears (presence of sickle-shaped cells and target cells), and erythrocyte sedimentation rate (elevated).

5. **Answer: a**
While iron from red meat is the easiest for the body to absorb, the nurse must limit fast food consumption from the drive thru as they are also high in fat, fillers, and sodium. The other statements are correct.

6. **Answer: b**
The best response for a 7-year-old is to use distraction and involve him in the infusion process in a developmentally appropriate manner. A 7-year-old is old enough to assist with the dilution and mixing of the factor. Asking for help with the band-aid would be best for a younger child. Teens should be taught to administer their own factor infusions. Telling him to be brave is not helpful and does
not teach.

7. **Answer: a**
The priority is to emphasize to the parents that they precisely measure the amount of iron to be administered in order to avoid overdosing. The other instructions are accurate, but the priority is to emphasize precise measurement.

8. **Answer: c**
Symmetrical swelling of the hands and feet in the infant or toddler is termed dactylitis; aseptic infarction occurs in the metacarpals and metatarsals and is often the first vaso-occlusive event seen with sickle cell disease. Symmetrical swelling of the hands and feet are not typically seen with the other conditions listed.

9. **Answer: b**
This response answers the parent's questions. In the nonsevere form, the granulocyte count remains about 500, the platelets are over 20,000, and the reticulocyte count is over 1%. The other responses do not address what the parents are asking and would block therapeutic communication.

10. **Answer: c**
Laboratory evaluation will reveal decreased hemoglobin and hematocrit, decreased

reticulocyte count, microcytosis and hypochromia, decreased serum iron and ferritin levels, and increase FEP level. The other findings do not point to iron deficiency anemia.

11. **Answer: d, c, a, b**
RATIONALE: The bone marrow releases a stem cell. Thrombopoietin acts on the cell to help turn it into a myeloid cell. Erythropoietin acts on the cell and it turns into a megakaryocyte. The megakaryocyte becomes an erythrocyte (red blood cell).

12. **Answers: a, c, d, e**
RATIONALE: This girl's erythrocyte count is below normal, which indicates she is anemic. The mean corpuscular hemoglobin concentration is below normal which indicates that her cells are hypochromic with a diluted amount of hemoglobin available. The mean corpuscular volume of the erythrocytes are decreased which indicates her cells are microcytic or smaller than normal.

13. **Answers: a, c, d, e**
RATIONALE: The caregivers should seek medical treatment promptly for any clinical manifestations associated with an infection. The child should receive prophylactic antibiotics. The child should be provided with immunization against the following organisms: *Streptococcus pneumoniae, Neisseria meningitidis,* and *Haemophilus influenzae* type B. The child should be taught techniques to reduce the transmission of infection. The child should wear his medic alert bracelet all the time.

14. **Answers: b, d**
RATIONALE: Iron supplements should not be mixed in milk because it reduces absorption. Iron supplements may make the child constipated. All of the other options are correct.

15. **Answer: 36 milligrams**
RATIONALE: 47.3 pounds $\times$ 1 kg/2.2 pounds = 21.5 kg

21.5 kg $\times$ 5 mg/1 kg = 107.5 mg/day
107.5 mg/3 doses = 35.8333 mg/dose

when rounded to the nearest whole number = 36 mg

Answers

CHAPTER 48

SECTION I: ASSESSING YOUR UNDERSTANDING

Activity A FILL IN THE BLANKS

1. Self-antigens
2. Chemotaxis
3. Bone marrow
4. Butterfly
5. Peanuts
6. Maculopapular
7. T-helper

Activity B MATCHING

1. e **2.** d **3.** b **4.** a **5.** c

Activity C SEQUENCING

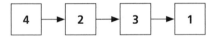

Activity D SHORT ANSWERS

1. The complement system is a series of blood proteins whose action is to augment the work of antibodies by assisting with destruction of bacteria, production of inflammation, and regulation of immune reactions.
2. The enzyme-linked immunosorbent assay (ELISA) method detects only antibodies so results may remain negative for several weeks up to 6 months (false negative). A false-positive result may occur with autoimmune disease.
3. Delayed hypersensitivity reactions are mediated by T-cells rather than antibodies. An infant's skin test response is diminished most likely due to the infant's decreased ability to produce an inflammatory response.
4. If a child acquires HIV infection "vertically" this means the disease was transmitted perinatally, either in utero or through breast milk. Transmission of the disease "horizontally" refers to transmission by nonsterile, HIV-contaminated needles or through unprotected sexual contact; less frequent is contaminated blood product transmission.

5. Avascular necrosis is an adverse effect of long-term use or high dosages of corticosteroids, causing tissue damage to a joint due to lack of blood supply to the joint. Any child receiving long-term or high-dose corticosteroids as treatment, such as a child with systemic lupus erythematosus (SLE), would be at an increased risk of developing this complication.

SECTION II: JAI APPLYING YOUR KNOWLEDGE

Activity E CASE STUDY

1. The discussion should include the following: A CBC, which may show a decreased hemoglobin and hematocrit, decreased platelet count, and low white blood cell count. Complement levels, C3 and C4, will also be decreased. Antinuclear antibody (ANA), though not specific to SLE, is usually positive in children with SLE.
2. The discussion should include the following: There is currently no single laboratory test that can confirm whether a person has lupus. In addition, since many of the symptoms with lupus come and go and tend to be vague, lupus can be difficult to diagnose. The physician will look at the entire medical history along with the results from the laboratory tests to determine whether your daughter has lupus.
3. The discussion should include the following: Education will focus on the importance of a healthy diet, regular exercise, and adequate sleep and rest. Teach the girl to apply sunscreen (minimum SPF 15) to her skin daily to prevent rashes resulting from photosensitivity. Administer NSAIDs, corticosteroids, and antimalarial agents as ordered. If the girl develops severe SLE or frequent flare-ups of symptoms she may require high-dose (pulse) corticosteroid therapy or medication with immunosuppressive drugs. Teach her to protect against cold weather by layering warm socks and wearing gloves when outdoors in the winter. If she is outside for extended periods during the winter months, educate her about the importance of inspecting her fingers and toes for discoloration. Ensure that yearly vision screening and ophthalmic examinations are performed in

order to preserve visual function should any changes occur. Refer the girl and her family to support services such as the Lupus Alliance of America and the Lupus Foundation of America.

SECTION III: PRACTICING FOR NCLEX

Activity F NCLEX-STYLE QUESTIONS

1. **Answer: c**
   Children with Wiskott–Aldrich syndrome should not be given rectal suppositories or temperatures since these children are at a high risk for bleeding. Tub baths are not contraindicated. Pacifiers are not contraindicated in Wiskott–Aldrich but should be kept as sanitary as possible to avoid oral infections.

2. **Answer: d**
   Premedication with diphenhydramine or acetaminophen may be indicted in children who have never received intravenous immunoglobulin (IVIG), have not had an infusion in over 8 weeks, have had a recent bacterial infection, or have history of serious infusion-related adverse reactions. The nurse should first premedicate, and then obtain a baseline physical assessment. Once the infusion begins, the nurse should continually assess for adverse reaction.

3. **Answer: c**
   The EpiPen Jr.® should be jabbed into the outer thigh, as this is a larger muscle, at a 90 degree angle, not into the upper arm. The other statements are correct.

4. **Answer: d**
   The ELISA test will be positive in infants of HIV-infected mothers because of transplacentally received antibodies. These antibodies may persist and remain detectable up to 24 months of age, making the ELISA test less accurate in detecting true HIV infection in infants and toddlers than the polymerase chain reaction (PCR). The PCR test is positive in infected infants over the age of 1 month. The erythrocyte sedimentation rate would be ordered for an immune disorder initial workup or ongoing monitoring of autoimmune disease. Immunoglobulin electrophoresis would be ordered to test for immune deficiency and autoimmune disorders.

5. **Answer: a**
   Older children and adolescents with allergic reactions to fish, shellfish, and nuts usually continue to have that concern as a life-long problem. The other statements are correct.

6. **Answer: d**
   Alopecia and the characteristic malar rash (butterfly rash) on the face are common clinical manifestations of SLE. Rhinorrhea, wheezing, and an enlarged spleen are not hallmark manifestations of SLE. Petechiae and purpura are more commonly associated with hematological disorders, not SLE.

7. **Answer: b**
   The parents must understand that their child cannot consume any part of an egg in any form. The other statements are accurate.

8. **Answer: b**
   Lip edema, urticaria, stridor, and tachycardia are common clinical manifestations of anaphylaxis.

9. **Answer: c**
   The nurse should instruct children and their families to avoid foods with a known cross-reactivity to latex, such as bananas.

10. **Answer: a**
    Polyarticular juvenile idiopathic arthritis is defined by the involvement of five or more joints, frequently the small joints, and affects the body symmetrically. Pauciarticular juvenile idiopathic arthritis is defined by the involvement of four or fewer joints. Systemic juvenile idiopathic arthritis presents with fever and rash in addition to join involvement at the time of diagnosis. The child with juvenile idiopathic arthritis is not at greater risk for anaphylaxis.

11. **Answers: b, c, d, e**
    RATIONALE: The following are common signs and symptoms of anaphylaxis: tongue edema, urticaria, nausea, vomiting, and syncope. Typically, the child who has developed anaphylaxis will be tachycardic.

12. **Answers: a, e**
    RATIONALE: Intravenous immune globulin (IVIG) should be given only intravenously and should not be given as an intramuscular injection. IVIG cannot be mixed with other medications. The nurse should closely monitor the child's vital signs during the infusion of the IVIG. The child may require an antipyretic and/ or an antihistamine during infusion to help with fever and chills.

13. **Answers: b, c, e**
    RATIONALE: The following children may have a primary immunodeficiency: a child with a persistent case of oral candidiasis, a child who has been diagnosed with pneumonia at least twice during the previous year, and a child who has taken antibiotics for 2 months or longer with little effect.

14. **Answers: c, d**
    RATIONALE: If a child has had a severe reaction to penicillin in the past, then this child should not receive penicillin or cephalosporins. Desensitization involves administration of increasingly larger doses of penicillin in an intensive care setting.

15. **Answers: a, c**
    RATIONALE: The child diagnosed with juvenile idiopathic arthritis should not take the oral form of methotrexate with dairy products. The approximate time to benefit from methotrexate is typically 3 to 6 weeks. The child will need blood tests to determine renal and liver function during treatment. Children with juvenile idiopathic arthritis usually find swimming to be a useful exercise for them because it helps maintain joint mobility without placing pressure on the joints. Sleep may be promoted by a warm bath at bedtime.

Answers

CHAPTER 49

SECTION I: ASSESSING YOUR UNDERSTANDING

Activity A FILL IN THE BLANKS

1. Langerhans
2. Exophthalmos
3. Polyuria

4. Tetany
5. Kussmaul
6. Deficiency
7. Hyperthyroidism

Activity B LABELING

Areas on the body corresponding with insulin injection sites.

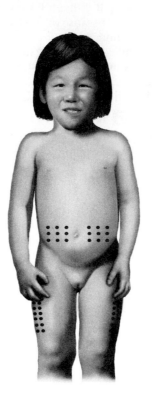
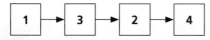
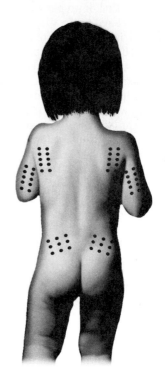

Activity C MATCHING

1. e   **2.** c   **3.** b   **4.** a   **5.** d

Activity D SEQUENCING

$$1 \rightarrow 3 \rightarrow 2 \rightarrow 4$$

Activity E SHORT ANSWERS

1. Diet should be low in fats and concentrated carbohydrates. Lists of foods high in carbohydrates, protein, and fat should be provided. The parents need to understand the need to plan for periods of rapid growth, travel, school parties, and holidays. Referring the parents to a nutritionist with diabetes expertise will be helpful. There should be a plan for three meals and two snacks per day in order to maintain blood glucose levels. Regular exercise should be encouraged, as well as participation in age-appropriate sports. The parents should be reminded of the importance of monitoring the insulin dose, food and fluid intake, and hypoglycemic reactions when exercising.

2.

Hypothyroidism	Hyperthyroidism
Nervousness/anxiety	Tiredness/fatigue
Diarrhea	Constipation
Heat intolerance	Cold intolerance
Weight loss	Weight gain
Smooth, velvet-like skin	Dry, thick skin; edema on the face, eyes, and hands
	Decreased growth

3. Nursing implications when teaching, discussing, and caring for children with diabetes mellitus (DM) are as follows:
   a. Infants and toddlers: Attempt to achieve consistent dietary intake. Give the toddler foods to choose from. Help the toddler to find and use a word or phrase to describe feelings when hypoglycemic symptoms occur. Establish rituals/routines with home management.
   b. Preschoolers: Use simple explanations and play therapy when instructing or preparing for a procedure or situation related to the disorder.
   c. School age: Use concise and concrete terms when instructing. Allow children to proceed at their own rate. Assist the family to incorporate the testing and injections into the school day and plan for field trips. Use the school nurse's assistance and help with the school plan.
   d. Adolescents: Care can be slowly turned over to an adolescent with minor supervision from family. Watch for depression in this age group.
4. *Healthy People 2020* recommends screening all children periodically to identify early signs of overweight or obesity based on CDC guidelines. In addition, families should receive education regarding appropriate diet and exercise early during the toddler years in an attempt to prevent obesity, thus decreasing the likelihood of diabetes.
5. The nurse should instruct the family to report headaches, rapid weight gain, increased thirst or urination, or painful hip or knee joints as possible adverse reactions.

SECTION II: APPLYING YOUR KNOWLEDGE
Activity F CASE STUDY

1. The discussion should include the following:
   In the past, DM type 2 occurred in adults with only a small percentage of cases seen in childhood. Since the early 1990s, the incidence has increased significantly in children. Many of these children have a relative with type 2 DM or they have other risk factors such as being overweight, African American, Hispanic American, Asian American, or Native American heritage.
   Type 2 DM begins when the pancreas usually produces insulin but the body develops a resistance

to insulin or no longer uses the insulin properly. As the need for insulin rises, the pancreas gradually loses its ability to produce sufficient amounts of insulin to regulate blood sugar. Eventually, insulin production decreases with the result similar to type 1 DM.
2. The discussion should include the following:
   Nursing management will focus on regulating glucose control, monitoring for complications, and educating and supporting the child and family. Other important interventions involve nutritional guidelines and exercise protocols.
3. The discussion should include challenges related to educating children with diabetes:
   • Children lack the maturity to understand the long-term consequences of this serious chronic illness.
   • Children do not want to be different from their peers and having to make life style changes may result in anger or depression.
   • Families may demonstrate unhealthy behaviors making it difficult for the child to initiate change because of the lack of supervision or role modeling.
   • Family dynamics are impacted because management of diabetes must occur all day, every day.

SECTION III: PRACTICING FOR NCLEX
Activity G NCLEX-STYLE QUESTIONS

1. **Answer: d**
   Administering intravenous calcium gluconate, as ordered, will restore normal calcium and phosphate levels as well as relieve severe tetany. Ensuring patency of the IV site to prevent tissue damage due to extravasation or cardiac arrhythmias is an intervention for any child with an IV, and monitoring fluid intake and urinary calcium output are secondary interventions. Providing administration of calcium and vitamin D is an intervention for nonacute symptoms.
2. **Answer: b**
   Observing pubic hair and hirsutism in a preschooler indicates congenital adrenal hyperplasia. Auscultation revealing an irregular heartbeat and palpation eliciting pain due to constipation may be signs of hyperparathyroidism. Observing hyperpigmentation of the skin would suggest Addison's disease.
3. **Answer: a**
   This child may have syndrome of inappropriate antidiuretic hormone (SIADH). Priority intervention for this child is to notify the physician of the neurologic findings. Remaining interventions will be to restore fluid balance with IV sodium chloride to correct hyponatremia, set up safety precautions to prevent injury due to altered level of consciousness, and monitor fluid intake, urine volume, and specific gravity.

4. **Answer: c**
Monitoring blood glucose levels during this study is the priority task along with observing for signs of hypoglycemia since insulin is given during the test to stimulate release of growth hormone. Providing a wet washcloth would be more appropriate for a child who is on therapeutic fluid restriction, such as with SIADH. Monitoring intake and output would not be necessary for this test but would be appropriate for a child with diabetes insipidus. While it is important to educate the family about this test, it is not the priority task.

5. **Answer: b**
Observation of an enlarged tongue along with an enlarged posterior fontanel and feeding difficulties are key findings for congenital hypothyroidism. The mother would report constipation rather than diarrhea. Auscultation would reveal bradycardia rather than tachycardia, and palpation would reveal cool, dry, and scaly skin.

6. **Answer: a**
Observation of acanthosis nigricans in addition to the obesity and amenorrhea is a further indication of polycystic ovary syndrome. Complaint of blurred vision and headaches are signs and symptoms of DM. Auscultation revealing an increased respiratory rate points to diabetes insipidus. Palpation revealing hypertrophy and weakness is typical of hypothyroidism.

7. **Answer: a**
A history of rapid weight gain and long-term corticosteroid therapy suggests this child may have Cushing's disease, which could be confirmed using an adrenal suppression test. A round, child-like face is common to both Cushing's and growth hormone deficiency. Observing high weight to height ratio and delayed dentition are findings with growth hormone deficiency.

8. **Answer: c**
The primary nursing diagnosis would be deficient fluid volume related to electrolyte imbalance. It is important to increase the child's hydration to minimize renal calculi formation. Disturbed body image related to hormone dysfunction is a diagnosis for growth hormone deficiency. Imbalanced nutrition: more than body requirements would be important for a child with DM. Deficient knowledge related to treatment of the disease is appropriate for hyperparathyroidism, but it is not a priority diagnosis.

9. **Answer: b**
Instructing child to rotate injection sites to decrease scar formation is important, but does not focus on managing glucose levels. Teaching the child and family to eat a balanced diet, encouraging the child to maintain the proper injection schedule, and promoting a higher level of exercise all focus on regulating glucose control.

10. **Answer: d**
Side effects of hypothyroidism are restlessness, inability to sleep, or irritability and should be reported to the physician. Educating how to recognize vitamin D toxicity is necessary for a child with hypoparathyroidism. Teaching parents how to maintain fluid intake regimens is important for a child with diabetes insipidus. Teaching the child and parents to administer methimazole with meals is necessary for hyperthyroidism.

11. **Answer: 393 micrograms**
RATIONALE: The child weighs 72 pounds and 2.2 pounds = 1 kg.
72 pounds × 1 kg/2.2 pounds = 32.727 kg
32.727 kg × 12 μg/1 kg = 392.727 μg
rounded to the nearest whole number = 393 μg

12. **Answers: b, d, a, c**
RATIONALE: Lispro is a rapid-acting insulin. Humulin R is a short-acting insulin. Humulin N is an intermediate-acting insulin. Lantus is a long-acting insulin.

13. **Answer: 0.075 milligram per day**
RATIONALE: The child weighs 58 pounds and 2.2 pounds = 1 kg.
58 pounds × 1 kg/2.2 pounds = 26.3636 kg of body weight
26.3636 × 0.2 mg/1 kg = 0.5273 mg of growth hormone per week
0.5273 mg/ week × 1 week/ 7 days = 0.0753 mg/ day

14. **Answers: a, c**
RATIONALE: The child has delayed puberty if any of the following is true: the female has not developed breasts by the age of 13; the male has had no testicular enlargement by the age of 14. In females, pubic hair should appear before the age of 14. In males, pubic hair should appear before the age of 15 and scrotal changes by the age of 14.

15. **Answers: a, b, c**
RATIONALE: The following are signs and symptoms related to the development of thyroid storm: fever, diaphoresis, and tachycardia. Children who are patients are also typically restless and irritable.

CHAPTER 50

SECTION I: ASSESSING YOUR UNDERSTANDING

Activity A FILL IN THE BLANKS

1. Mediastinal
2. Leukocoria
3. Sepsis
4. Prevention
5. Limb-salvage
6. Leukemia
7. Clinical trial

Activity B LABELING

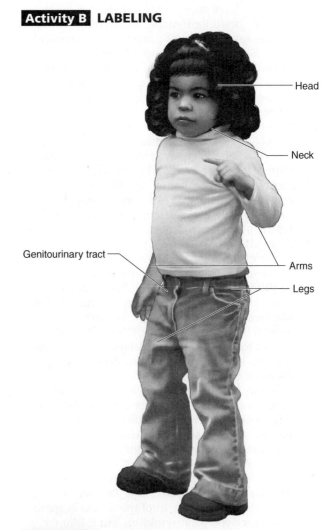

Head

Neck

Genitourinary tract

Arms

Legs

Activity C MATCHING

1. c   2. b   3. d   4. e   5. a

Activity D SEQUENCING

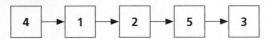

4 → 1 → 2 → 5 → 3

Activity E SHORT ANSWERS

1. Nine locations with presenting signs and symptoms from Table 50.6.
2. Answer can include any of the following types of drugs. Refer to Drug Guide 50.1 for more information on specific drugs, action/indications, and nursing implications.

    Antitumor antibiotics, antimetabolites, antimicrotubulars, mitotic inhibitors, topoisomerase inhibitors, corticosteroids, colony-stimulating factors, interleukins, tumor necrosis factor (protein cytokine), monoclonal anti-bodies, interferons, allopurinol, antibiotics (oral, parenteral), antiemetics, antifungal agents, immunosuppressant drugs, mesna, methotrexate antidote.
3. Chest X-ray, computed tomography (CT), magnetic resonance imaging (MRI), bone scan, and ultrasound. Refer to Common Laboratory and Diagnostic Tests 50.1.
4. There are a number of differences between childhood and adult cancer: Most common sites for childhood cancer are blood, lymph, brain, bone, kidney, and muscle. The most common sites for adult cancer are breast, lung, prostate, bowel, and bladder; Environmental factors have a strong influence on the cause of adult cancers versus minimal influence on childhood cancer; and childhood cancers are typically very responsive to treatment if diagnosed early enough, whereas adult cancers tend to be less responsive to treatment. Additional comparisons of childhood and adult cancer can be found in Comparison Chart 50.1.
5. Chemotherapy drugs are either cell cycle-specific or cell cycle-nonspecific. This is why protocols for chemotherapy treatment often use a combination of drugs to destroy cancer cells during various phases of the cell cycle.

SECTION II: APPLYING YOUR KNOWLEDGE
Activity F CASE STUDY

1. The discussion should include the following:
    The child, who has a low neutrophil count (neutropenia), is at a significant risk for developing a serious infection since neutrophils are the primary infection fighting cells.

    Neutropenia precautions need to be instituted for this child. Precautions related to neutropenia generally include:
    - Maintain hand hygiene prior to and following each child contact
    - Place child in private room
    - Monitor vital signs every 4 hours
    - Assess for signs and symptoms of infection at least every 8 hours
    - Avoid rectal suppositories, enemas or examinations, urinary catheterization, and invasive procedures

- Restrict visitors with fever, cough, or other signs/symptoms of infection
- No raw fruits or vegetables, no fresh flowers or live plants in room
- Place mask on the child when transporting outside of room
- Maintain dental care with soft toothbrush if platelet count is adequate

    Family and visitors must be educated regarding the need to restrict the child from contact with known infectious exposures and the importance of practicing meticulous hand hygiene. The family should also be educated on the importance of proper nutrition, hydration, and rest for the child.
2. The discussion should include the following:
    Teach the family to monitor for fever at home and report temperature elevations to the oncologist immediately (Seek medical care if temperature is 38.3°C (101°F) or greater). Family and visitors must practice meticulous hygiene. The child should avoid any known ill contacts, especially persons with chickenpox. If exposed to chickenpox notify the physician immediately. He should avoid crowded areas, and should not receive live vaccines. The child's temperature should not be taken rectally nor should he be given any medication rectally. Prophylactic antibiotics should be given as ordered by the physician.
3. The discussion should include the following:
    Children desire to be normal and in order to maintain appropriate growth and development; parents need to promote this normalization. The child should attend school whenever he is well enough and his white blood cell counts are not dangerously low. Other activities that he enjoys should be promoted if medically appropriate. Encourage him to play with his friends while remembering to avoid ill contacts. Special camps are available for children with cancer and offer the child an opportunity to experience a variety of activities safely and to spend time with many other youngsters who are experiencing the same challenges.

SECTION III: PRACTICING FOR NCLEX
Activity G NCLEX-STYLE QUESTIONS

1. **Answer: c**
    The parents should seek medical care immediately if the child has a temperature of 101°F or greater. This is because many chemotherapeutic drugs cause bone marrow suppression; the parents must be directed to take action at the first sign of infection in order to prevent overwhelming sepsis. The appearance of earache, stiff neck, sore throat, blisters, ulcers, or rashes, or difficulty or pain when swallowing are reasons to seek medical care, but are not as grave as the risk of infection.

2. **Answers: b, c, d**
Observation revealing a thick, yellow discharge is typical of infectious conjunctivitis, not retinoblastoma. Headaches and hyphema, a collection of blood in the anterior chamber of the eye, are associated with retinoblastoma as is leukocoria, "cat's eye reflex." Most children with retinoblastoma are diagnosed by 3 years of age.

3. **Answer: a**
The priority intervention is to monitor for increases in intracranial pressure because brain tumors may block cerebral fluid flow or cause edema in the brain. A change in the level of consciousness is just one of several subtle changes that can occur indicating a change in intracranial pressure. Lower priority interventions include providing a tour of the ICU to prepare the child and parents for after the surgery, and educating the child and parents about shunts.

4. **Answer: b**
Ewing's sarcoma may result in swelling and erythema at the tumor site. Common sites are chest wall, pelvis, vertebrae, and long bone diaphyses. Dull bone pain in the proximal tibia is indicative of osteosarcoma. Persistent pain after an ankle injury is not indicative of Ewing's sarcoma. An asymptomatic mass on the upper back suggests rhabdomyosarcoma.

5. **Answers: a, c, d, e**
Answer b would not be part of the teaching plan. It would be more accurate and appropriate for the nurse to stress that testicular cancer is one of the most curable cancers if diagnosed early. Self-examination is an excellent way to screen for the disease. Girls should know that they can take responsibility for their own sexual health by getting a Papanicolaou smear. All the children should understand that early intercourse, sexually transmitted disease (STDs), and multiple sex partners are risk factors for reproductive cancer. Information should be provided so the teen girls can discuss the benefits of receiving the human papilloma virus vaccine since many cervical cancers are attributed to human papillomavirus.

6. **Answer: c**
Giving medications as ordered using the least invasive route is a postsurgery intervention focused on providing atraumatic care and is appropriate for this child. Since the child has a stage I tumor, it can be treated by surgical removal, and does not require chemotherapy or radiation therapy. Applying aloe vera lotion is good skin care following radiation therapy. Administering antiemetics and maintaining isolation are interventions used to treat side effects of chemotherapy.

7. **Answer: d**
Increased heart rate, murmur, and respiratory distress are symptoms of hyperleukocytosis (high white blood cell count) which is associated with leukemia. Increased heart rate and blood pressure are indicative of tumor lysis syndrome, which may occur with acute lymphoblastic leukemia, lymphoma, and neuroblastoma. Wheezing and diminished breath sounds are signs of superior vena cava syndrome related to non-Hodgkin's lymphoma or neuroblastoma. Respiratory distress and poor perfusion are symptoms of massive hepatomegaly which is caused by a neuroblastoma filling a large portion of the abdominal cavity.

8. **Answer: a**
Coupled with the mother's complaints, observation of nystagmus and head tilt would suggest the child may have a brain tumor. Elevated blood pressure of 120/80 might be indicative of Wilm's tumor. Fever and headaches are common symptoms of acute lymphoblastic leukemia. A cough and labored breathing points to rhabdomyosarcoma near the child's airway.

9. **Answer: b**
Along with the symptoms reported by the mother, the fact that the child has Beckwith–Wiedemann syndrome suggests that the child could have a Wilm's tumor. Down syndrome would point to leukemia or brain tumor. Schwachman syndrome would suggest leukemia. A family history of neurofibromatosis is a risk factor for brain tumor, rhabdomyosarcoma, or acute myelogenous leukemia.

10. **Answer: c**
It would not be necessary for the nurse to inform the parents about postoperative care since this is not a treatment method for the disease. The treatment of choice for Hodgkin's disease is chemotherapy, but radiation therapy may be necessary; however, discussing the treatment methods may be overwhelming at this time. Upon first learning the diagnosis, it is most helpful for the nurse to explain that staging refers to the spread of the disease (stages I through IV, see Table 50.3); and that A means the child is asymptomatic, while B means that symptoms are present.

11. **Answers: a, c, d, e**
RATIONALE: Common adverse effects of chemotherapeutic drugs are: immunosuppression, alopecia, hearing changes, and nausea. Another common adverse effect is microdontia, not enlarged teeth.

12. **Answer: 0.99**
    RATIONALE: Square root of (height [cm] × weight [kg] divided by 3,600) = BSA
       The child is 130 cm tall and weighs 27 kg: 130 × 27 = 3,510; 3,510/3,600 = 0.975; and the square root of 0.975 is 0.9874. The BSA would be 0.987, when rounded to the hundredths place = 0.99.

13. **Answer: d, b, c, a**
    RATIONALE: During induction, the child receives oral steroids and IV vincristine. During consolidation, the child receives high doses of methotrexate and mercaptopurine. During maintenance, the child receives low doses of methotrexate and mercaptopurine. During central nervous system prophylaxis, the child receives intrathecal chemotherapy.

14. **Answer: 3,450**
    RATIONALE: (Bands + segs/100) × WBC = ANC
    14 + 9 = 23% = 23/100 = 0.23
    0.23 × 15,000 = 3,450

15. **Answers: a, b**
    RATIONALE: The child in neutropenic precautions should be placed in a private room. Prior to transportation to other areas of the hospital, the nurse should place a mask on the child before she leaves her room. The nurse should monitor the child's vital signs at least every 4 hours. The nurse should carefully assess for signs and symptoms of infection at least every 8 hours. The nurse should perform hand hygiene before and after contact with each child.

Answers

CHAPTER 51

SECTION I: ASSESSING YOUR UNDERSTANDING

Activity A FILL IN THE BLANKS

1. Alleles
2. Consanguinity
3. Phenotype
4. Heterozygous
5. Nondisjunction
6. Genome
7. Chromosome

Activity B MATCHING

1. d   **2.** e   **3.** a   **4.** c   **5.** b

Activity C SHORT ANSWERS

1. Complications of Down syndrome include cardiac defects, hearing or vision impairment, developmental delays, mental retardation, gastrointestinal disorders, recurrent infections, atlantoaxial instability, thyroid disease, and sleep apnea.
2. Building a relationship of trust, empathizing with and understanding the family's stresses and emotions, rejecting personal bias, encouraging open discussion.
3. Phenylketonuria excretions exhibit a mousy or musty order caused by a deficiency of the liver enzyme that processes phenylalanine; children with maple syrup urine disease have a maple syrup odor associated with a deficiency of the enzyme that metabolizes leucine, isoleucine, and valine; children with tyrosinemia have excretions with a rancid butter or cabbage like odor as a result of a deficiency of the enzyme that metabolizes tyrosine; and excretions have a rotting fish odor with the disorder trimethylaminuria, resulting from the body's inability to normally produce flavin (which breaks down trimethylamine).
4. Trisomy 21, also known as Down syndrome, occurs in 1 in 800 births across all maternal ages and socioeconomic levels, and 75% of trisomy 21 conceptions result in spontaneous abortion. It is the most common genetic defect that is linked with intellectual disability. The highest incidence of the disorder occurs in mothers who are over 35 years of age, with the likelihood of having a trisomy 21 baby 1 in 400 at the age of 35, 1 in 100 at the age of 40, 1 in 35 at the age of 45, and 1 in 12 at the age of 49.
5. The infant with trisomy 13 will likely display a microcephalic head with wide sagittal suture and fontanels. Other physical features include malformed ears, small eyes, extra digits, cleft lip and palate, and severe hypotonia. Severe intellectual disability will most likely be exhibited as the child ages.

SECTION II: APPLYING YOUR KNOWLEDGE

Activity D CASE STUDY

1. The discussion should include the following:
   Newborn screening is done to detect disorders before symptoms develop. Recent developments in screening techniques allow many metabolic disorders or inborn errors of metabolism to be detected early. Chloe's test results tell us that additional testing is needed to rule out a false positive or confirm the diagnosis. Most inborn errors of metabolism presenting in the neonatal period are lethal or can result in serious complications such as mental retardation if specific treatment is not initiated immediately. This is why it is so important that you came in today for additional testing.
2. The discussion should include the following:
   In fatty acid oxidation disorders (such as medium-chain acyl-CoA dehydrogenase deficiency) the goal is to prevent or avoid prolonged fasts and to provide frequent feedings. Special consideration during illness is very important. If Chloe is unable to tolerate food she needs to be seen by a physician immediately; intravenous dextrose may be required. Supplementation with specific vitamins may also be important in the treatment and a dietician and the physician will work with you. Strict adherence to frequent meals is necessary to prevent complications from arising.
   Nursing management will focus on education and support for the family and caregivers. Ensure they have thorough knowledge about medium

chain acyl-CoA dehydrogenase deficiency and its management. Refer the family to a dietician and other appropriate resources, including support groups. Monitor the developmental progress of Chloe and initiate therapies if concern arises.

SECTION III: PRACTICING FOR NCLEX
Activity E NCLEX-STYLE QUESTIONS

1. **Answers: b, c, e**
   Numerous café au lait spots on the trunk of the child, a slightly larger head size due to abnormal development of the skull, and abnormal curvature of the spine (especially scoliosis) are clinical signs of this disorder. A first-degree relative rather than a second-degree relative having had neurofibromatosis is clinical sign of the disorder, and freckles in the child's axilla and groin, not the lower extremities, are symptoms of the disorder. Two or more clinical signs and symptoms of the disorder must be present for a diagnosis to be made.

2. **Answers: b, c, d, e**
   Although children with Marfan syndrome have a number of physical problems, respiratory conditions are not one of them, so it would not be appropriate to arrange in home respiratory therapy. The other interventions are needed for children with Marfan syndrome, because they do have ophthalmologic, orthopedic, and cardiac problems.

3. **Answer: d**
   Angelman syndrome is characterized by jerky ataxic movements, similar to a puppet's gait. Hypotonicity is a symptom of Angelman syndrome as well as Prader Willi syndrome, and Cri du chat. Cleft palate is a symptom of velo-cardiofacial/DiGeorge syndrome.

4. **Answer: b**
   This disorder is not X-linked. Either father or mother can pass the gene along regardless of whether their mate has the gene or not. The only way that an autosomal dominant gene is not expressed is if it does not exist. If only one of the parents has the gene, then there is a 50% chance it will be passed on to the child.

5. **Answer: b**
   The priority intervention is to assess the family's ability to learn about the disorder. The family needs time to adjust to the diagnosis and be ready to learn for teaching to be effective. Screening to determine current level of functioning, explaining the care required due to the disorder, and educating the family about available resources are interventions that can be taken once the family is ready.

6. **Answer: c**
   Children with phenylketonuria will have a musty odor to their urine, as well as an eczema-like rash, irritability, and vomiting. Increased reflex action and seizures are typical of maple sugar urine disease. Signs of jaundice, diarrhea, and vomiting are typical of galactosemia. Seizures are a sign of biotinidase deficiency or maple sugar urine disease.

7. **Answer: d**
   The nurse would likely find records of corrective surgery for anal atresia because it is a symptom of VATER association. The nurse may observe that the child has a hearing deficit, underdeveloped labia, and a coloboma, along with heart disease, retarded growth and development, and choanal atresia if the child had CHARGE syndrome. See Table 51.6 for more information.

8. **Answer: a**
   A major anomaly is an anomaly or malformation that creates significant medical problems and requires surgical or medical management. Café au lait macules are a major anomaly. Polydactyly, or extra digits, syndactyly, or webbed digits, and protruding ears are minor anomalies. Minor anomalies are features that vary from those that are most commonly seen in the general population but do not cause an increase in morbidity in and of themselves.

9. **Answer: b**
   Galactosemia is a deficiency in the liver enzyme needed to convert galactose into glucose. This means the child will have to eliminate milk and dairy products from her diet for life. Adhering to a low phenylalanine diet is an intervention for phenylketonuria. Eating frequent meals and never fasting is an intervention for medium-chain acyl-CoA dehydrogenase deficiency. Maple sugar urine disease requires a low-protein diet and supplementation with thiamine.

10. **Answer: c**
    Children with Sturge–Weber syndrome will have a facial nevus, or port wine stain, most often seen on the forehead and one eye. While the child may experience seizures, retardation, and behavior problems, they are not definitive findings.

11. **Answers: a, b, d**
    RATIONALE: The following are risk factors for genetic disorders: oligohydramnios, paternal age over 50, a family history of genetic disorders, positive alpha-fetoprotein test, and multiple births.

12. **Answers: c, d, e**
    RATIONALE: Boys with Klinefelter syndrome may have learning disabilities, underdeveloped testes, and gynecomastia. Typically, they have long legs and short torsos and are taller than their peers.

13. **Answers: c, d, e**
    RATIONALE: Babies born with trisomy 18 may have been born with a congenital cardiac defect, webbing between digits and low-set ears. Microcephaly and the development of extra digits are not associated with trisomy 18.

14. **Answers: a, b, c**
    RATIONALE: Monogenic disorders (caused by a single gene that is defective) include autosomal dominant, autosomal recessive, X-linked dominant and X-linked recessive disorders. Mitochondrial inheritance and genomic imprinting are considered multifactorial disorders (caused by multiple gene and environmental factors).

15. **Answers: b, c, d, e**
    RATIONALE: The following people should receive genetic counseling: paternal age over 50, the presence of consanguinity, parents of African descent, and those parents who have a child at home who was born blind or deaf. A mother-to-be over the age of 35 may also benefit from genetic counseling.

Answers

CHAPTER 52

SECTION I: ASSESSING YOUR UNDERSTANDING

Activity A FILL IN THE BLANKS

1. Bowel
2. 6
3. Dyslexia
4. Stocking
5. Neglect
6. Münchausen syndrome by proxy (MSbP)
7. Autism spectrum disorder (ASD)

Activity B

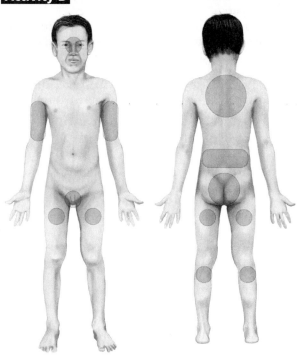

Common nonaccidental injury sites

Activity C MATCHING

1. b   2. a   3. d   4. e   5. c

Activity D SHORT ANSWERS

1. Behavior management techniques include the following:
   - Set limits with the child, holding him responsible for his behavior
   - Do not argue, bargain, or negotiate about the limits once established
   - Provide consistent caregivers (unlicensed assistive personnel and nurses for the hospitalized child) and establish the child's daily routine
   - Use a low-pitched voice and remain calm
   - Redirect the child's attention when needed
   - Ignore inappropriate behaviors
   - Praise the child's self-control efforts and other accomplishments
   - Utilize restraints only when absolutely necessary
2. Building a relationship of trust, empathizing with and understanding the family's stresses and emotions, rejecting personal bias, encouraging open discussion.
3. Generalized anxiety disorder (GAD) is characterized by unrealistic concerns over past behavior, future events, and personal competency. Social phobia may result in which the child or teen demonstrates a persistent fear of formal speaking, eating in front of others, using public restrooms, or speaking to authorities.
4. Obtain a health history from the adolescent and his parents separately. Assess for a history of recent changes in behavior, alterations in school, changes in peer relationships, withdrawal from previously enjoyed activities, sleep disturbances, changes in eating behaviors, and an increase in accidents or sexual promiscuity. Ask about potential stressors, conflicts with parents or peers, school concerns, dating issues, and abusive events. If possible utilize a standardized depression screening questionnaire.

   Assess for history of weight loss. Observe for apparent apathy. Inspect the entire body surface for the presence of self-inflicted injuries which may or may not be present.

Assess for risk factors of suicide including a change in school performance, changes in sleep or appetite, disinterest in former preferred activities, expressing feeling of hopelessness, depression, thoughts of suicide, and any previous attempts at suicide.

5. The most common classifications of medication used for the management of ADHD include psychostimulants, nonstimulant norepinephrine reuptake inhibitors and/or alpha-agonist antihypertensive agents. The goal of treatment with medication is to help increase the child's ability to pay attention and to increase the ability to control impulsive behavior. Medications for ADHD do not cure the disorder.

SECTION II: APPLYING YOUR KNOWLEDGE
Activity E CASE STUDY

1. The discussion should include the following:
   ASD is a developmental disorder that has its onset in infancy or early childhood. Autistic behaviors may be first noted in infancy as developmental delays or between 12 months and 36 months when the child loses previously acquired skills. Children with ASD demonstrate impairments in social interactions and communication. The exact cause of autism is unknown; it is believed to be linked to genetics, brain abnormalities, altered chemistry, a virus, or toxic chemicals. The spectrum of the disorder ranges from mild to severe.
2. The discussion should include the following:
   Warning signs of autism that may be seen with infants and toddlers include: no babbling and no pointing or using gestures by 12 months of age; by 16 months of age the child is not using single words and by 24 months of age is not using any two-word phrases; and the child exhibits loss of language or social skills at any age.

SECTION III: PRACTICING FOR NCLEX
Activity F NCLEX-STYLE QUESTIONS

1. **Answer: b**
   The nurse should pay particular attention to reports of a child spending hours in a repetitive activity, such as lining up cars rather than playing with them. Most 3-year-olds are very busy and would rather play than sit on a parent's lap. The other statements are not outside the range of normal and do not warrant further investigation.
2. **Answer: c**
   The nurse should encourage the family to explore with their physician the option of one of the newer extended-release or once daily attention deficit/hyperactivity disorder medications. The other statements are not helpful and do not address the mother's or boy's concerns.

3. **Answer: b**
   Sudden, rapid, stereotypical sounds are a hallmark finding with Tourette's syndrome. Toe walking and unusual behaviors such as hand-flapping and spinning are indicative of ASD. Lack of eye contact is associated with ASD but is also noted in children without a mental health disorder.
4. **Answer: c**
   The nurse should emphasize the importance of rigid unchanging routines as children with ASD often act out when their routine changes. The other statements would not warrant additional referral or follow-up.
5. **Answer: b**
   An IQ of 35 to 50 is classified as moderate. An IQ of 50 to 70 is classified as mild. An IQ of 20 to 35 is classified as severe, and an IQ less than 20 is considered profound.
6. **Answer: b**
   It is important to continue the usual routine of the hospitalized child, particularly of children with intellectual disability. By asking an open-ended question about a typical day, the nurse can identify the routine activities that can potentially be duplicated in the hospital. Telling the girl she will be going home soon or asking about art supplies does not address her concerns. Asking whether she has talked to her parents is unhelpful at this time.
7. **Answer: a**
   The nurse should be aware that rapid nutritional replacement in the severely malnourished can lead to refeeding syndrome. Refeeding syndrome is characterized by cardiovascular, hematologic, and neurologic complications such as cardiac arrhythmias, confusion, and seizures. Orthostatic hypotension, hypertension, and irregular and decreased pulses are complications of anorexia but do not characterize refeeding syndrome.
8. **Answer: a**
   The nurse should be sure to carefully assess the mouth and oropharynx for eroded dental enamel, red gums, and inflamed throat from self-induced vomiting. The other findings are typically noted with anorexia nervosa.
9. **Answer: b**
   Typical facial features include a low nasal bridge with short upturned nose, flattened midface, and a long filtrum with narrow upper lip. Microcephaly rather than macrocephaly is associated with fetal alcohol syndrome. Clubbing of fingers is associated with chronic hypoxia.
10. **Answer: c**
    It is important to remind the parents that medications for the management of ADHD are not a cure but help to increase the child's ability to pay attention and decrease the level of impulsive behavior. The other statements are correct.

11. **Answers: d, e**
    RATIONALE: Children diagnosed with dyslexia and dysgraphia experience difficulty with reading, writing, spelling, and producing written words.

12. **Answers: a, b, c**
    RATIONALE: An 18-month-old toddler should have babbled by 12 months. He should be using gestures and using single words to communicate. The use of sentences to communicate and the ability to jump rope would be expected later.

13. **Answers: b, d, e**
    RATIONALE: Common side effects related to the use of psychostimulants are: headaches, irritability, and abdominal pain. Children typically exhibit a decreased appetite and may have difficulty with insomnia.

14. **Answers: a, b**
    RATIONALE: The parents should use a calm, low-pitched voice when communicating with her. They should ignore inappropriate behaviors. The parents should not argue or bargain with the child about set limits. They should praise the child for accomplishments and help the child see the importance of accountability for her own behavior.

15. **Answers: a, b, d**
    RATIONALE: Altered sleep patterns, weight loss, and problems at school are commonly found in children with mental health disorders. There also may be alterations in friendships and changes in extracurricular activity participation.

CHAPTER 53

SECTION I: ASSESSING YOUR UNDERSTANDING

Activity A FILL IN THE BLANKS

1. Pediatric
2. "LEAN"
3. Airway
4. Pupil
5. Cyanosis
6. Jaw-thrust
7. Femoral

Activity B LABELING

Figure A shows sinus tachycardia
Figure B shows supraventricular tachycardia
Figure C shows ventricular tachycardia
Figure D shows coarse ventricular fibrillation

Activity C MATCHING

1. c　　2. a　　　　3. b　　　　4. e　　　　5. d

Activity D SEQUENCING

4 → 5 → 1 → 3 → 2

Activity E SHORT ANSWERS

1. **Infant:**
   - One-person CPR: 30 compressions to two breaths; Hand placement: two fingers placed one finger breadth below the nipple line
   - Two-person CPR: 15 compression to two breaths; Hand placement: two thumbs encircling the chest at the nipple line

   Child:
   - One-person CPR: 30 compressions to two breaths; Hand placement: heel of one hand or two hands (adult position in larger child) pressing on the sternum at the nipple line
   - Two-person CPR: 15 compressions to two breaths; Hand placement: heel of one hand or two hands (adult position in larger child) pressing on the sternum at the nipple line

2.

	SVT	Sinus Tachycardia
Rate (beats/minute)	Infants >220, children >180	Infants <220, children <180
Rhythm	Abrupt onset and termination	Beat to beat variability
P-waves	Flattened	Present and normal
QRS	Narrow (less than 0.08 seconds)	Normal
History	Usually none significant	Fever, fluid loss, hypoxia, pain, fear

3. Choose an appropriate size bag and mask using a Broselow tape or referring to the code reference sheet. Connect the bag valve mask (BVM) via the tubing to the oxygen source and turn on the oxygen. Set the flow rate at approximately 10 L/minute for infants and small children, and 15 L/minute for an adolescent who is adult-sized. Check to make sure that the oxygen is flowing through the tubing to the bag. Open the airway. Place the mask over the child's face. Use the thumb and index finger of one hand to hold the mask on the child's face, and the other hand to squeeze the resuscitator bag. Use upward pressure on the jaw angle while pressing downward on the mask below the child's mouth to keep the mouth open.

4. Cricoid pressure may be used during the ventilation portion of resuscitative efforts to prevent gastric distention, possibly leading to vomiting and aspiration, during ventilation. Pressure is used to occlude the esophagus so that air does not entire the stomach during ventilation.

5. The mnemonic is used to assist in determining a worsening respiratory status of a child who is intubated. Each letter represents possible problems that require further assessment:
   D: Displacement of the tracheal intubation tube
   O: Obstruction of the tracheal intubation tube from mucus of other sources

P: Pneumothorax
E: Equipment failure

SECTION II: APPLYING YOUR KNOWLEDGE
Activity F CASE STUDY

1. The discussion should include the following:
   The use of AEDs on children was not recommended by the AHA until 2005. If the child is over 1 year of age and the emergency is a sudden witnessed collapse, the AHA suggests the use of an AED; this recommendation comes from the result of studies indicating that the AED can be sensitive and specific for detecting and treating arrhythmia by defibrillation in this population.

2. The discussion should include the following:
   The chain of survival for children differs from the adult chain of survival due to the common causes of pediatric versus adult cardiopulmonary arrest. These differences affect the priority of steps during an emergency. The pediatric chain of survival begins with prevention of cardiac arrest and injuries, followed by early CPR, then early access to the emergency response system, and ends with early advanced care. The adult chain of survival begins with activation of the EMS, followed by early CPR, then early defibrillation, and ends with early access to advanced care.

SECTION III: PRACTICING FOR NCLEX
Activity G NCLEX-STYLE QUESTIONS

1. **Answer: c**
   The AHA emphasizes the importance of cardiac compressions in pulseless clients with arrhythmias, making this the priority intervention in this situation. Current AHA recommendations are for defibrillation to be administered once followed by five cycles of CPR. The AHA now recommends against using multiple doses of epinephrine because they have not been shown to be helpful and may actually cause harm to the child.

2. **Answer: a**
   The nurse would be suspicious of a 7-month-old climbing out of his crib, since it is not consistent with his developmental stage. Other areas of concern are if the parents have different accounts of the accident and if the injury is not consistent with the type of accident.

3. **Answer: a**
   Due to the potentially devastating effects of drowning-related hypoxia on a child's brain, airway interventions must be initiated immediately. The child's airway should be suctioned to ensure patency. Other interventions such as covering the child with blankets, inserting a nasogastric tube, and assuring that the child remains still during X-ray are interventions that are appropriate once airway patency is achieved and maintained.

4. **Answer: b**
   Unilateral absent breath sounds are associated with foreign body aspiration. Dullness on percussion over the lung is indicative of fluid consolidation in the lung as with pneumonia. Auscultating a low-pitched, grating breath sound suggests inflammation of the pleura. Hearing a hyperresonant sound on percussion may indicate pneumothorax or asthma.

5. **Answer: b**
   An adolescent, not a 9-year-old, would most likely require an oxygen flow rate of 15 L/minute for effective ventilation. A flow rate of 10 L/minute is appropriate for infants and children. All other options are valid for preparing to ventilate with a bag valve mask.

6. **Answer: c**
   Decrease skin turgor is a late sign of shock. Blood pressure is not a reliable method of evaluating for shock in children because they tend to maintain normal or slightly below normal blood pressure in compensated shock. Equal central and distal pulses are not a sign of shock. Delayed capillary refill with cool extremities are signs of shock that occur earlier than changes in skin turgor.

7. **Answer: d**
   Once the ABCs have been evaluated, the nurse will move on to "D" and assess for disability by palpating the anterior fontanel for signs of increased intracranial pressure. Observing skin color and perfusion is part of evaluating circulation. Palpating the abdomen for soreness and auscultating for bowel sounds would be part of the full-body examination that follows assessing for disability.

8. **Answer: b**
   Inserting a small, folded towel under shoulders best positions the infant's airway in the "sniff" position as is recommended by AHA Basic Cardiac Life Support (BCLS) guidelines. The hand should never be placed under the neck to open the airway. The head tilt chin lift technique and the jaw-thrust maneuver are used with children over the age of 1 year.

9. **Answer: b**
   Exhaled CO_2 monitoring is recommended when a child has been intubated. It provides quick, visual assurance that the tracheal tube remains in place and that the child is being adequately ventilated. When moving the child, maintaining tube placement would be crucial. The other interventions would also be appropriate but not as essential as monitoring the child's exhaled CO_2 level. Unlike the other interventions, exhaled CO_2 monitoring can provide an early sign of a problem.

10. **Answer: c**
    Attaining central venous access is the priority intervention for a child in shock who is receiving respiratory support. Gaining access via the femoral route will not interfere with CPR efforts.

Peripheral venous access may be unattainable in children who have significant vascular compromise. Blood samples and urinary catheter placement can wait until fluid is administered.

11. **Answer: 6 millimeters**
    RATIONALE: The following formula should be used to calculate the correct tracheal tube size for a child: Divide the child's age by 4 and add 4 = size in millimeters

    $$(8 \text{ years old}/4) + 4 = 6 \text{ mm}$$

12. **Answer: 5,700**
    RATIONALE: Cardiac output (CO) is equal to heart rate (HR) times ventricular stroke volume (SV). That is, CO = HR × SV.

    $$76 \text{ beats per minute} \times 75 \text{ mL} = 5,700$$

13. **Answer: 25 milliliters per hour**
    RATIONALE: 56 pounds × 1 kg/2.2 pounds = 25.455 kg of body weight.

    $$25.455 \text{ kg} \times 1 \text{ mL/kg} = 25.455 \text{ mL/hour}$$

    The child must produce 25 mL/hour

14. **Answer: 709 milliliters**
    RATIONALE: 78 pounds × 1 kg/2.2 pounds = 35.455 kg × 20 mL/kg = 709.1 mL. When rounded to the nearest whole number = 709 mL.

15. **Answer: 84**
    RATIONALE: Use the following formula (according to PALS):

    $$70 + (2 \text{ times the age in years})$$

    Hence, the minimal systolic BP of a 7-year-old is 70 + (2 × 7) = 84.